Developments in Cardiovascular Medicine

VOLUME 161

The titles published in this series are listed at the end of this volume.

Coronary Bypass Surgery in the Elderly

Coronary Bypass Surgery in the Elderly

Ethical, Economical and Quality of Life Aspects

Edited by

PAUL J. WALTER

Department of Cardiovascular Surgery,
University Hospital Antwerp, Antwerp, Belgium

With a foreword by

Nanette K. Wenger

Emory University School of Medicine,
Atlanta, Georgia, USA

SPRINGER-SCIENCE+BUSINESS MEDIA, B.V.

Library of Congress Cataloging-in-Publication Data

```
Coronary bypass surgery in the elderly : ethical, economical, and
  quality of life aspects / edited by Paul J. Walter.
      p.   cm.
  Includes index.
  Based on a conference held March 9-11, 1994 in Antwerp, Belgium.
  ISBN 978-94-010-4093-8     ISBN 978-94-011-0209-4 (eBook)
  DOI 10.1007/978-94-011-0209-4
    1. Coronary artery bypass--Decision making--Congresses.  2. Aged-
  -Surgery--Decision making--Congresses.  3. Coronary artery bypass-
  -Economic aspects--Congresses.  4. Coronary artery bypass--Moral and
  ethical aspects--Congresses.  5. Quality of life--Congresses.
  I. Walter, P. J. (Paul J.), 1935-    .
    [DNLM: 1. Coronary Artery Bypass--in old age--congresses.
  2. Coronary Artery Bypass--economics--congresses.  3. Ethics,
  Medical--congresses.   W1 DE997VME v. 161 1995 / WG 169 C8219 1995]
  RD598.35.C67C686   1995
  617.4'12059'0846--dc20
  DNLM/DLC
  for Library of Congress                                    94-37708
  ISBN 978-94-010-4093-8
```

Printed on acid-free paper

Table of Contents

List of Contributors   ix

Preface   xiii

Foreword by Nanette K. Wenger   xix

Part One: Demographics and health policy

1. Demographic and economic trends in Europe and the need for
   coronary bypass surgery   3
   Markus Schneider

2. Do growing proportions of elderly mean more cardiovascular
   diseases?   13
   Hans Hoffmeister and Lee Muecke

Part Two: Favourable clinical results of CABG in the elderly

3. Isolated CABG in the elderly: Operative results and risk factors over
   the past three decades   27
   Wilbert J. Keon

4. Combined valve and coronary bypass surgery in the elderly   41
   Janos Szécsi, Paul Herijgers, Ilse Scheys and Willem Flameng

5. Cardiac surgery in the octogenarians: Perioperative results and
   clinical follow-up   55
   Francis Fontan, Alain Becat, Guy Fernandez, Nicolas Sourdille,
   Pascal Reynaud and Paul Montserrat

6. Coronary artery bypass grafting and use of the LIMA in
   octogenarians   61
   Gideon Sahar, Ehud Raanani, Itzhak Hertz, Ron Brauner and
   Bernardo A. Vidne

Part Three: Health care costs of elderly CABG patients

7. Age-specific costs of heart surgery and follow-up treatment in
   Germany   71
   Detlef Chruscz and Wolfgang König

Part Four: Clinical, economical and ethical controversies

8. Opportunities to improve the cost-effectiveness of CABG surgery   79
   William B. Stason

9. Who gets bypass surgery – should the doctor, patient or computer
   decide?   91
   John Kellett

10. The economics of treatment choice. Making choices in coronary
    bypass surgery in the elderly   101
    Alan Maynard

11. The role of age and life expectancy in prioritising health care   111
    John Harris

12. When does the cost of living exceed the return on our investment?
    The social and economic consequences of coronary bypass surgery
    in the elderly   121
    Roger W. Evans

**Part Five: The heart of the matter: Health-related quality of life after CABG
in the elderly**

13. Coronary artery bypass surgery and health-related quality of life:
    Data from the National Health and Nutrition Examination Survey   137
    Pennifer Erickson

14. The selection of health-related quality of life measures for older
    adults with cardiovascular disease   145
    Sally A. Shumaker and Roger Anderson

15. Survival and health-related quality of life of elderly patients
    undergoing cardiac surgery   155
    Noreen Caine, Susan Tait and John Wallwork

16. Health-related quality of life after coronary revascularization in
    older patients   167
    Paul D. Cleary, Edward Guadagnoli and John Z. Ayanian

17. Longitudinal health-related quality of life assessment in five years
    after coronary artery bypass surgery – does benefit continue with
    advancing age?   179
    Ravinder Mohan, Paul J. Walter and Erik van Hove

18. Health-related quality of life five years after coronary bypass surgery
    at age 75 or above: A research approach to item selection   195
    Paul J. Walter, Ravinder Mohan and Chris Cornelissen

Part Six: Rehabilitation

19. Rehabilitation following coronary artery bypass graft surgery at
    elderly age   213
    Nanette K. Wenger

Discussions   223

Index   259

List of contributors

Noreen Caine
Director of Research and Development, Papworth Hospital NHS TRUST,
Papworth Everard, Cambridge CB3 8RE, U.K.
Co-authors: Susan Tait and John Wallwork

Paul D. Cleary
Department of Health Care Policy, Harvard Medical School, Parcel B, 25
Shattuck St., Boston, MA 02115, U.S.A.
Co-authors: Edward Guadagnoli and John Z. Ayanian

Detlef Chruscz
BKK BV, Koperschaft des Offenliches Rechts, Kronprinserstr. 6, D-45128
Essen, Germany
Co-author: Wolfgang König

Pennifer Erickson
Clearinghouse on Health Indexes, QA EHP, National Center for Health
Statistics, Room 730, 6525 Belcreast Road, Hyattsville, MD 20782, U.S.A.

Roger W. Evans
Head, Section of Health Services Evaluation, Department of Health Sciences
Research, Mayo Clinic, 200 First Street, Rochester, MN 55905, U.S.A.

Willem Flameng
Department of Cardiac Surgery, Gashuisberg University Clinic, University
Hospital of Louvain, Herestraat 49, B-3000 Louvain, Belgium
Co-authors: Janos Szécsi, Paul Herijgers and Ilse Scheys

Francis Fontan
Department of Cardiovascular Surgery, Clinique Saint-Augustin, 114 Avenue
D'Ares, F-33000 Bordeaux Cedex, France
Co-authors: Alain Becat, Guy Fernandez, Nicolas Sourdille, Pascal Reynaud
and Paul Montserrat

P.J. Walter (ed.), Coronary Bypass Surgery in the Elderly, pp. ix–xi.

John Harris
The Centre for Social Ethics and Policy, University of Manchester, Humanities Building, Oxford Road, Manchester M13 9PL, U.K.

H. Hoffmeister
Director, Institute for Social Medicine, & Epidemiology, German Institute of Health, P.O. Box 33 00 13, D-14191 Berlin, Germany
Co-author: L. Muecke

John Kellett
Consultant Physician, Nenagh General Hospital, Nenagh, County Tipperary, Ireland

Wilbert J. Keon
Division of Cardiovascular and Thoracic Surgery, University of Ottawa Heart Institute, 1053 Carling Avenue, Ottawa, Ontario, Canada KIY 4E9

Alan Maynard
Centre for Health Economics, University of York, Heslington, York Y01 5DD, U.K.

Ravinder Mohan
Department of Cardiovascular Surgery, University of Antwerp, Wilrijkstraat 10, B-2650 Antwerp/Edegem, Belgium
Co-authors: Paul J. Walter and Erik Van Hove

Markus Schneider
Director BASYS, Advisory Bureau For Applied System Research, Reisingerstrasse 25, D-86159 Augsburg, Germany

Sally A. Shumaker
Department of Public Health Sciences, The Bowman Gray School of Medicine, Wake Forest University, Medical Center Boulevard, Winston Salem, NC 27157, U.S.A.
Co-author: Roger Anderson

William B. Stason
29 Sandy Pond Road, Lincoln, MA 01773, U.S.A.

Bernardo A. Vidne
Division of Cardiothoracic Surgery, Sackler School of Medicine, Beinson Medical Center, Tel-Aviv University, 49100 Petah-Tikva, Israel
Co-authors: Gideon Shar, Ehud Raanani, Itzhak Hertz and Ron Brauner

Paul J. Walter
Department of Cardiovascular Surgery, University Hospital of Antwerp, Wilrijkstraat 10, B-2650 Antwerp/Edegem, Belgium
Co-authors: Ravinder Mohan and Chris Cornelissen

Nanette K. Wenger
Division of Cardiology, Emory University School of Medicine, Grady Memorial Hospital, 69 Butler Street, S.E., Atlanta, GA 30303, U.S.A.

Preface

Coronary artery bypass surgery in the elderly:
Too often or too seldom?

It is a testimony to scientific advances that raising a simple inquiry today, such as whether coronary artery bypass surgery is done too often or too seldom in elderly patients, requires an exploration of what views one might hold on several medical as well as non-medical issues. Unlike earlier years when doctors were clinically free to decide what should be done with a patient, health has become an expensive human right, decisions about which also involve the patient, the epidemiologist, the health policy administrator, politicians, the exchequer, and the philosopher. In its broadest definition health has come to mean the core of well-being and, therefore, the goal of any socio-economic system.

Until only a decade ago, medical opinion regarding how often coronary artery bypass surgery (CABG) was indicated or useful was unclear. Because of multi-organ senescence, the elderly were expected to have a higher rate operative morbidity and mortality and, having crossed an advanced life span, might not live very long after the operation. Decision making on medical grounds first depends on knowing if a patient can survive an operation compared to how long they would survive without it, i.e. is the operation required to save life? What are the chances of operative complications leading to a situation worse than that before the operation? Could medication or a less invasive procedure save the life and/or alleviate anginal complaints with greater safety? Can the operation really prolong life in the long term? And, even life saved or life prolonged may not be very desirable if it continues to be crippled in some way. Besides these medical issues, concerns such as whether freedom from angina would allow elders to perform activities of daily living more easily, e.g. bathing, without dependence on others could be of peripheral interest to the cardiologist, but not to the gerontologist. Even if objective capacity was adequately restored, lack of patient perceived benefit could mean failure in realising the operation's goal and reason for considering whether resources spent on the operation were wasted. Do patients feel less disabled or dependent and more energetic to be able to enjoy family relationships and a fuller social life, or has the family come under heavy emotional and financial strain due to the operation?

Equal availability to the right to treatment further complicates what we may

P.J. Walter (ed.), Coronary Bypass Surgery in the Elderly, pp. xiii–xvii.
© 1995 *Kluwer Academic Publishers, Dordrecht.*

be asking. About 30 years ago emerging concern for health as a human right legalised health insurance systems in the industrialised world to secure health for all. This idyll has evaporated in recent years, as spiralling health costs have made economists question how a market commodity such as health can be provided as a right and whether the burden of disease must fall more on the patient's pocket. Scarcity of health budgets and the high cost of coronary operations may force both the surgeon and the health planner to choose between patients and management options according to their cost. These considerations, instead of those of medical need and the benefit of intervention raise important ethical controversies. The issue of whether we must try to prolong life after the age of, say, 75, is related to the question if one has the right to judge who must live and who can die. Statistically, elderly patients who undergo an operation are found to have significantly more extensive coronary disease, more unstable angina and more urgent operations than younger patients; such a situation is likely to have arisen only because of prior refusal of the operation and allowing the spread of the disease. This may occur due to physician perceived notions that advanced chronological age, per se, as opposed to physiological age, can entail too great a risk for the operation. It may also be because surgeons may believe that younger patients, with expectations of longer, active and productive lives, with dependents to look after in their 'prime' of life, must get first preference and are better surgical candidates. Acting on this attitude, surgeons may not give priority to the elderly. As urgent operations carry even greater risk and greater postoperative morbidity, physician prejudices can unwittingly discriminate against older patients.

Of larger relevance in our inquiry is society's decision whether elderly people have an equal right to expensive, life-saving and possibly life-improving treatment. Often sick, the elderly consume the largest share of the health budget; it is argued if this amount would not be better spent on maximising infant lives in a pediatric intensive care. Doctors may find themselves incompetent to deal with such a choice, however, due to centuries of their unquestioned authority and commitment to impartiality, they find it difficult to become quasi-involved bystanders to the debate between health economists and philosophers of medical ethics. The key to these questions, indeed to the usefulness of all health-related expenditure in society, is beginning to be provided by outcome analysts and 'quality of life' specialists. However, as it is doctors who have a direct relationship with a patient, are most aware of the physiological effects of disease and treatment, and have a personal responsibility towards the outcome of their treatment, it would probably be most appropriate if their decision-making role came to lead in the division of the health budget. This would, however, require their better understanding of non-medical issues such as patient psychology and social well-being, as well as health economics.

This book is concerned with the ageing of society and its health-related economics, a demographic change that will explode into the next century. Current life expectancy has doubled from 47 years in 1900 to above 75 years for Belgium, Germany and the United States, and above 80 years for Sweden,

France and Japan [1–4]. In the U.S.A. the rise in people aged 65 years or older will increase from 28.6 million people in 1985 to 34.9 million by 2000 and 64.6 million by 2030; the number of people 85 years and older was expected to rise from 2.7 million in 1985 to 8.6 million in 2030 [5]. Associated with ageing is the disproportionate amount of health care services consumed by the elderly. Utilisation of these services increases their life expectancy and, therefore, their potential for re-demanding the services in the future. Age-related multiorgan-system senescence requires hospitalised, institutionalised and home care because of disease and dependence. Thus, managing the current and future-projected expense of old-age health is now emerging as the most serious contender to demand a restructuring of existing health policies.

Attitudes towards becoming old are also changing, because increased life span primarily means that after reaching age 60, there are not a few years of crippled life remaining, but possibly a new era lasting 20 to 30 years. According to Fries, with careful health planning by both the individual and the state, projected statistics show that not only is a normal maximum human life span of 115 years attainable, but the last years of life shall be spent with minimal or 'compressed' morbidity [6]. The retirement age of 65 has long served as a borderline but has become devoid of meaning, since for many this is the time to *begin* a new, long and satisfying era of self-discovery. With crucial life responsibilities behind people, this becomes a period of calm and rest, individualism, a position of respect in society, time for hobbies and gentle outdoor recreation, time to spend with loved ones, in other words, a period of active as opposed to passive involvement. The awareness that time is limited opens a new meaning to the duration and gift of life. Such a full and enjoyable life has become possible because some consequences of biological decline in organ function can effectively be combated by medical intervention. On the other hand, if society is uncaring or unwilling to spend on the health of old people, illness and dependence can indeed make old age an agonising and miserable wait for the end, the spectre for which it is dreaded. Especially because old people have served their full time in this world, it therefore behooves society to take care of its aged, not to keep decrepit bodies alive at all costs, but to bring them a life vibrantly alive, a good life as long as possible and, finally, a dignified death.

Because of this new understanding there is an increasing trend to conduct diagnostic or theraputic procedures which would have been considered too invasive at such ages only two decades ago. The upper age limit of coronary bypass surgery in the seventies was 60 years and the mean age in Belgium in 1972 was 48 years, whereas 50% of all patients undergoing coronary bypass surgery in 1989 in New York State were older than 65 years [7], and the mean patient age in Belgium in 1990 was 64 years [8]. At the Cleveland Clinic, the median age of coronary bypass patients was 50 years; in 1986 the median age was 62 years and 40% of patients were older than 65 years [9]. In several centres, advanced age, per se, is not considered a contraindication [10]. In recent years, publications have appeared considering that operations on patients 80 and even 96 years of age [11] do not appear to constitute a strict limit. Several reasons encourage the accelerating increase of surgical and interventionist medical treatment for coronary disease in older patients. These are:

a) increasing technical confidence in operating on sicker (and older) patients;
b) spreading confidence in society regarding the safety and desirability of a coronary operation;
c) evidence of a variety of controlled clinical trials showing that the benefit of surgery over medical treatment increases in proportion with severity of angina and coronary disease, and elderly coronary operation patients typically have these characterstics;
d) the significantly more extensive disease of the elderly is often not amenable to PTCA;
e) unstable angina and impending myocardial infarction because of more extensive coronary disease makes urgent operation unavoidable to save life; and
f) the rapidly increasing elderly population.

Because medicine has been such a substantial help in alleviating misery in old age, because 'health' has become a social ideal, and especially because health is likely to suffer in the elderly, health in old age is increasingly demanded as a basic human right. Both health services and social services are involved in providing this right, with considerable overlap. The question is, at what cost? The question is raised because of two 'recent' realisations, namely, that (a) *life is finite* and (b) *resources are limited*. Coronary artery bypass surgery consumed 1.5% of the U.S. health care budget in 1989 [12]. In 1993, Newsweek magazine reported that coronary bypass surgery had increased 2800% since 1970, and its current budget was close to $12 billion, i.e. exceeding the budget of the National Institutes of Health [13].

The obvious answer to this ethical predicament is to first gauge the operative risk and, second, the long-term quality of life benefit irrespective of cost. Only then can cost-appropriateness be considered. Although several reports of operative results exist in literature, data on long-term (> 1 year) quality of life (in all its dimensions) after coronary bypass surgery do not exist. Therefore, we invited renowned experts in each of the issues of this many-sided question to a conference (March 9–11, 1994, Antwerp, Belgium) and there presented some results of our recent investigations. This book comprises the presentations and discussions which took place at the conference. As an introduction to the reader, I would like to dwell on what 'quality of life' has meant in recent research. Can one measure a vast, amorphous and elusive concept, an intangible cluster of ideas which comprise our whole consciousness, and indeed the 'goodness' of the everday process of living? To capture such a boundless entity 'under the same roof' [14], or even give it a value or number would appear impossible, and to some extent that remains the case. Bergner gave a list of quality of life domains suggested as relevant outcomes of health and medical care at a workshop sponsored by the National Heart, Lung and Blood Institute [14]. These were: symptoms, functional status (self-care, mobility, physical activity), role activities (work, household management), social functioning (personal interactions, intimacy, communications interactions), emotional status (anxiety, stress, depression, locus of control), spiritual well-being, cognition, sleep and rest, health perceptions and, lastly, general satisfaction. The definition of 'Health-related Quality of Life' used by various authors in this book was coined by Patrick [15] which broadly covers these domains.

I would like to thank Dr. Nanette K. Wenger for agreeing to write the Foreword for this book, and to all the contributors, without whose contributions this book would not be possible, I express my deep gratitude. Also, I thank Kluwer Academic Publishers for putting this book into print in such a thoughtful way.

PAUL J. WALTER

References

1. World Health Organization. World Health Statistics 1990. Genèva: WHO, 1990.
2. Council for Europe. Recent demographic developments in Europe and North America. Straatsburg: The Council, 1993.
3. Coleman D. Lange levensduur – steeds langer. Spectrum Internationale 1993; 36: 2–8.
4. CNN. Factoid, 26 November, 1993.
5. United States Bureau of Census. Washington, DC: US Bureau of Census, 1984.
6. Fries JF. Aging, natural death and compression of morbidity. N Engl J Med 1980; 303: 130–5.
7. Hannan EL, et al. Coronary artery bypass surgery: the relationship between in-hospital mortality rate and surgical volume after controlling for risk factors. Med Care 1991; 29: 1094–1107.
8. Sergeant P. Changing pattern in age distribution of coronary bypass patients and their possible early influence on early and late events. Proceedings of the 3rd World Congress of the International Society of Cardiothoracic Surgeons; 1993 Jan 25–27; Salzburg, 1993: 79.
9. Loop FD, Lytle BW, Cosgrove DM, et al. Coronary artery bypass surgery in the elderly. Cleve Clin J Med 1988; 55: 23–4.
10. Bashour TT. Coronary bypass grafting in the over 80 population. Prog Cardiol 1993; 5(1): 117–29.
11. Glower PD. Performance status and outcome after coronary artery bypass grafting in persons aged 80 to 93 years. Am J Cardiol 1992; 70: 567–71.
12. Preston TA. Assessment of coronary bypass surgery and percutaneous transluminal coronary angioplasty. Int J Assess Hlth Care 1989; 5: 431.
13. Cowley G. What high tech can't accomplish. Newsweek 1993; Oct 4: 34.
14. Bergner M. Quality of life, health status and clinical research. Med Care 1989; 27: S148–56.
15. Patrick DL, Erickson P. What constitutes quality of life? Concepts and dimensions. J Clin Nutr 1988; 7: 53–63.

Foreword

The worldwide graying of coronary bypass graft surgery

As we plan for medical care in the twenty-first century, the aging of the population worldwide poses scientific, economic, and ethical challenges, both to medical professionals and to formulators of health care-related public policy. The burgeoning of the elderly population, owing to a virtual doubling of life expectancy during the past century, has engendered an escalation in health care costs. As more people live to elderly age, they have increased needs for and more extensive use of medical services. Economic issues have, in turn, resulted in proposals for age-based limitations of access to medical care. Age-based prioritization of health care resources is ethically inappropriate; availability of medical services must be assured to all patients for whom comparable benefit from an intervention has been demonstrated.

Among the sectors highlighted for these restrictions are the high-technology, costly components of contemporary cardiac care, prominent among which is coronary artery bypass graft surgery (CABG). Currently, almost half of all diagnostic and therapeutic cardiovascular procedures in the U.S. are performed on patients older than 65 years of age. Worldwide, reported series of CABG surgical patients have progressively increased in age from those involving patients in their 60s and 70s to octogenarians and nonagenarians. The feasibility of performing CABG surgery, event at very elderly age, has clearly been demonstrated. The development of guidelines for the selection of appropriate elderly patients for this procedure warrants high priority and requires expansion of our current clinical date base to enable this ascertainment; a compelling need in this regard is delineation of the resulting quality of life following CABG surgery at elderly age.

Most contemporary CABG surgery at advanced age is undertaken for severely symptomatic coronary heart disease, which is unresponsive or poorly responsive to medical therapies. Typically, the coronary anatomy is deemed unsuitable for coronary angioplasty (PTCA); or CABG may have been occasioned by a failed PTCA procedure. A high percentage of CABG operations at elderly age are thus performed on an urgent or emergency basis. Elective CABG, in one series of patients older than age 75 years, entailed a 3.6% operative mortality, in contrast to a 14.9 operative mortality rate for urgent or

P.J. Walter (ed.), Coronary Bypass Surgery in the Elderly, pp. xix–xx.
© 1995 *Kluwer Academic Publishers, Dordrecht.*

emergency CABG surgery. Should indications for earlier evaluation and risk stratification among elderly patients be expanded in an effort to improve their operative risk? To what extent does this approach have the potential to postpone servere and debilitating manifestations of coronary disease at even more elderly age? How is this counterbalanced by the extent and duration of morbidity and dependency that detract from the patient's comfort and sense of well-being following invasive procedures? Elderly patients undergoing CABG surgery have a high likelihood of requiring a protracted hospital stay (including prolonged time spent in an intensive care unit); greater requirement for ventilatory and inotropic agent support, for temporary or permanent pacemakers, and intra-aortic balloon counterpulsation; increased likelihood of early re-operation, often for bleeding complications; and greater predisposition to postoperative stroke, myocardial infarction, wound infection, sepsis, and other complications of CABG surgery. Nevertheless, octogenarian survivors of CABG surgery are characteristically pain-free, and their 5-year survival differs little from comparably-aged populations free of clinical manifestations of coronary heart disease.

But only marginal life-extending benefits can be anticipated from any intervention in very elderly coronary patients. The pivotal issue, and the appropriate focus of therapeutic interventions, is therefore the extent to which the contemplated procedure, in this instance CABG surgery, can lessen or postpone disability. Limited information and consideration uncertainty about the assessment of functional status at elderly age hamper these determinations and constitute an unmet need. Instruments validated at younger age do not appear to target the functions relevant for impaired elderly patients or to be responsive to the modest improvements characteristic among elderly patients. Of concern are numerous studies documenting that elderly patients consider the severity of their impairments less and the quality of their lives significantly better than do their treating physicians. Similarly, elderly patients define their functional status as substantially better than do their treating physicians. Also, elderly patients define their functional status as substantially better than do their family members, nurses, or other caretakers. These perceptions buttress the observations that many elderly and very elderly coronary patients, with a major burden of illness, both continue to value living and continue to actively seek those treatments, including surgery, that appear likely to effect symptomatic and functional improvements.

Clinical and societal judgments, guided by elderly patients' preferences, must be incorporated into recommendations for CABG surgery at advanced age. Given the marked heterogeneity of the population at elderly age, unequivocally not solely age-based criteria, but rather the interrelationships among the patients' symptomatic and functional limitations; independence, vigor and alertness of the pre-interventional status; level of operative and postoperative risk; and likelihood of restoration and maintenance of a meaningful and personally satisfying lifestyle are appropriate determinants of elderly candidates suitable for CABG surgery.

NANETTE KASS WENGER

PART ONE

Demographics and health policy

1. Demographic and economic trends in Europe and the need for coronary bypass surgery

MARKUS SCHNEIDER

Introduction

During the last 26 years, since the first reporting of CABG by Favorolo [1], considerable demographic and economic changes have taken place within the twelve Member States of the European Community. The share of the elderly has risen from 11% to nearly 15% of the population. At the same time, the gross national product per capita per year has increased from 1800 ECU to 16000 ECU in constant prices. Life expectancy has increased approximately 5 years or 70 days per year. Furthermore, expansion of economic development has been observed in all health care systems. Especially in the hospital sector considerable changes have taken place. The average length of stay in acute hospitals has fallen by about 8 days, from 19 to 11 days. Many more patients can now be treated despite a reducing number of beds and cost containment policies. The dominant factor of these changes has been medical technical progress: improvements in diagnostic and surgical procedures, pharmaceuticals and support functions. CABG is an excellent example of this technological development.

According to forecasts for the next 26 years, similarly huge changes can be expected. The share of elderly will increase by nearly 20%. As chronological age is the most significant risk factor for coronary atherosclerosis, a further increase in the need for CABG might be expected. Even though new technologies may replace CABG in 10 or 15 years, the need for re-operation has to be considered.

In discussing the future need for CABG in Europe it is useful to distinguish the following questions:
1. How has CABG developed in Europe and how does it vary among countries?
2. What economic and demographic trends can be expected in future?
3. What role would medical technical progress play, especially regarding the development of new technologies and improvements in operation techniques?
4. What conclusions can be drawn for the need for CABG?

P.J. Walter (ed.), Coronary Bypass Surgery in the Elderly, pp. 3–12.
© 1995 *Kluwer Academic Publishers, Dordrecht.*

Variations in bypass surgery

For the past 20 years similar developments could be observed in all European countries: a steady increase of cardiac operations and a steady increase in the age of patients as expressed [2–9].

Analyzing the present situation in Europe, we find a great variation of capacities for cardiac surgery and delivered procedures (see Figure 1.1). Obviously, the need for coronary bypass surgery differs in the opinion of doctors, patients and health politicians in Europe.

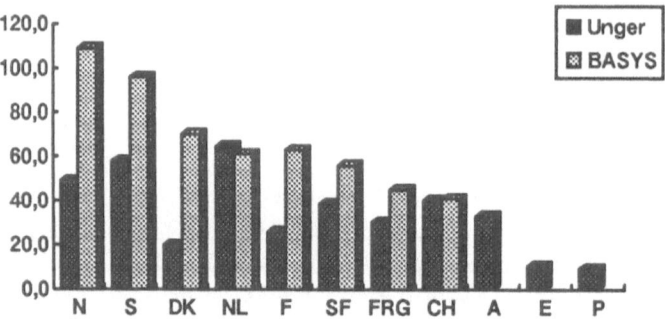

Figure 1. Variation of CABG in Europe: CABG per 100.000 capita in 1991.

According to the European Survey on Open Heart Surgery by Felix Unger of the University of Innsbruck, approximately 27 coronary bypass operations per 100,000 people were performed in 1990 in the Member States of the European Community [10, 11]. The highest figures have been reported for the Netherlands, Sweden and Belgium, the lowest for the southern Mediterranean countries and the former socialist countries.

Compilations of the BASYS Institute, based on national statistics of surgical procedures, exhibit much higher figures for most of the countries. However, independent of the statistical differences, in general, high rates of operations seem to exist in the Nordic countries as well as in the middle European states, i.e. the Netherlands, Belgium, France, Germany, Switzerland and Austria, which have incomes per capita above the European average. The lower ratio in the U.K. corresponds to lower capacities in the whole acute-bed sector and the regulation of scarce resources by waiting lists.

Demographic development

Analyzing demographic forecasts in detail – although demographic forecasting seems to be easier than economic forecasting – we see that those projections deliver only a candle in the darkness of the future. Depending on assumptions for the future development of fertility, life expectancy and migration, great variations in possible demographic developments are projected. In a low population scenario, the European Statistical Office (EUROSTAT) forecasts 338 million inhabitants by the year 2020, in a high scenario, nearly 400 million [12] (Table 1.1).

For the elderly's share of the population the EUROSTAT forecasting model predicts more stable results. The share of people aged 65 years and older will increase from 15.2% in 1995 to 19.2–19.5% by 2020. But this means an increase of 42% in the high scenario and 24% in the low scenario. In the high scenario, which assumes a further significant increase in male and female life expectancy, the number of elderly will be 76 million by 2020. In the low scenario, with a low increase in life expectancy, approximately 10 million less elderly are predicted. For the whole population, this deviation amounts to 58 million people. By the year 2020, the numbers are 338 million in the low scenario and nearly 400 million in the high scenario.

Still higher variations exist in the prediction of the very elderly, aged 80 years and older. The high scenario predictions suggest a 64% increase in the very elderly by 2020, from 13.4 million in 1995 to 22.0 million in 2020, confirming that the oldest age groups are those growing the most rapidly. Data from the U.S. Bureau of Census and Japan's Economic Planning Agency confirm similar trends for their respective countries. In the low scenario, the number of this age group will increase 24%, from 13.4 million in 1995 to 16.6 million in 2020.

The different assumptions of the development of life expectancy in the high and low forecast models of EUROSTAT imply different developments in lifestyles and economic growth, as well as health care provision. Presently there is no forecast model available that allows to tackle these complex interdependencies, especially the feedback between the health care sector and

Table 1.1. Population projection for Europe

	Low scenario population[a]		High scenario population[b]	
	In 1000	In %	In 1000	In %
Total				
1995	349,013	100	353,366	100
2020	337,899	100	396,111	100
65 and older				
1995	53,194	15.2	53,610	15.2
2020	65,925	19.2	76,095	19.5
80 and older				
1995	13,207	3.8	13,384	3.8
2020	16,690	4.9	21,925	5.5

[a] Total fertility rate 1.51 (1995) and 1.50 (2019), life expectancy males 73.0 (1995) and 73.3 (2019), life expectancy females 79.3 (1995) and 79.6 (2019), net external migration 250,000 (1995 and 2019).
[b] Total fertility rate 1.72 (1995) and 2.00 (2019), life expectancy males 73.7 (1995) and 78.0 (2019), life expectancy females 79.9 (1995) and 83.0 (2019), net external migration 750,000 (1995 and 2019).
Source: EUROSTAT 1993.

life expectancy. Increased longevity does not necessarily mean long life in good health, that is, life expectancy free of major disability. Available indicators on health expectancy provide some insight that life expectancy has been prolonged more than time of incapacity [13]. Sweden has reported the most improvements in health status among the elderly [14].

It can be expected that the future increase in the number of elderly will be accompanied by a major change in morbidity and mortality pattern. However, what is important regarding the future need for CABG, is that mortality and morbidity will not move in the same direction. Although decreasing mortality in cardiovascular diseases can be expected, chronological age is the most significant risk factor of coronary atherosclerosis.

Population structure and the components of demographic change are of major importance for designing and implementing health care services. Investigations of the health situation have invariably shown that the nature and extent of coronary heart diseases differ widely among population subgroups. The representation of these groups in the total population depends, in turn, on previous levels and trends of fertility, mortality and geographical variation. Even within such a comparatively demographic region as Europe, where most countries have completed the process of demographic transition a long time ago, significant intercountry variations of demographic behaviour can be found.

The future increase in mortality may also be accompanied by a major change in morbidity and mortality pattern. Decreasing cardiovascular diseases and increasing cancer can be expected. Chronological age is the most significant risk factor for coronary atherosclerosis [15], therefore, despite decreasing mortality, an increasing share of the population would suffer from coronary diseases. This result is projected by Dutch RIVM, which has discussed the development of

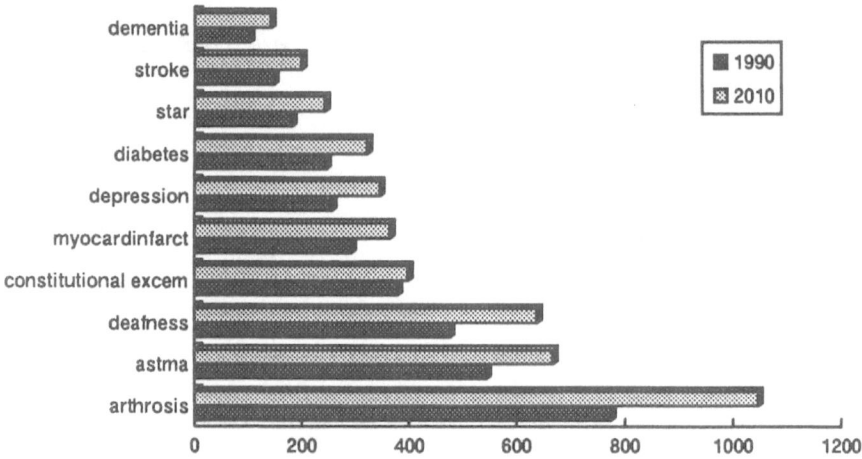

Figure 1.2. Patients with the 10 diseases with the highest prevalence, NL 1990 and 2010. Source: RIVM 1993, Volksgezondheid Toekomst Verkenning.

morbidity and mortality in the Dutch population in a comprehensive study for the period 1950 until 2020 [16].

According to the RIVM study, mortality by reason of cardiovascular diseases will diminish by approximately 47% until the year 2010 (Figure 1.2). This is the highest reduction among the most important causes of mortality. Nevertheless, coronary heart diseases contribute the most to lost-life years in the year 2010. This corresponds to the fact that, at the same time, the prevalence of coronary heart diseases will rise 38.9% among the top leading diseases.

Economic development

Similar to demographic development, great changes have also taken place in the economic field. In the long run, we observed a decline in economic growth from an average of 4.8% in the sixties, to 3% in the seventies, and 2.3% in the eighties (see Table 1.2). In a worst case scenario, the Commission extrapolated a growth of 1.8% for the nineties. Corresponding to the decrease in economic growth, an increase in unemployment was observed, from 2% in the sixties to over 10% in the eighties.

According to the Commission of the European Communities, an average growth rate of 2% or higher within the community can only be reached by massive structural investments consolidating public budgets and modest wage increases. This policy inevitably requires cost containment in health care.

A main cause for the increase of economic growth rates is reduced capital formation. It is not so much the behaviour of people who prefer travelling to saving free incomes as the behaviour of public institutions. The loss of capital formation by the government is the central problem. Therefore, rationalization of public administration and reduction of public deficits must be of the highest priority.

There are many economists who see the ageing of the total population negatively for economic growth. In the Commission's Annual Economic Report of 1991–1992, we can find the following meaning: 'as regards the labour market,

Table 1.2. Economic growth, unemployment and capital formation in the EC, 1960–2000

	Economic growth (%)	Unemployment (%)	Capital formation (%)
1961–1970	4.8	2.0	23.0
1971–1980	3.0	4.0	22.6
1981–1990	2.3	8.7	19.9
1991–2000 low scenario	1.8	10.2	
1991–2000 high scenario	2.7	8.4	

Source: EC: Annual Economic Report for 1993.

opinions converge towards a net negative impact of ageing by a general loss of dynamism, entrepreneurial spirit and willingness to take risks'. Apart from this argument of inflexibility, a second argument is directed to the increasing burden of labour costs caused by financing higher social benefits for the elderly [17, 18].

In the eighties strong cost containment policies were implemented in Ireland, the Netherlands, Denmark, Germany and Sweden. As a consequence of expected low economic growth as well as the nominal convergence criteria in the Maastricht Agreement, it can be expected that in the future cost containment policies will be enforced in all European States. Cost containment policies will be a central element of all European health care systems. Nevertheless, economic growth and medical technological progress would allow increases in the treatment of coronary diseases. Experience from the United States and several European Countries show decreasing relative prices of CABG.

Now we have to ask how to manage the increasing prevalence of cardiovascular disease within the framework of reduced economic growth and increasing cost containment pressure. From an economic point of view, there are two approaches to tackle this problem without rationing coronary bypass surgery.

The first is to reduce the costs of CABG.

The second is to encourage methods which are more cost-efficient.

The first approach means a decrease in the relative price of CABG and in length of stay. For example, for Medicare patients the relative prices of CABG (DRG code 107), that is, price for CABG in relation to average costs per DRG, diminished from 4.8 in 1983 to 3.11 in 1990 [19]. Furthermore, a decrease in length of stay for CABG could be observed in all European countries.

Medical progress

From an economic point of view, the resource allocation process between competing procedures is directed by their marginal costs and benefits. The choice for CABG always implies a decision against other technologies, e.g. PTCA. The contraindications for angioplasty are sclerosis of the stenosis, total closure and unfavourable location of the vessel.

Health care is sometimes described as a half-way technique. Turning to the evolution of medical technology, the biomedical scientist and physician Lewis Thomas has noted the following successive stages of managing disease: non-technology; half-way technology and advanced technology [20]. Early on, the cause was obscure and doctors had no effective therapy for diseases but felt obliged to provide some recommendation such as bedrest, which was not inexpensive. Today this still applies in many areas, such as late stage cancer treatment and the management of the degenerative diseases of old age. Half-way technologies are not based on a thorough understanding of the biological processes causing a disease, but go some way towards restoring the functions lost as a result of the disease. These replacement processes are often the most expensive. According to Lewis Thomas, truly advanced technologies are not the methods using the most expensive equipment and skills directly on patients. Advanced technologies are specific therapeutic solutions that are simple to administer and follow preventive strategies. These are invariably the most cost effective.

In cardiovascular diseases, palliative low-tech approaches (leeches) were replaced by half-way technologies (transplants, bypass grafts). Pioneering results of major epidemiological studies with thoughtful meta-analysis have helped to identify both patients at risk and risk factors. This should usher in a new wave of cost-effective pharmaceutical solutions and preventive strategies. But less invasive procedures such as PTCA are increasing rapidly. Alternative less invasive techniques will probably become more important in the future. Certainly, the rapid increase in research knowledge and new scientific information attest to the further progress of treatment of coronary artery disease.

With emphasis on hospitals and specialists, heart diseases are more often tackled in hospitals and ambulatory care than by prevention-oriented strategy. Preventive policies that focus on risk factors (hypertension, high cholesterol, smoking) and at-risk patient subsets (diabetes) as primary targets might reduce the incidence of cardiovascular disease in lower age-groups, but, probably, will postpone it in higher ages, too.

Today, coronary-artery surgery is a billion-ECU growth industry. That bypass surgery improves symptoms and enhances the quality of life, at least in the short term, is well established. The improvement of surgical techniques, especially the life span of grafts, as well as the therapy to inhibit platelet aggregation has also favourably influenced long-term survival rates. Investigators at Duke University have argued that surgical techniques have advanced more rapidly than medical therapy and that surgical outcome progressively has become better [21].

Need or necessaries of bypass surgery

Need involves the idea of instrumentality: if a particular service is a necessary condition of the accomplishment of a desired end state, then that service is needed. Classical economists, such as Smith and Ricardo in particular, used the term 'necessaries' to indicate the commodities which are indispensably necessary for the support of life, and also 'whatever the custom of the country renders it indecent for creditable people, even of the lowest order, to be without' [22]. Thus the term 'necessaries' includes both a purely physical element (the goods which are strictly required for the survival of workers and their families) and a sociological one (the commodities which by habit and custom are regarded as 'necessary to the lowest rank of people'). In this classical view necessaries are distinguished from luxuries, which are all the goods that are not strictly required to guarantee the workers a decent standard of living.

The difference between necessaries and luxuries is often discussed in connection with the medical goods and the health care system [23]. If medical goods would be necessaries, the so-called elasticity of demand would be lower than one. This means that a rise in price would not affect demand of medical goods very much. Beyond all doubt, under certain conditions CABG is a prerequisite for life and quality of life. Therefore, with the increasing prevalence of coronanry artery diseases a further rise in CABG may be expected, independent of cost containment policies in health care. Unfortunately, there is little information on this point. A comparison of Medicaid patients with private fee-for-service patients shows the opposite. The frequency of coronary revascularization in California in 1983 was nearly twice as high for patients with private fee-for-service insurance as for patients enrolled in HMOs or Medicaid recipients [24].

There are two components of the future need for CABG: primary operations and re-operations. While the need for primary operation is mainly determined by the prevalence of certain heart diseases, alternative treatment methods and the social value of CABG for society, re-operations depend on the life expectancy after primary operation and the lifespan of grafts.

In the United States and Europe there is a greatly increasing incidence of second CABG surgery (re-operation). The cumulative incidence of patients undergoing a second CABG procedure in the United States is approximately 30% at 15 years after the primary procedure [25]. Projecting these data to the U.S. population at large, Cosgrove of the Cleveland Clinical Foundation estimates there will be 55,000 coronary re-operations annually, making it the second most common cardiac surgical procedure performed in the U.S.A. As age increases, operative mortality in re-operation also increases, with nearly a five-fold increase in re-operative mortality in those aged 75 years and older as compared with patients aged 55 years or younger. Among the elderly population, operative mortality is significantly higher after re-operation than after primary CABG surgery [26].

The age of the coronary artery bypass candidate is gradually increasing, reflecting our ageing population. Many studies confirm the efficacy of CABG surgery in the elderly as an effective means of improving symptoms, long-term survival and quality of life. Impressively, longevity following CABG surgery exceeds that of the U.S. population matched for age and gender. CABG surgery will no doubt be an important operation for the elderly, as the population continues to age and those in this age category desire an ever-improving quality of life.

Conclusions

The discussion has focused on a few central aspects of the need for CABG. Certainly the selection of these subjects cannot reflect all the different developments in the European Member States. Nevertheless, some conclusions can be drawn.

1. The increase of the elderly within a range of 24–64% by 2020 will raise the prevalence of coronary diseases probably within a comparable range.
2. The ageing of society and the reduction of public debts pressed by the convergence criteria of the Maastricht agreement, as well as pressure on labour costs to rise international competitiveness will enforce cost containment in health care.
3. The 'necessary' nature of medically beneficial CABG will further increase the demand for CABG, although cost containment policies will restrict demand.
4. The share of re-operations within the total volume of CABG will increase with further increase in longevity.
5. Medical progress in CABG as well as in alternatives will help to cope with increasing need. Rationing does not seem inevitable if rationalization in delivering CABG is improved.
6. Different conclusions exist for the Member States with low capacities and different demographic structures at present, as well as for the Central and Eastern European States with insufficient income to expand CABG.

References

1. Favorolo R.G. Saphenous vein autograft replacement of severe segmental coronary artery occlusion. Ann Thorac Surg 1968; 5: 334–9.
2. Bruckenberger E. Fünfter Bericht des Krankenhausausschusses der Arbeitsgemeinschaft der Leitenden Medizinalbeamten (AGLMB) zur Situation der Herzchirurgie 1992 in Deutschland. Hannover: Niedersächsisches Sozialministerium, 1993.
3. Department of Health. Hospital episode statistics, NHS hospitals. Volume 1, England 1992/93, London: Government Statistical Service.
4. Danish Hospital Institute (DHI). Hyertekirurgi i Danmark – Behov, kapacietet og organisation, Copenhagen: DHI, 1991.
5. Kalmar P, Irrgang E. Cardiac surgery in Germany during 1992. The thoracic and cardiovascular surgeon No 3 Vol 41. Hamburg: Department of Cardiovascular Surgery, University Hospital Eppendorf, 1993, 202–4.
6. Ministère de la Santé. Direction des hopitaux, rapport d'activité de 72 services de chirurgie cardiaque. Paris: Ministère de la Santé, 1992.
7. Nordic Medico-Statistical Committee (NOMESKO). Health statistics in the Nordic countries 1991. Copenhagen: NOMESKO, 1993.
8. SIG. Zorginformatie, jaarboek ziekenhuizen, kliniek, dagverpleging en polikliniek, gebaseerd op de gegevens uit de landelijke medische registratie. Utrecht: SIG, 1991.
9. Vereinigung Schweizerischer Krankenhäuser (VESKA). Medizinische Statistik – Diagnosen und Operationen. Aarau: VESKA, 1993.
10. Unger F. European survey on open heart surgery, 1990, vol 2. Report of the Institute for Cardiac Survey. Ann – Acad Sci Artium Eur 1991.
11. Unger F. European survey on open heart surgery, interventional cardiology and PTCA in 1991, vol 4. Report of the Institute for Cardiac Survey. Ann – Acad Sci Artium Eur 1992.
12. EUROSTAT. Population projection [manuscript]. Luxembourg: EUROSTAT, 1993.
13. Wilkins R, Adams OB. Tendances de l'espérance de santé au Canada, 1951–1986. In: Robine JM, Blanchet M, Dowd J, editors. Espérance de santé. Paris: Inserm, 1992: 210–6.
14. Statistica Centralbyran. Pensionärer 1980–1989, Stockholm: Statistica Centralbyran, 1993.
15. Kannel WB, Vokonas PS. Primary risk factors for coronary heart disease in the elderly: the

Framinghame Study. In: Wenger NK, Furberg CD, Pitt E, editors. Coronary heart disease in the elderly. New York: Elsevier Science, 1986: 60–95.

16. Rijksinstituut voor Volksgezondheid en Milieuhygiene (RIVM). Volksgezondheid toekomst verkenning: de gezondheidstoestand van de Nederlandse bevolking in de periode 1950–2010. Den Haag, The Netherlands: Sdu Uitgeverij, 1993.

17. Commission of the European Communities. Annual economic report for 1992. Euro Econ 1992; 51.

18. Commission of the European Communities, Annual economic report for 1993. Euro Econ 1993; 54.

19. Helbing Ch. Hospital insurance short-stay hospital benefits. In: Health care financing review, Medicare and Medicaid statistical supplement, 1992 Annual Supplement: 55–96.

20. Thomas LG. The lives of a cell. New York: Viking Press, 1974.

21. Pryor DB, Harrell FE Jr, Rankin JS, et al. The changing survival benefits of coronary revascularization over time. Circulation 1987; 76(suppl V): 13–21.

22. Smith A. An inquiry into the nature and causes of wealth of nations, vol 2. Oxford: Oxford University Press, 1776: 869–70.

23. Rice T. An alternative framework for evaluating welfare losses in the health care market. J Health Econ 1992; 11: 86–92.

24. Langa KM, Sussman EJ. The effects of cost-containment policies on rates of coronary revascularization in California. N Engl J Med 1993; 329: 1784–9.

25. Cosgrove DM. Surgical myocardial revascularization. Cardiology in the Elderly 1993; 193(1): 71–6.

26. Keon WJ, Menzies SC. Morbidity and mortality after myocardial revascularization in patients with ischemic heart disease. In: Walter PJ, editor. Quality of life after open heart surgery, Dordrecht, The Netherlands: Kluwer Academic Publishers, 1992: 107–14.

2. Do growing proportions of elderly mean more cardiovascular diseases?

HANS HOFFMEISTER and LEE MUECKE

Introduction

As we approach the end of this century and prepare to enter a new millenium, we find that our many medical advances provide us with the longest life expectancies ever known. Western societies are now faced with larger numbers of these 'survivors' than ever before. But is it a clear victory for society to increase the longevity of its people? Or, as some critics might claim, are we merely prolonging life without consideration of its diminished quality: the pain and limitations of chronic disease.

We can begin to answer these complex questions by looking at epidemiological data to provide objective measures on which to base such decisions. In the case of cardiovascular diseases, we can demonstrate an overall increase in disease-free years by comparing data on mean age of cardiovascular mortality. This provides an overall improvement in quality of life in society at large.

First, some important aspects of cardiovascular morbidity and mortality in the elderly will be discussed. Secondly, I will try to elucidate the influence that improved lifestyle has had on health and longevity, and discuss the role of cardiovascular interventions in prolonged life expectancy.

Mortality: Structure in developed countries and their consequences

Life expectancy provides a meaningful reflection of a population's health status. Figure 2.1 gives an overview of life expectancy among newborns in European and other industrialized nations in 1990. The presence of a net increase or decrease since 1970 is indicated for each country [1] for both males (Figure 2.1a) and females (Figure 2.1b).

The enhancement of life expectancy is the main cause for an increasing proportion of elderly in most countries. In this respect, Japan is the most successful country, and many European countries have also progressed over the past two decades. Only the East European countries were less successful.

13

P.J. Walter (ed.), Coronary Bypass Surgery in the Elderly, pp. 13–23.
© 1995 *Kluwer Academic Publishers, Dordrecht.*

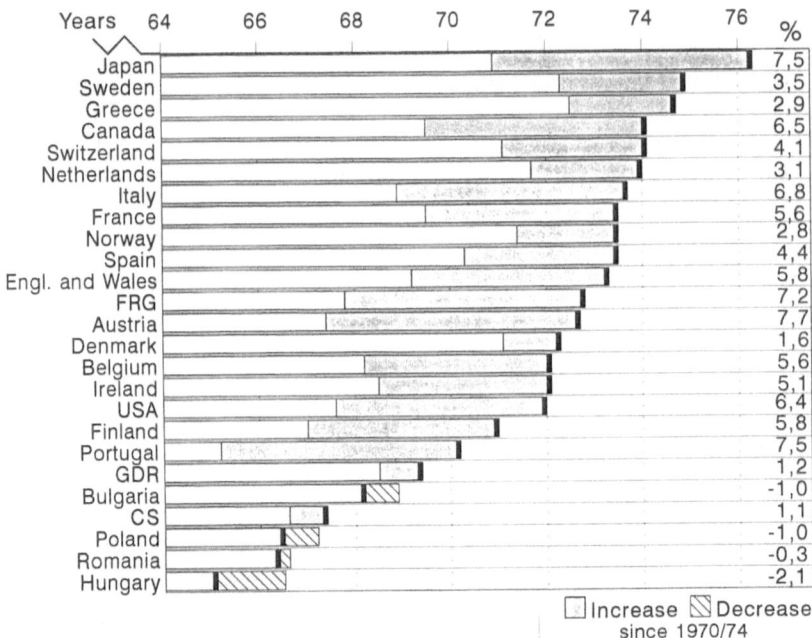

Figure 2.1a. Mean life expectancy for males, 1990 (Sweden, Italy, Spain, U.S.A., Finland 1989; Belgium 1987; Romania 1988).

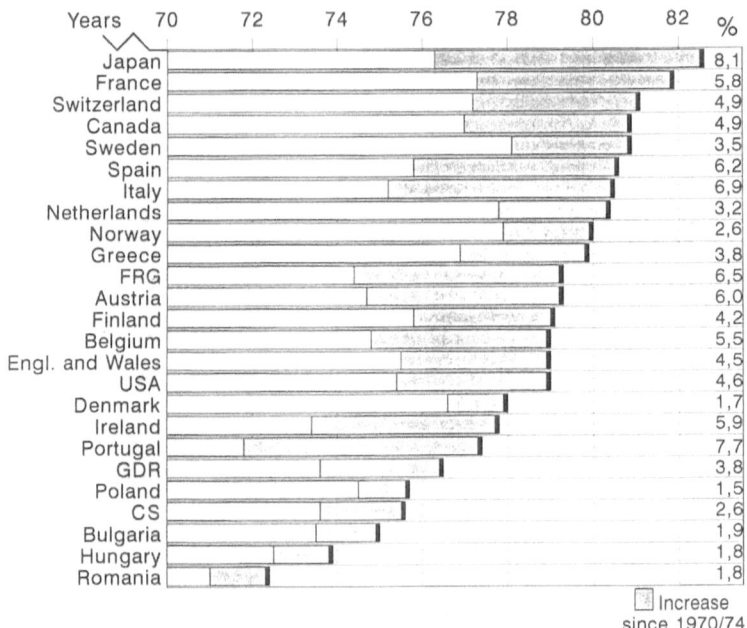

Figure 2.1b. Mean life expectancy for females, 1990 (Sweden, Italy, Spain, U.S.A., Finland 1989; Belgium 1987; Romania 1988).

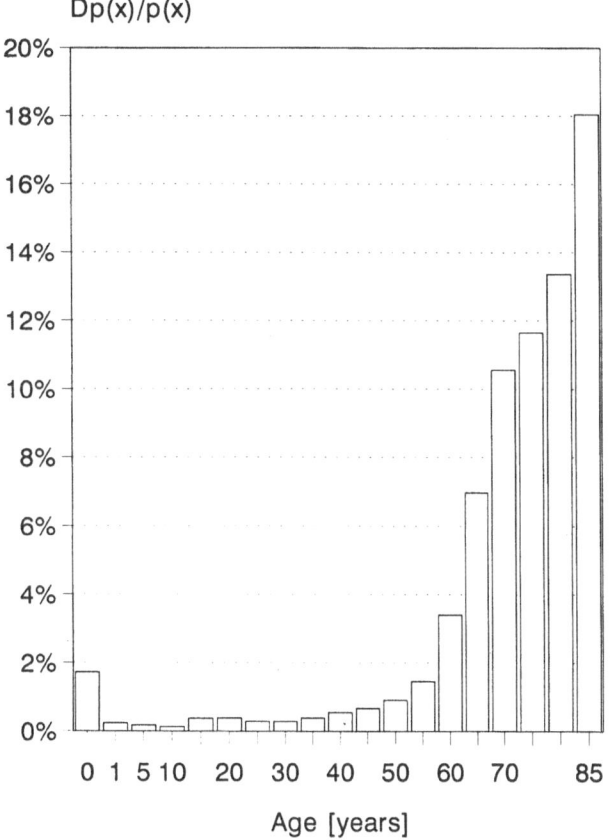

Figure 2.2. Relative increase of age-specific life expectancy; Germany (West) 1971–1987.

Today, our increased life expectancy can be primarily attributed to increased survival among the elderly sector of society rather than decreases in infant mortality. In Figure 2.2, the West German trends of age-specific gains in years of life over the last two decades demonstrate this convincingly. Clearly the largest gains in survival steadily increase with increasing age, with the most aged members of society benefiting the most.

Together with low birth rates, this development will lead to growing proportions of elderly in industrialized countries. Figure 2.3 contains the results of a prognostic model for population growth in Germany [2]. The graph shows that in the year 2030, there will be double the number of people over age 60, compared with the group aged 20 or younger. Today, these two age groups are roughly the same size. New prognoses from EUROSTAT and the U.N. Population Prospects give similar figures for other European countries as well.

Does this predicted population distribution imply that there will be a corresponding increase in cardiovascular disease? And, if so, will there be an

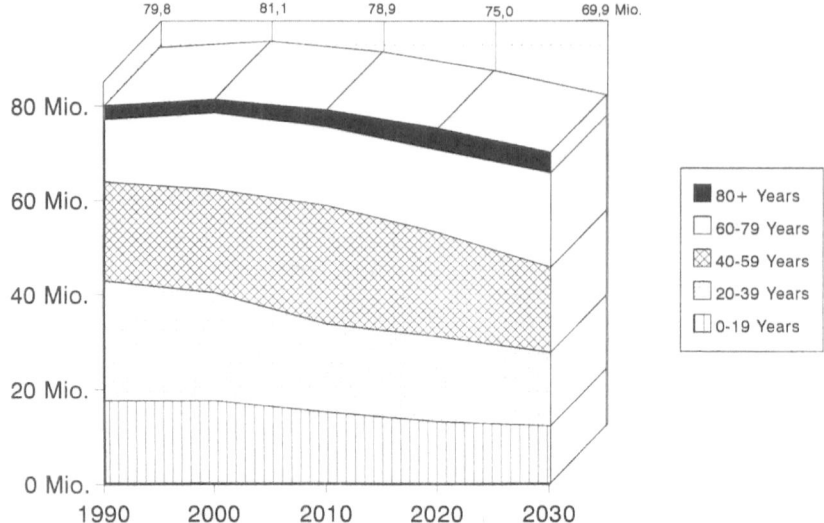

Figure 2.3. Predicted trend of the German population (Statistisches Bundesamt 31.12.1989).

increased need for cardiovascular surgery and associated health care expenses? This assumption is not valid upon closer examination.

It is well known that cardiovascular disease is the leading cause of death in western societies. Normally, the proportion of cardiovascular death is higher than 50%. In Figure 2.4, we see the rates for Germany in 1990 [3]. Figure 2.5

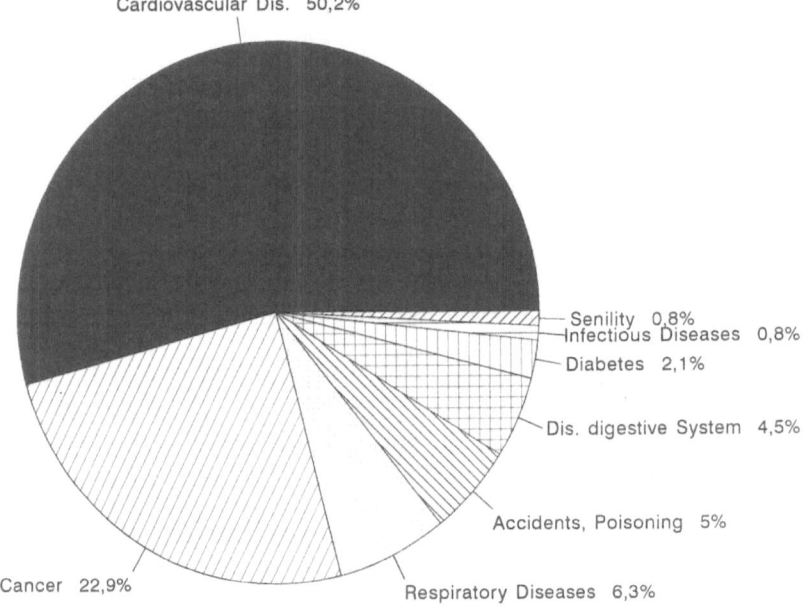

Figure 2.4. All causes of death, Germany (West) 1990.

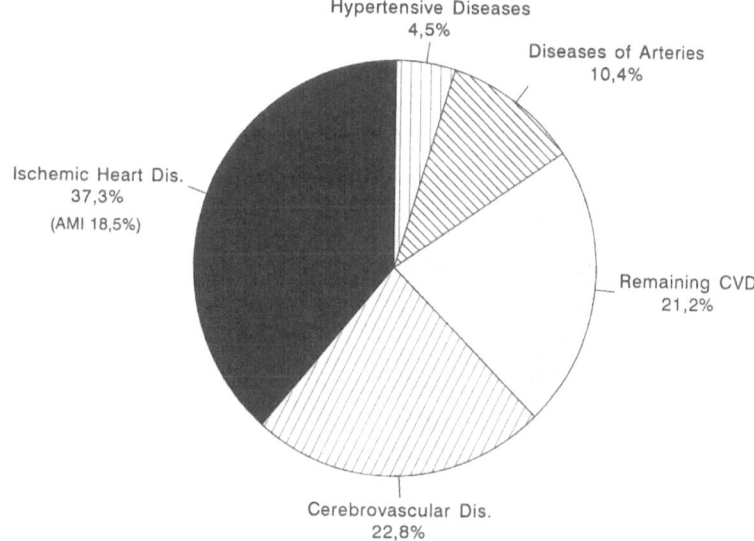

Figure 2.5. Specific causes of death, Germany (West) 1990 – cardiovascular diseases.

shows that among all cardiovascular deaths, ischemic heart disease is most common (nearly 40%) while cerebrovascular disease accounts for 23% of deaths, and other heart diseases comprise the balance. But a mortality structure like this

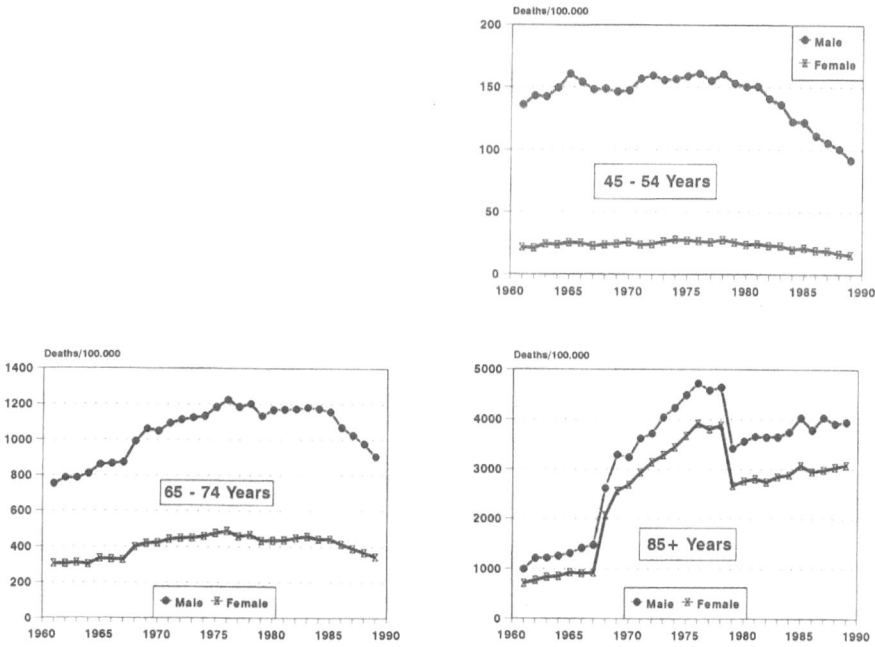

Figure 2.6. Ischemic heart diseases ICD 410–414 Germany (West).

is often misunderstood. The dominance of these diseases in a society is not alarming but, on the contrary, provide an indication of superior health status and medical care [4].

Although we have managed to prolong our life expectancy to record lengths, it is inevitable that the majority of very elderly people will be afflicted with chronic disease and many will die from cardiovascular disease. Clearly, this sector of society will require significant medical care. What is important, however, is that early onset of disease, and its associated increase in mortality, is avoided. With this in mind, a look at age-specific mortality rates provides some interesting insights.

In many western countries, there is a prolonged downward trend in cardiovascular mortality rates among all age groups below age 75. Figure 2.6 demonstrates the trends in Germany over the last thirty years for selected age groups and for the diagnosis of ischemic heart disease. The past two decades have shown a steady decrease among those under 75 years of age (men greater than women). As a consequence of decreasing rates in the 'younger groups', the age-specific mortality rates in those over 85 years are growing. In Figure 2.7, similar trends for myocardial infarction can be seen. A more complete set of age-specific mortality data is published elsewhere [2].

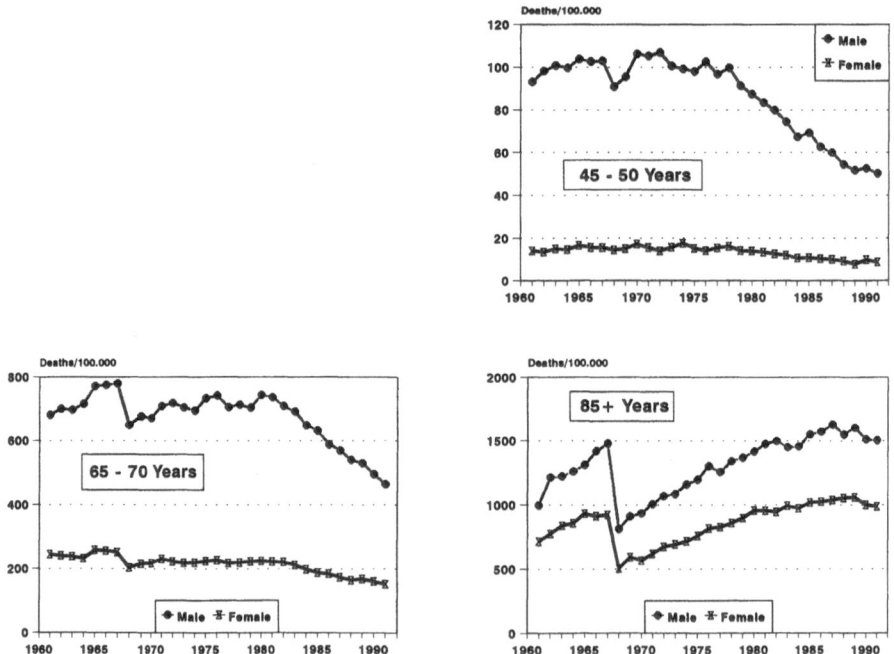

Figure 2.7. Acute myocardial infarction ICD 410 Germany (West).

Morbidity trends

Do the morbidity data reflect the same downward trends seen in age-specific mortality for those under age 75? The German National Health surveys [5, 6] show di fferent trends for cardiovascular morbidity. Data on self-reported cardiovascular disease, including angina pectoris and MI, from three national representative samples of the German population demonstrate there was no significant increase in prevalence of these diseases over the last decade (Table 2.1). This finding, however, is inconsistent with current worldwide trends in cardiovascular hospitalizations [7]. One must use caution in interpreting this apparent contradiction.

Table 2.1. Prevalence of ischemic heart diseases Germany (West), age 25–69.

	Men		Women	
Disease (self-reported)	1984	1991	1984	1991
Angina pectoris	10.8 %	11.0 %	10.9 %	9.1 %
Acute myocardial infarction	3.6 %	4.1 %	1.5 %	1.5 %

Indeed, there is a tremendous increase in hospital admissions for all cardiovascular diseases, both acute and chronic. This is illustrated by comparing representative German data from 1979 with 1991 for men and, to a lesser degree, women (Table 2.2). These data were derived from repeated clinical surveys of the hospitalized German population performed by Infratest, and are age standardised [8]. However, concurrent with this increase in prevalence, the average length of a hospital stay became several days shorter than a decade before. This is the first hint that perhaps hospital admissions do not provide an

Table 2.2. Hospital prevalence and mean stay in hospital Germany (West), age 60+.

	Hospital prevelance patients/1000				Mean stay in hospital days/patient			
	Men		Women		Men		Women	
Disease ICD 8	1979	1991	1979	1991	1979	1991	1979	1991
Cardiovasc. Diseases 390–459	591	991	452	633	21.1	16.1	24.9	16.8
Ischemic Heart Dis. 410–414	158	335	85	127	23.7	14.6	25.2	14.9
Other Heart Diseases 390–398, 415–429	192	277	182	221	19.5	17.6	23.6	18.2
Acute myocard. Infarc. 410	87	133	34	45				

accurate picture of true disease prevalence, although they may reflect other issues such as improved access to care, increased public awareness and technological advances allowing earlier detection.

Public health campaigns regarding early detection of disease have been part of an overall secular trend towards valuing one's health. Members of western societies are no longer willing to bear their pain in silence and now actively seek out sophisticated therapies, all of which serves to increase health care utilization and costs. Such attitudinal changes have been documented by analyzing the data on subjective health feeling and satisfaction with life conditions in German National Health surveys over the last decade.

A deeper insight into the morbidity data reveals another dimension of the complex issue of evaluating true morbidity. It is important to determine whether the age at onset of cardiovascular disease shows the same or similar trends as mortality. Unfortunately there are no representative, population-based data in the literature to answer this question. Even in the MONICA-projects of the World Health Organization, which registers cardiovascular morbidity and mortality in many places of the world, such data are unavailable. In Germany, the previously mentioned data base from Infratest is available for this purpose [8]. In these national representative samples, hospital admissions and diagnoses are recorded for every year since 1978.

Table 2.3 contains age-standardized, comparable data on the mean age of hospitalized patients. Although subject to secular influences, this statistic can serve as a rough marker for the more severe clinical onset of different diseases. As seen in Table 2.3, the average age of patients with cardiovascular diseases was approximately two years higher in 1991 as compared to the mean age in 1979. Clearly, this is strong evidence for later onset of disease. This delay in onset of cardiovascular morbidity can be seen throughout all cardiovascular disease, including heart infarction (+3.2 years) (Table 2.3). This trend reflects

Table 2.3. Indices for morbidity and mortality in Germany (West).

Disease ICD 9	Mean age of hospitalized patients (years)			Mean age of death (years)					
				Men			Women		
	1979	1991	Diff.	1979	1989	Diff.	1979	1989	Diff.
Cardiovasc. Dis. 390–459	62.3	64.3	+ 2.0	76.9	77.7	+ 0.8	80.3	81.2	+ 0.9
Ischemic Heart Dis. 410–414	62.5	64.0	+ 1.5	73.5	75.5	+ 2.0	78.2	79.7	+ 1.5
Other Heart. Dis. 390–398, 415–429	65.1	68.0	+ 2.9						
Acute myocard. Inf. 410	63.2	66.4	+ 3.2	71.1	73.3	+ 2.2	75.5	77.3	+ 1.8

a decreased risk for early myocardial infarction in 1991 relative to 10 years earlier.

A side-by-side comparison of both 1979 and 1989 values for mean age at death for cardiovascular diseases is also provided in Table 2.3. These data show a net increase among men, ranging from 0.8 years for all cardiovascular disease, to 2.2 years for acute M.I. The later onset of morbidity in conjunction with increased life span results in a net increase in disease-free years.

How can these apparent improvements in morbidity and mortality be explained? Two questions must be answered. First: Are there preventive effects which have delayed the mean age for onset of cardiovascular disease and mortality? Second: What role has medical intervention, including surgical techniques, played in this trend?

The answer to the first question is not easy. In Table 2.4, trends in prevalence of classic cardiovascular risk factors among the German population are shown from 1984 to 1991 [6]. Hypercholesterolemia, hypertension and obesity are more prevalent in our population in the early 1990s than they were ten years earlier. There is also minimal change to be seen in overall smoking prevalence over this period, with the subgroup of young women showing a small increase while older men showed a decrease.

The overall risk for cardiovascular deaths, from these four classic risk factors, calculated by multiple logistic regression, indicates this risk is higher in Germany today than it was 10 years ago [4].

Why is there a sustained decrease of all cardiovascular diseases in men and women under these circumstances? One possible explanation is that there are

Table 2.4. Prevalence of risk factors and health behaviour – National Health surveys, Germany (West).

	Trends 1984–1991			
	Men		Women	
Parameter	Age 25–69	Age 60–69	Age 25–69	Age 60–69
Body Mass Index ≥ 30 kg/m^2	+ 13 %	+ 17 %	+ 15 %	+ 8 %
Total cholesterol ≥ 250 mg/dl^{-1}	+ 12 %	+ 12 %	+ 1 %	− 5 %
HDL-Cholesterol ≤ 35 mg/dl^{-1}	− 35 %	− 107 %	± 0 %	− 49 %
Hypertension $\geq 160/95$ mmzhg^{-1}	− 11 %	+ 4 %	+ 8 %	+ 15 %
Proportion of smokers	− 5 %	− 15 %	+ 6 %	− 3 %
Mean pulse rate 1 min^{-1}	− 4 %	− 4 %	− 4 %	− 4 §
Intak of antioxidants as medication	+	++	+	++

other important influences reducing the risk, a few of which are included in Table 2.4. HDL-Cholesterol has continued to improve over the past ten years and, along with a significant lowering of mean pulse rate, may reflect increased social awareness and participation in regular physical activity.

Also, there is mounting evidence for the role of anti-oxidants in reducing cardiovascular disease [9]. Evidence from the nutritional and drug consumption components of the German National surveys indicates that the intake of antioxidants, both in the diet and as medication, has increased over the past decade (unpublished data).

Concerning the second question, there is no simple picture. As seen in Table 2.4, medical intervention for hypertension has been largely unsuccessful in Germany over the past decade (and longer). Also, the growing role of PTCA and the use of CABG cannot alone explain the delay in cardiovascular mortality [10]. Further studies are required to fully evaluate the efficacy of intervention PTCA, which has undergone phenomenal growth in Germany from 2,809 cases in 1984 to 56,967 in 1992. As the aging population of industrialized nations continues to grow, we will inevitably see increased cardiovascular morbidity among the elderly. But what does this really mean? A growing amount of cardiovascular intervention in the elderly, along with associated high cost of health care, reflects nothing less than having successfully avoided cardiovascular and other diseases in younger years. Therefore we should be pleased with our progress, while at the same time, we continue to investigate all aspects of cardiovascular disease, including both etiology and prevention. But one fact is certain: the elderly segment of society is growing, and this elderly segment will need intervention techniques such as CABG and PTCA more than ever. This prolonged longevity and delay in morbidity represents a significant gain in our overall quality of life.

References

1. World Health Organization. World Health statistics annual, 1993. Geneva: WHO, 1993.
2. Statistisches Bundesamt. Internal report, Wiesbaden, 1989.
3. Statistisches Bundesamt (Hrsg.). Fachserie 12, Reihe 4: Todesursachen, 1960–1993. Stuttgart: Metzler-Poeschel-Verlag, 1960; 1961.....1993.
4. Hoffmeister H. Gesundheitszustand und Krankheitsspektrum als Basis der Gesundheitsvorsorge. In: Zukunftsaufgabe Gesundheitsvorsorge, Verlag für Gesundheitsförderung, Hamburg: Bundesministerium für Gesundheit (Hrsg.), 1993: 4–18.
5. Hoffmeister H, Hoeltz J, Schön D, Schröder E, Güther B. Nationaler Untersuchungs-Survey der DHP, DHP-Forum, Bd. I. Bonn: Wissenschaftliches Institut der Ärzte Deutschlands, 1988.
6. Bundesgesundheitsministerium (Hrsg.): Daten des Gesundheitswesens, Bd. 25. Baden-Baden: Nomos Verlagsgesellschaft, 1993: 93–121.
7. Bonneux L, et al. Estimating clinical morbidity due to ischemic heart disease and congestive heart failure: the future rise of heart failure. Am J Public Health 1994; 84(1): 20–7.

8. Infratest-Gesundheitsforschung. Umfang von Fehlbelegungen in Akutkrankenhäusern bei Patienten aller Altersklassen. In: Forschungsbericht Gesundheitsforschung. Bonn: Bundesministerium für Arbeit und Sozialordnung (Hrsg.), 1989.

9. Kardinaal AFM, et al. Antioxidants in adipose tissue and risk of myocardial infarction: the EURAMIC study. The Lancet 1993; 342: 1379–84.

10. Gleichmann U, Mannebach H, Lichtlen P. Bericht über Struktur und Leistungszahlen der Herzkatheterlabors in der Bundesrepublik Deutschland. Z Kardiol 1994; 83: 74–8.

PART TWO

Favourable clinical results of CABG in the elderly

3. Isolated CABG in the elderly: Operative results and risk factors over the past three decades

WILBERT J. KEON

Introduction

It is well established that coronary artery bypass graft (CABG) surgery performed on patients with severe angina leads to lessening of symptoms in a majority of cases [1, 2] and prologation of life in certain patient subsets. With an ageing population, increased safety of surgical procedures, and improvements in post-operative care, coronary artery bypass grafting is being performed on an increasing number of elderly patients [3]. However, because of the reported increased mortality and morbidity in the elderly [4–11], many patients with severely symptomatic coronary atherosclerotic heart disease are not considered for surgery (or younger patients are given precedence).

The aim of this study was to compare perioperative mortality and morbidity of patients, 70 years of age and over, with patients 69 years of age and younger undergoing CABG surgery. In addition, patients who underwent isolated bypass surgery at the University of Ottawa Heart Institute during three separate time periods (1970–1973, 1980–1983 and 1990–1993) were analysed so that trends in these parameters could be assesed over the past three decades.

The results of this study indicate that with current techniques, coronary bypass can be performed in the elderly with mortality and morbidity rates which are only slightly higher than those in younger patients. Therefore, patients aged 70 years and older should not be denied coronary bypass surgery on the basis of age alone.

Methods

Patients

The population for the first part of this study included all patients who underwent isolated coronary arterial bypass surgery at the University of Ottawa Heart Institute from 1990–1993. Patients aged 70 years of age or older (70+ years) were analyzed separately from those less than 70 years of age (< 70

27

P.J. Walter (ed.), Coronary Bypass Surgery in the Elderly, pp. 27–40.
© 1995 *Kluwer Academic Publishers, Dordrecht.*

Table 3.1. Risk factors for isolated CABG patients

	< 70 years		70+ years		
	N	(%)	N	(%)	*p*
Number	246		54		
Mean age (± SD)	56.9 ± 8.8		73.3 ± 2.3		
Female	45	(18)	17	(32)	0.030
Smoking	64	(26)	1	(1.9)	< 0.001
Hyperlipidemia	27	(11)	1	(1.9)	0.037
Hypercholesteremia	59	(24)	6	(11)	0.038
Family history	100	(41)	8	(15)	< 0.001
PVD	17	(6.9)	1	(1.9)	NS
Diabetes	41	(17)	6	(11)	NS
MI (< 3 months)	38	(15)	9	(17)	NS
MI (> 3 months)	8	(35)	14	(26)	NS
COPD	14	(5.7)	5	(9.3)	NS

Comparative results in a consecutive series of 300 patients during the time period 1990–1993.
PVD, peripheral valve disease; MI, myocardial infarction; COPD, coronary obstructive pulmonary disease.

years). The number, mean age and sex of patients in each age group are summarized in Table 3.1.

For the analysis of trends over time, data from the following time periods were used: 1970–1973, 1980–1983 and 1990–1993. For this analysis, patients aged 65 years of age or older (65+ years) were analyzed separately from those less than 65 years of age (< 65 years). The number of patients, mean age and sex of patients in each age group for each time period are summarized in Table 3.2.

Table 3.2. Risk factors and procedural variable for isolated CABG patients (trends over time)

	1970–1973				1980–1983				1990–1993			
	< 65		65+		< 65		65+		< 65		65+	
	N	(%)	N	(%)	N	(%)	N	(%)	N	(%)	N	(%)
Number	334		7		1574		228		1452		997	
Mean age	48.9		65.7		52.3		68.2		54.6		69.9	
Female	22	(6.6)	1	(14)	234	(15)	74	(32)	225	(16)	256	(26)
Emergency	36	(11)	1	(14)	96	(6.1)	23	(10)	58	(4)	42	(4.3)
Urgent									78	(5.4)	82	(8.4)
Repeat operation	2	(0.6)	0		80	(5.1)	5	(2.2)	178	(12)	94	(10)
LIMA/RIMA	4	(1.2)	0		7	(0.04)	2	(0.09)	921	(63)	504	(52)
Endarterectomy	62	(19)	1	(14)	329	(21)	50	(22)	195	(13)	172	(18)
Mean – grafts	1.9		1.9		3.1		3.1		3.0		2.9	

LIMA/RIMA, left/right interior thoracic (mammary) artery.

Patients having concomitant surgical procedures were excluded from the study.

Definitions

Congestive heart failure is defined in our institute as clinical pulmonary or peripheral edema and dyspnea necessitating the use of diuretics. Patients undergoing emergency surgery exhibited cardiogenic shock, acute unstable myocardial infarction and pre-infarctional angina requiring immediate revascularization. Urgent surgery is defined as requiring revascularization within the same admission (Provincial Adult Cardiac Care Network definition). Patients were classified functionally according to the New York Heart Association (NYHA) guidelines: asymptomatic (Class I), symptomatic on moderate exertion (Class II), symptomatic on mild exertion (Class III) or symptomatic at rest (Class IV). For angiographic classification of ventricular contractility, the left ventricle was divided into four segments. Class I function indicates hypokinesia, akinesia or dyskinesia in one segment; Class IV indicates dysfunction in all four segments.

Surgical methods

Because this study covers surgery over the past three decades, there were a number of differences in the surgical methods used. During the 1970s, all operations were performed under conditions of normothermic, anoxic cardiac arrest. During the 1980s, hearts were K^+-arrested with cold (5 °C) crystalloid cardioplegia using one of four cardioplegia solutions was used: Plegisol (no additives); St. Thomas concentrate; Plegisol buffered with 10 meq $NaHCO_3$; or, St. Thomas reconstituted and buffered with 5 meq $NaHCO_3$. Myocardial temperature was maintained between 0 and 5 °C with topical cooling. During the 1990s, hearts were K^+-arrested with cold (5 °C) St. Thomas solution containing 19.57 mmol KCl and myocardial temperature was maintained at 12 °C with topical cooling.

Every effort was made to use the internal mammary artery for one graft because of its improved patency rate.

Statistics

Univariate statistical analysis was performed by means of Student's t-test for continuous variables, and a χ^2 or Fisher's exact test (where appropriate) when comparing frequencies.

Results

Detailed comparison between young (< 70 years) and elderly (70+ years) CABG patients

A consecutive series of 300 patients who underwent isolated coronary artery bypass grafting as of 1 April 1990 were analyzed. A series of 54 patients aged 70+ years was compared with a consecutive series of 246 patients under the age of 70 who underwent the same surgical procedure during the same period. Preoperative, operative and post-operative data were analyzed.

Preoperative data
Preoperative data are summarized in Table 3.1. The patients aged 70+ were more often female (p = 0.030), had a lower incidence of hyperlipidemia (p = 0.037) and hypercholesteremia (p = 0.038), were less likély to have a family history of heart disease (p < 0.001) and were less likely to smoke (p < 0.001). Differences in peripheral vascular disease, diabetes, previous myocardial infarction and coronary obstructive pulmonary disease between age groups were not significant.

As with younger patients, moderate to severe angina pectoris was the main indication for bypass surgery. Significantly more elderly patients exhibited

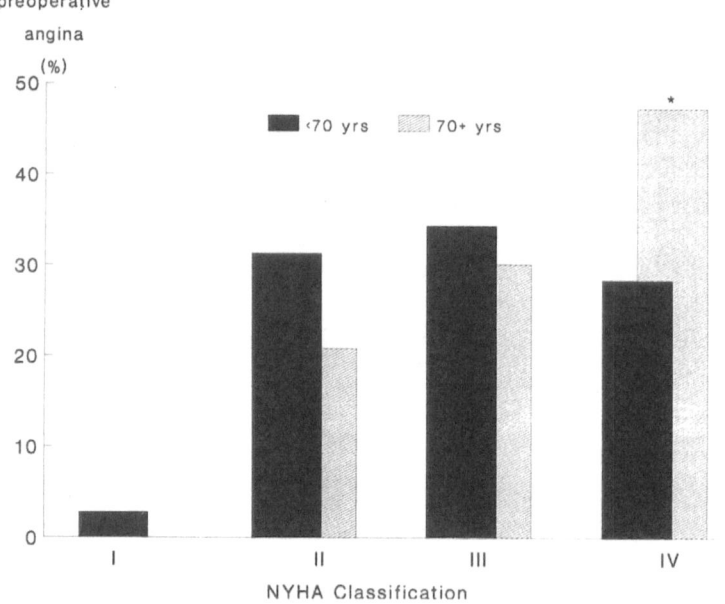

Figure 3.1. Preoperative angina in elderly isolated CABG patients. Data were obtained from a consecutive series of 300 patients. The number of patients 70 years of age and older exhibiting Class IV angina was significantly higher (p < 0.05) in comparison with younger patients undergoing the same surgical procedure.

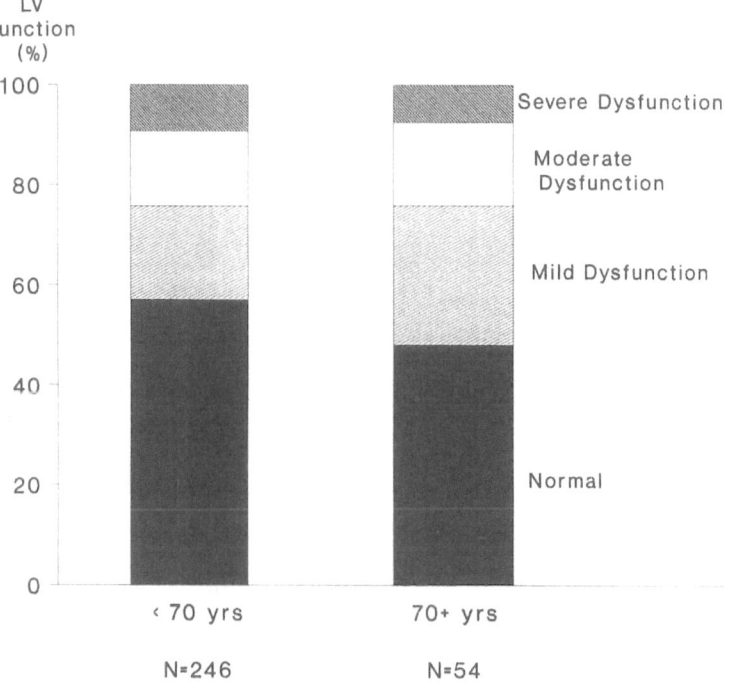

Figure 3.2. Preoperative left ventricular classification in isolated CABG patients. Data were obtained from a consecutive series of 300 patients. There were no significant differences in levels of left ventricular dysfunction between age groups.

severe preoperative angina (NYHA Class IV, $p < 0.05$ relative to the younger patients) (Figure 3.1) (see Methods for details of classification). The majority of patients in both groups exhibited normal left ventricular function. Mild, moderate and severe dysfunction was seen to a lesser degree in both groups (Figure 3.2) (see Methods for details of classifications). The number of patients exhibiting each level of ventricular dysfunction was not significantly different between age groups.

Operative data
Mean post-operative hospital stay was significantly higher in the elderly ($p = 0.006$) but differences in other procedural variables were not significant (Table 3.3). Number of grafts required, anoxic time and bypass time were all comparable between age groups.

Post-operative data
In this study, hospital mortality (defined as within 30 days of surgery) was not significantly different between age groups (Table 3.4). Significantly more patients aged 70+ years required reopening ($p < 0.037$) relative to < 70 years and leg wound complications were significantly higher in the 70+ group

Table 3.3. Procedural variables for isolated CABG patients

	< 70 years		70+ years		
	N	(%)	N	(%)	*p*
Number	246		54		
Repeat surgery	32	(13)	3	(5.6)	NS
Urgent surgery	32	(13)	4	(7.4)	NS
Emergency surgery	18	(7.3)	7	(13)	NS
LIMA/RIMA	152	(66)	32	(59)	NS
Endarterectomy	22	(8.9)	4	(7.4)	NS
IABP	11	(4.5)	2	(3.7)	NS
	Mean		Mean		
No. grafts	2.8 ± 0.8		3.0 ± 0.9		NS
Anoxic time (min)	40.4 ± 13.6		38.5 ± 13.3		NS
Bypass time (min)	85.2 ± 31.9		82.4 ± 26.5		NS
Post-op hospital stay (days)	10.8 ± 6.7		14.0 ± 12.7		0.006

Comparative results in a consecutive series of 300 patients during the time period 1990 – 1993. LIMA/RIMA, left/right interior thoracic (mammary) artery; IABP, intraaortic balloon.

Table 3.4. Mortality and complications in isolated CABG patients

	< 70 years		70+ years		
	N	(%)	N	(%)	*p*
	246		54		
Hospital mortality[a]	4	(1.6)	3	(3.7)	NS
Reopening	5	(2.0)	4	(7.4)	0.037
Renal failure	4	(1.6)	3	(5.6)	NS
Peri-operative MI	7	(2.8)	2	(3.7)	NS
Stroke	3	(1.2)	1	(1.9)	NS
Leg wound complications	21	(8.5)	8	(15)	0.003
Atrial fibrillation/flutter	129	(12)	5	(9.3)	NS
Sternal wound complications	6	(2.4)	6	(11)	NS
Other infection	8	(3.2)	2	(3.7)	NS
Pulmonary complications	10	(4.1)	2	(3.7)	NS
Ventricular rhythm disturbances	7	(2.8)	2	(3.7)	NS
Heart block	3	(1.2)	0		NS
Urology complications	1	(0.4)	1	(1.8)	NS
Other[b]	4	(1.6)	2	(3.7)	NS

Comparative results in a consecutive series of 300 patients during the time period 1990–1993.
[a] Within 30 days.
[b] Tracheitis, coagulopathy, gangrene or excess bleeding in patients < 70 years of age; graft thrombosis or phrenic nerve palsy in patients 70+ years.

(p = 0.003). All other major and minor post-operative complications, including cardiac and non-cardiac complications, were comparable between groups (Table 3.4).

Trends in preoperative, operative and post-operative parameters over the past three decades

A consecutive series of patients (65 years of age and older) who underwent isolated coronary artery bypass grafting at the University of Ottawa Heart Institute were analyzed for three separate time periods: 1970–1973, 1980–1983 and 1990–1993. Preoperative, operative and post-operative data were analyzed for a total of 4592 patients.

Preoperative
Over the past three decades, the number of female patients has increased for both age groups (Table 3.2). Although the number of patients undergoing emergency isolated CABG tended to be higher for the elderly patients (65+ years) in comparison with the younger patients for all time periods, only the data for 1980–1983 was significantly different (p = 0.02). The number of elderly patients undergoing surgery classified as urgent was significantly higher than

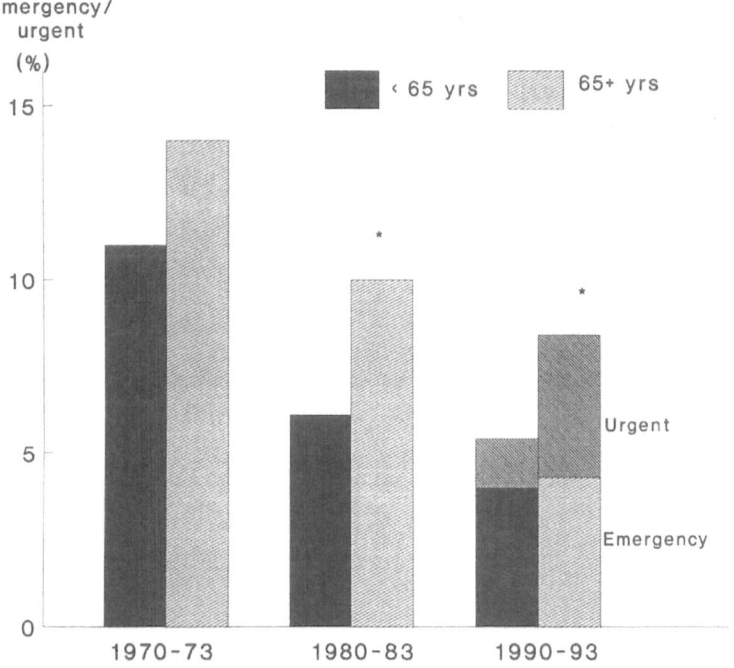

Figure 3.3. Trends in the number of young (< 65 years of age) and elderly (65 years of age and older) patients undergoing emergency isolated CABG surgery during the three time periods of study. For the final time period, both emergency and urgent surgery are shown.

for younger patients ($p = 0.004$) and the sum of urgent and emergency surgery was also higher ($p = 0.01$) (Table 3.2 and Figure 3.3). The number of patients undergoing emergency surgery has decreased for both groups over time ($p < 0.001$ for < 65 years and $p = 0.001$ for 65+). However, when the data for urgent and emergency surgery were combined, the decrease was not significant in the elderly.

The number of patients undergoing repeat CABG surgery has increased dramatically over time for both age groups (Table 3.2). In the first time period (1970s) < 1% of the younger patients and no elderly patients underwent repeat surgery. This had increased to 5.1% of < 65 years of age and 2.2% of 65+ years of age by the 1980s, and 12% of < 65 and 10% of 65+ by the 1990s.

Operative
The incidence of surgery utilizing the right/left internal thoracic (mammary) artery (RIMA/LIMA) was low for both age groups (< 2%) during the 1970s and 1980s and increased dramatically for both age groups during the 1990s (63% for < 65 and 52% for 65+ years of age) (Table 3.2). Endarterectomies remained essentially constant for both age groups over the time periods studied.

Post-operative
Mortality for younger patients (< 65 years of age) showed a small but significant decrease over the past three decades ($p < 0.001$) (Figure 3.4). In comparison, our data indicates that mortality for the elderly patients decreased significantly from the 1970s to the 1980s and continued to decrease into the 1990s ($p < 0.001$). For all time points, mortality for the elderly was higher than for the younger patients, but as discussed above, the differences are not

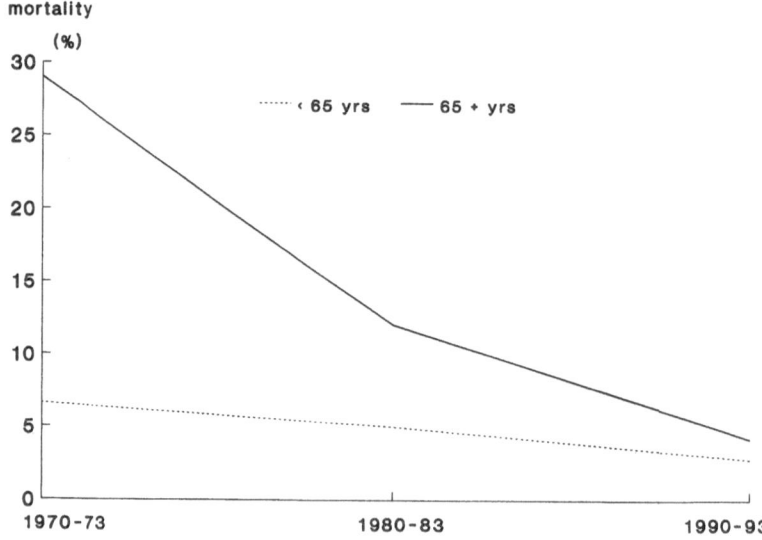

Figure 3.4. Trends in post-operative mortality of isolated CABG patients over the past three decades. Mortality for young and elderly patients during 1990–1993 were not significantly different.

significant for the most recent set of data (data obtained during 1990–1993) (1970s, $p = 0.002$; 1980s $p = 0.008$; 1990s, NS).

Discussion

Persons aged 70 years or over have the highest incidence of coronary heart disease [12], the highest incidence of acute myocardial infarction [13] and the highest cardiovascular death rate in the country [14]. Because this age group is increasing relative to the rest of the population, the use of open heart surgical techniques in this age group is also increasing [15]. However, early studies [4] reported a 21% hospital mortality rate in 1977 for patients aged 70 to 80 years and an exponential relationship between hospital mortality and age for patients 70 years or older. Based on this data, the use of CABG surgery for the management of heart disease in the elderly has been questioned [16]. Our study was undertaken to determine the operative risks and benefits of CABG surgery in elderly patients by analyzing a large body of data (a total of 4592 patients) obtained over three decades at the University of Ottawa Heart Institute.

Comparison with data reported by other centres

To assess the risk associated with isolated CABG, a group of 54 consecutive patients, aged 70 years or more at the time of operation, was studied and compared with 246 consecutive younger patients who underwent the same surgical procedure. These data were then compared with similar data reported by other centres.

As shown in Figures 3.5–3.9, there is a high degree of variability between data reported by different researchers. However, the percentage of patients aged 70 years or older exhibiting specific risk factors (sex, diabetes, hypertension, smoking, COPD) (Figure 3.6), procedural variables (repeat surgery, emergency surgery, LIMA/RIMA and IABP) (Figure 3.7), perioperative complications (MI, reopening, atrial fibrillation/flutter, renal failure, wounds and stroke) (Figure 3.8) reported in this study all fall within the maximum and minimum limits reported by other researchers. The preoperative coronary status (number of diseased vessels, congestive heart failure, degree of stenosis, left ventricular dysfunction and severe angina) (Figure 3.9) also fall within the maximum and minimum limits.

Perhaps the highest degree of variability between ages and between centres is in the reported mortalities of young and elderly CABG patients, as shown in Figure 3.5. Comparison of these data with those reported previously indicate that mortality ranges from < 1% to 5% for young patients and < 2% to 12% for elderly patients. In contrast to early studies [4], 7 of 14 researchers, including the present study, report no significant difference in mortality between young and elderly patients.

As reported previously, non-cardiac complications are more common in the

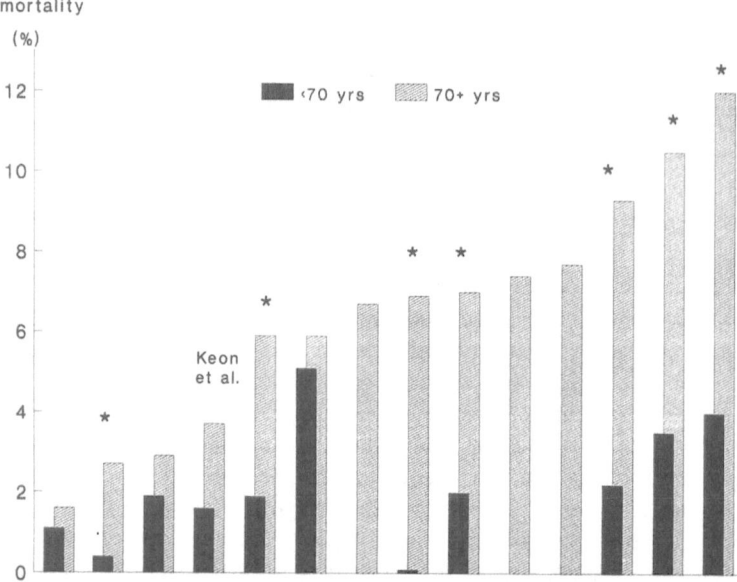

Figure 3.5. Comparison of current and previously reported mortalities for young (< 70 years of age) and elderly (70 years of age and older) CABG patients [5–11, 15, 17–20].

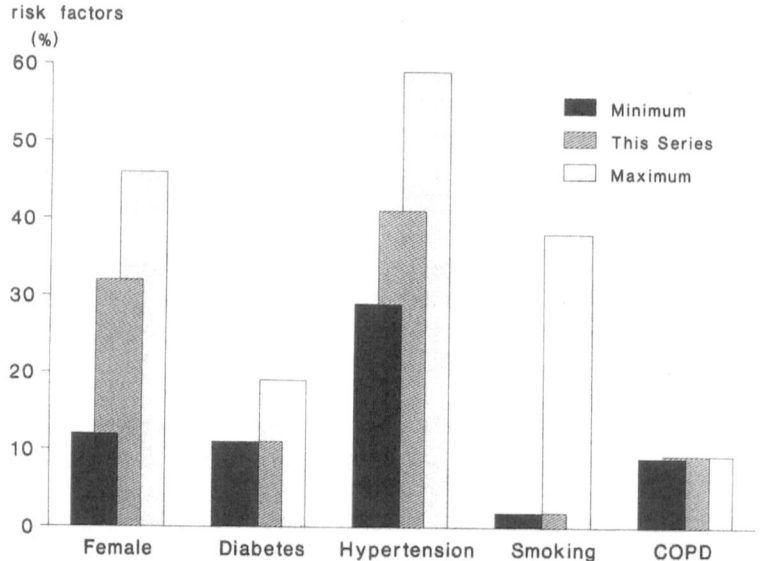

Figure 3.6. Risk factors for elderly isolated CABG patients. Data shown are those from the current study as well as maximum and minimum values from the literature.

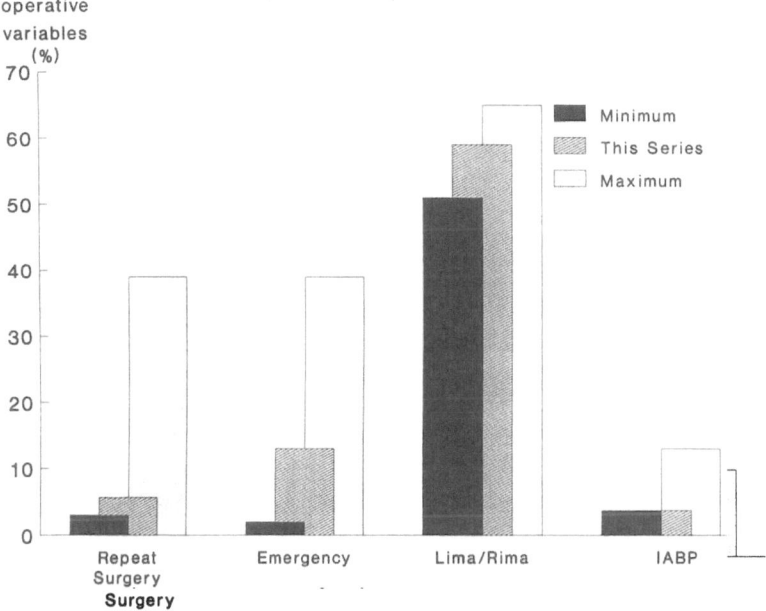

Figure 3.7. Operational variables for elderly isolated CABG patients. Data shown are those from the current study as well as maximum and minimum values from the literature.

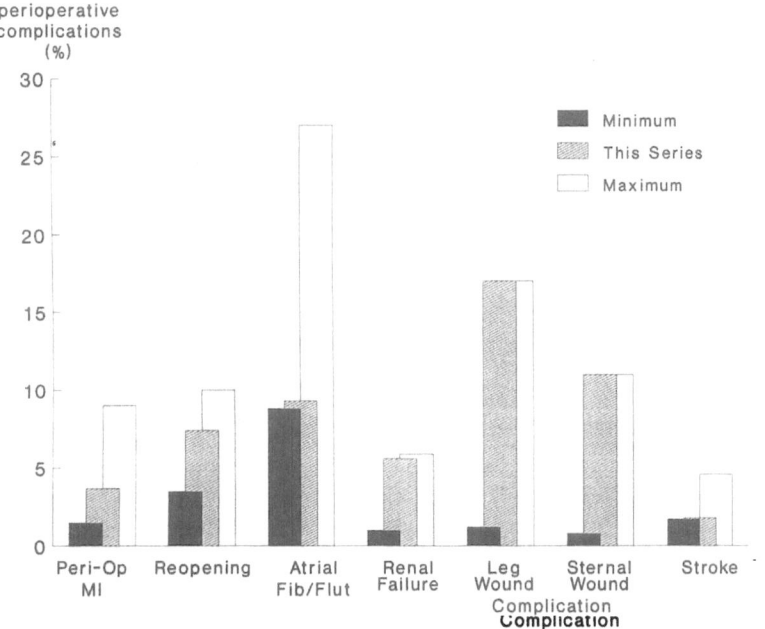

Figure 3.8. Perioperational complications for elderly isolated CABG patients. Data shown are those from the current study as well as maximum and minimum values from the literature.

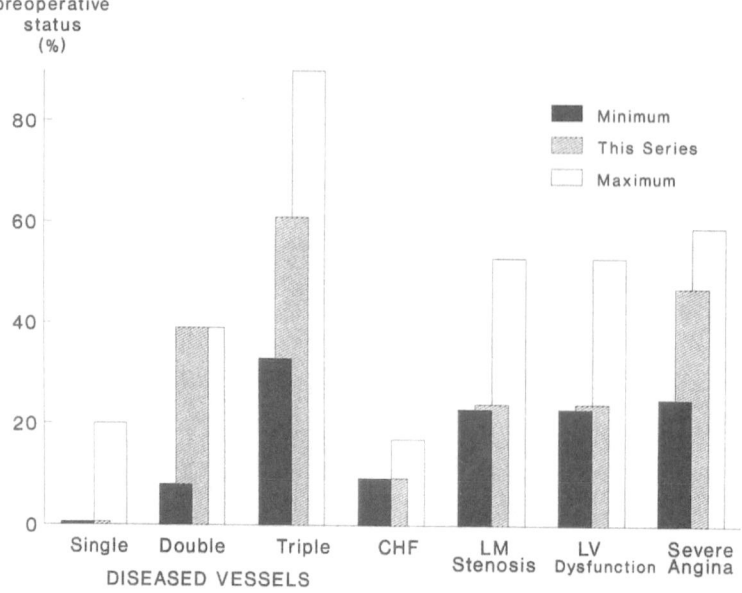

Figure 3.9. Perioperational coronary status for elderly isolated CABG patients. Data shown are those from the current study as well as maximum and minimum values from the literature.

older patients. Ennabli [8] and Montague [15] reported higher cerebral, sternal and respiratory complications and argued that patients with non-cardiac disorders should not be considered for surgery. However, in this study the requirement for reopening and leg wound complications were increased significantly relative to younger patients.

Trends over the past three decades

Our data obtained since 1970 indicate a slight decrease in mortality in the younger patients but a significant decrease in mortality for patients over 70 years. This decrease can be attributed to at least three factors: 1) improved surgical techniques, including the use of cold cardioplegia solutions for heart preservation; 2) improved post-operative care and experience dealing with the elderly; and 3) more careful selection of candidates for surgery, based on determined risk factors [21]. In comparison with operations on younger patients, operations on the elderly were more likely to be emergency or urgent (Figure 3.3), although this has decreased since the 1970s and 1980s. This observation is consistent with previous studies and can probably be attributed to postponement of the surgery until the disease becomes more extensive and the angina more severe. This delay in surgery arises from the belief of higher mortality and morbidity in the elderly and from age bias by which younger, active, employed patients with family responsibilities are treated preferentially.

Conclusions

As with younger patients, disabling angina pectoris is the main indication for bypass surgery. Our data show that where post-operative mortality rates have remained relatively constant for younger patients, rates have decreased dramatically for elderly patients. Our recent data show no significant differences between age groups. Reopening rates and leg wound complications are higher in elderly patients, but no other complications are significantly different. Thus, with improved surgical techniques and post-operative care, mortality and morbidity rates for CABG surgery in the elderly are acceptable and age should not be considered a contraindication for surgery.

References

1. Buccino RA, McIntosh HD. Aortocoronary bypass grafting in the management of patients with coronary artery disease. Am J Med 1979; 66: 651–66.
2. Loop RF, Sheldon WE, Rencon G, et al. Surgical treatment of coronary artery disease: pure graft operations. Prog Cardiovasc Dis 1975; 18: 237–53.
3. Hannan EL. Coronary artery bypass surgery: the relationship between inhospital mortality rate and surgical volume after controlling for clinical risk factors. Medical Care 1991; 29: 1094–107.
4. Kirklin JW, Kouchoukow NT, Blackstone EH, Oberman A. Research related to surgery treatment of coronary artery disease. Circulation 1979; 60: 1613–8.
5. Gann D, Colin C, Hildner FJ, Samet P, Yahr WZ, Greenberg JJ. Coronary artery bypass surgery in patients seventy years of age and older. J Thorac Cardiovascular Surg 1977; 2: 237–41.
5. Horneffer PJ, Gardner TJ, Manolio TA, et al. The effects of age on outcome after coronary bypass surgery. Circulation 1987; 76(V): 6–12.
6. Acinapura AJ, Rose DM, Cunningham JN, Jacobowitz IJ, Kramer MD, Zisbrod Z. Circulation 1988; 78: 179–84.
7. Rose DM, Gelbfish J, Jacobowitz IJ, et al. Analysis of morbidity and mortality in patients 70 years of age and over undergoing isolated coronary bypass surgery. Am Heart J 1985; 110: 341–6.
8. Ennabli K, Pelletier C. Morbidity and mortality of coronary artery surgery after the age of 70 years. Ann Thorac Surg 1986; 42: 197–200.
9. Faro RS, Golden MD, Javid H, et al. Coronary revascularization in septuagenarians. J Thorac Cardiovasc Surg 1983; 86: 616–20.
10. Hochberg MS, Levine FH, Daggett WM, Akins CW, Austen WG, Buckley MJ. Isolated coronary artery bypass grafting in patients seventy years of age and older – early and late results. J Thorac Cardiovasc Surg 1982; 84: 219–23.
11. Edwards FH, Taylor AJ, Thompson L, et al. Current status of coronary artery operation in septagenarians. Soc Thorac Surgeons 1991; 52: 265–9.
12. Rodstein M. Heart disease in the aged. In: Rossman I, editor. Clinical Geriatrics. Philadelphia: JB Lippincott, 1979: 181–203.
13. Blorck G. The biology of myocardial infarction. Circulation 1968; 37: 1071–85.
14. Kovar MG. Elderly people – the population 65 years of age and over: health United States 1976–1977, DHEW Pub. HRA 77-1232. Washington DC: Government Printing Office, 1977: 9.
15. Montague NT, Kouchoukos NT, Wilson TAS, et al. Morbidity and mortality of coronary bypass grafting in patients 60 years of age and older. Ann of Thorac Surg 1985; 39: 552–7.
16. Kellett J. The outcome of coronary artery bypass surgery as predicted by decision analysis: the influence of age, disease, severity and ventricular function. Thor Surg 1992; 7: 57–75.

17. Knapp WS, Douglas JS, Craver JM, et al. Efficacy of coronary artery bypass grafting in elderly patients with coronary artery disease. Am J Cardiology 1981; 47: 923–30.
18. Huysmans HA, van Ark E. Predictors of perioperative mortality, morbidity and late quality of life in coronary bypass surgery. E Heart J 1989; 10: 10–2.
19. Janusz MT, Jamieson WRE, Causton N, Burr LH, Allen P, Munro AI. Coronary artery bypass in patients over 65 years of age. Can J Surg 1983; 26: 186–8.
20. Noyez L, van de Wal HJ. Perioperative morbidity and mortality of coronary artery surgery after the age of 70 years. Cardiovas Surg 1989; 30: 981–4.
21. Meyer J, Wukasch DC, Seybold-Epting W, et al. Coronary artery bypass in patients over 70 years of age: indications and results. Am J Cardiol 1975; 36: 342–5.

4. Combined valve and coronary bypass surgery in the elderly

JANOS SZÉCSI, PAUL HERIJGERS, ILSE SCHEYS and
WILLEM FLAMENG

Introduction

The general ageing of the population is paralleled by the increasing proportion
of elderly among patients referred to open heart surgery. When having an
operation for a valvular heart disease, more people should undergo combined
valve and coronary bypass graft (CABG) surgery, since ischemic heart disease
also becomes more frequent with advanced age. Cardiac surgery in the elderly
demands an increasing part of limited health care resources. Therefore, a better
understanding of the surgical risk and long-term prognosis of this special
subgroup of cardiosurgical patients is warranted by socio-economic as well as
medical reasons. The objective of this study was to analyse our early and late
results of combined valve and CABG surgery in the elderly in comparison with
younger patients who were operated on in the same period at our institution.

Patients and methods

A total of 205 combined valve and CABG operations were performed in
patients who were at least 70 years or older at the time of surgery (old group)
between 1980 and 1992 at the Katholieke Universiteit Leuven. In the same
period, 535 younger patients (young group, < 70 years old) underwent the same
type of surgery and served as a control group for this study. Aortic valve
replacement (AVR) was the most frequent procedure (134 and 314 patients),
followed by mitral valve replacement (MVR) (44 and 135 patients), while
multiple valve replacement (MtpVR) was performed in an additional 18 and 44
patients in the old and the young group, respectively.

Nine patients in the old group and 42 patients in the young group had valve
plasties or plasties and valve replacement in combination with CABG. Elderly
patients preferably received biological valves (72%), and mechanical prostheses
were mainly used for the younger patients (83%). The most frequently
implanted biological valves were the Ionescu-Shiley low profile, Carpentier-
Edwards pericardium and Mitral-flow valves. Among the mechanical devices,

P.J. Walter (ed.), Coronary Bypass Surgery in the Elderly, pp. 41–53.
© 1995 *Kluwer Academic Publishers, Dordrecht.*

Bjork-Shiley Monostrut, Bjork-Shiley convex-concave and St. Jude Medical were predominantly used.

During the first five years of the study, only veins were applied as bypass conduits, but later internal mammary arteries were used for an increasing proportion of patients. A total of 20.5% of the old group and 28.4% of the young group received at least one internal mammary artery alone or in combination with veins. Operations were performed in moderate hypothermia (25°C oesophageal temperature) and with crystalloid cardioplegia. Since 1988, myocardial protection has been promoted by lidoflazine pretreatment (1 mg

Table 4.1. Preoperative variables

	Old group (205)		Young group (535)		
	n	%	n	%	p
Mean age	73.2 ± 2.9		61.2 ± 6.2		
Gender					0.0005
Male	101	(48.3)	380	(71)	
Female	104	(50.7)	155	(29)	
NYHA[a]					0.024
I	0	(0)	1	(0.2)	
II	49	(23.9)	155	(29)	
III	100	(48.8)	239	(44.7)	
IV	45	(22)	129	(24.1)	
V	10	(4.9)	10	(1.9)	
Etiology					n.s.
Degenerative	92	(44.9)	224	(41.9)	
Rheumatic	68	(33.2)	85	(34.6)	
Ischemic	30	(14.6)	70	(13.1)	
Endocarditis	2	(1)	6	(1.1)	
Prosthetic valve endocarditis	4	(2)	10	(1.9)	
Left ventricle function					n.s
Normal	131	(63.9)	340	(63.6)	
Mild↓	37	(18.1)	93	(17.4)	
Moderate ↓	25	(12.2)	64	(12)	
Severe ↓	6	(2.9)	22	(4.1)	
Extent of CAD[b]					0.044
One-vessel disease	75	(36.6)	240	(33.3)	
Two-vessel disease	69	(33.7)	180	(33.3)	
Three-vessel disease	61	(29.8)	115	(33.3)	
Left main disease	21	(29.8)	26	(33.3)	n.s.
Associated diseases					n.s.
AMI[c]	40	(19.5)	136	(33.3)	
Diabetes	15	(7.3)	38	(33.3)	
Renal insufficiency	4	(2)	11	(33.3)	
Respiratory insufficiency	2	(1)	13	(33.3)	

[a] New York Heart Association class.
[b] coronary artery disease.
[c] acute myocardial infarction.

kg^{-1} iv. prior to cardiopulmonary bypass) [1]. In most of the procedures distal anastomosis was done first, followed by valve surgery during one period of cardioplegic arrest. (In the initial phase of the study, the distals were constructed applying intermittent aortic cross-clamping and the valve procedure was then done in a period of cold cardioplegia.)

The following preoperative variables were collected retrospectively (Table 4.1): age, gender, New York Heart Association (NYHA) functional class, valve lesion (stenosis, insufficiency, mixed), aetiology of valve disease (rheumatic, degenerative, ischemic, congenital, endocarditis, other), associated diseases, extent of coronary artery disease (CAD), left ventricular (LV) ejection fraction (EF), LV end diastolic pressure (EDP), LV regional wall motion (RWM), cardiac rhythm (sinus, non-sinus, pacemaker), previous operation (redo yes/no). Coronary bypass grafting was performed if $\geq$ 50% stenosis was documented by the angiography. Extent of CAD was categorised as one-, two- or three-vessel disease, left main disease (LM) was considered separately. LV function was defined according to the following rules: *normal* – if EF $\geq$ 50%, or LV EDP < 15 mmHg with RWM being normal [2]; *mildly impaired* – if 40% $\leq$ EF < 50% or 15 mmHg < LV EDP $\leq$ 20 mmHg with RWM being mildly impaired; *moderately impaired* – if 30% $\leq$ EF < 40%, or 20 mmHg < LV EDP $\leq$ 25 mmHg with RWM being moderately impaired; *severely impaired* – if EF < 30%, LV EDP > 25 mmHg with RWM severely depressed.

The recorded operative and post-operative variables were as follows: date of surgery, surgeon, type of valve prosthesis, type of conduit for CABG, number and place of bypasses, duration of aortic cross-clamp time and extracorporeal circulation (ECC), outcome of surgery (mortality within 30 days and in-

Table 4.2. Operative characteristics

	Old group (205)		Young group (535)		
	n	%	n	%	p
Type of valve replacement					n.s.
Aortic	134	(65.4)	314	(58.7)	
Mitral	44	(21.5)	135	(25.5)	
Multiple	18	(8.8)	44	(8.2)	
Biological valve used					< 0.05
Aortic	110	(82)	85	(27)	
Mitral	24	(54)	27	(20)	
Use of IMA[a]	42	(20.5)	152	(28.4)	n.s.
Duration of ECC[b] (min)	136.5 ± 35.1		134.6 ± 40.1		n.s.
Duration of Aoxclamp[c] (min)	80.5 ± 21.6		78.3 ± 24.8		n.s.
Mean number of distals	2.4 ± 1.2		2.1 ± 1.2		n.s.

[a] internal mammary artery.
[b] extracorporal circulation.
[c] aortic crossclamp.

hospital), cardiac complications (low cardiac output syndrome (LCO), perioperative infarction (AMI), rhythm disturbances, pacemaker implantation, reoperation for bleeding, tamponade, use of intraaortic balloon pump (IABP) or ventricular assist device (VAD), LV dissection), valve-related complications (transient ischemic attack (TIA), cerebrovascular accident (CVA), peripheral emboli, anticoagulation-related (AC) bleeding, paravalvular leak, hemolysis, endocarditis), general complications (respiratory and renal insufficiency, sepsis,

Table 4.3. Early results

	Old group (205)		Young group (535)		
	n	%	n	%	p
30-day mortality	22	(10.7)	38	(7.1)	n.s.
Hospital mortality	29	(14.2)	40	(7.5)	0.037
Cardiac complications					
Total	90	(43.9)	175	(32.7)	0.011
LCO[a]	49	(23.9)	85	(15.9)	0.019
AMI[b]	3	(1.5)	14	(2.6)	n.s.
Rhythm disturbances	50	(24.4)	109	(20.4)	n.s.
PM implantation	5	(2.4)	6	(1.1)	n.s.
Reoperation bleeding	14	(6.8)	22	(4.1)	n.s.
IABP[c]	7	(3.4)	16	(3)	n.s.
LVAD[d]	3	(1.5)	3	(0.6)	n.s.
Heart standstill	3	(1.5)	3	(0.6)	n.s.
Left ventricle dissection	0	(0)	1	(0.2)	n.s.
Tamponade	2	(1)	5	(0.9)	n.s.
Valve-related complications					n.s.
Total	11	(5.4)	18	(3.4)	n.s.
TIA/CVA[e] '	4	(2)	10	(1.9)	n.s.
Peripheral emboli	1	(0.5)	3	(0.6)	n.s.
AC-bleeding[f]	1	(0.5)	1	(0.2)	n.s.
Endocarditis	1	(0.5)	1	(0.2)	n.s.
Paravalvular leak	1	(0.5)	1	(0.2)	n.s.
Hemolysis	5	(2.4)	0	(0)	n.s.
General complications					
Total	58	(28.3)	115	(21.5)	0.027
Respiratory insufficiency	32	(16.6)	46	(8.6)	0.029
Renal insufficiency	22	(10.7)	28	(5.2)	0.033
Sepsis	99	(4.4)	16	(3)	n.s.
MOF[g]	5	(2.4)	7	(1.3)	n.s.
Mediastinitis	2	(1)	4	(0.8)	n.s.
Decubitus	4	(2)	11	(2.1)	n.s.
Wound problems	1	(0.5)	17	(3.2)	0.029
Coma	2	(1)	2	(0.4)	n.s.

[a] low cardiac output.
[b] acute myocardial infarction.
[c] intraaortic balloon pump.
[d] left ventricular assist device.

[e] transient ischemic attack/cerebrovascular accident.
[f] anticoagulation related bleeding.
[g] multiple organ failure.

multiple organ failure (MOF), mediastinitis, decubitus, wound infection, coma). The operative characteristics of the patients are shown in Table 4.2; the early results and hospital morbidity are presented in Table 4.3. A follow-up was conducted through March 1993 by letter or telephone contact to the patient or their general practitioner. The mean duration was 47.7 ± 39.8 months and it was 97.3% complete. Events during the follow-up were defined according to the guidelines on reporting complications after valve operations [3]. Survival analysis considered any deaths during follow-up, including hospital mortality. Ischemic complications comprised return of angina, AMI and reoperations or PTCA due to return of ischemic symptoms. Valve-related complication is defined as a sum of all thromboembolic events, severe AC-related bleeding (i.e. necessitating hospitalisation), endocarditis, external and internal malfunction, degeneration, and reoperations due to valve-related complications. Death was considered cardiac and valve-related when it resulted from AC bleeding, CVA, endocarditis, sudden death, or death at reoperation. It was classified as cardiac but non-valve related when it was due to AMI, decompensation or rhythm disturbances. Non-cardiac death comprised malignancies, pneumonia, accidents. The total of all valve-related, ischemic complications and hospital as well as late mortality was referred to as total complications. Activity status (partial or full-time return to work, household activity, invalidity due to cardiac or non-cardiac reasons) was also recorded. Patients were asked to compare their general condition to that which they had preoperatively (better, same, worse, much worse). Activity, general condition and NYHA functional class were used to describe quality of life at the time of follow-up.

Statistical methods

Values of continuous variables (e.g., age, duration of ECC or aortic cross-clamping) were expressed as mean ± SD. Discrete variables (e.g., gender, etiology of valve disease, complications) were given as percentages. Pre-, intra- and post-operative variables were tested by univariate analysis: continuous variables were analysed with Wilcoxon 2-sample test, discrete variables were compared with χ^2 analysis or by Fischer's exact test [4], $p < 0.05$ was considered significant. Survival and event-free survival curves were constructed with the Kaplan-Meier life table method. Differences between survival curves were analysed by Wilcoxon test.

Early results

Elderly patients had significantly higher hospital mortality in general (14.2% versus 7.5%), and in the AVR (11.9% versus 5.7%) and MVR (13.6% versus 5.2%) groups as well. MtpVR was accompanied by a slightly lower risk in the old group (16.7% versus 20.5%). Hospital mortality was consistently higher than

30-day mortality in both groups (Table 4.3). The lowest hospital mortality was observed after AVR, the highest in the MtpVR group, with the MVR patients falling in between. A total of 53% of the elderly and 42% of the young patients had at least one complication during their hospitalization. Cardiac complications were seen in 43.9% of the old group and 32.7% of the young group ($p = 0.011$). The significant difference was mainly due to the more frequent occurrence of low cardiac output syndrome in the aged population (23.9% versus 15.9%). Higher rates of post-operative respiratory and renal insufficiency were observed among the elderly, which led to the significant difference between the two groups concerning general complications. All valve-related complications, except haemolysis, which was more frequent in the elderly patients, occurred in similar percentages of the two groups (Table 4.3.)

Late results

Kaplan-Meier survival of the patients at 1, 5 and 10 years post-operatively (including hospital mortality) was 81%, 68% and 29% in the old group and 88%, 77% and 46% in the young group, respectively ($p = 0.0002$, Figure 4.1). The statistically significant difference originates from the first 3 post-operative months, when the elderly were affected by substantially higher mortality (30.7% versus 23.7%). All cases of death, including in-hospital mortality, are depicted in Figure 4.2. There was no significant difference between the old and the young patients concerning total valve-related and ischemic complications (Figure 4.3), only TIA and valve degeneration occurred significantly more in the old patients than in the young ones. Freedom from all complications at 1, 5 and 10 years

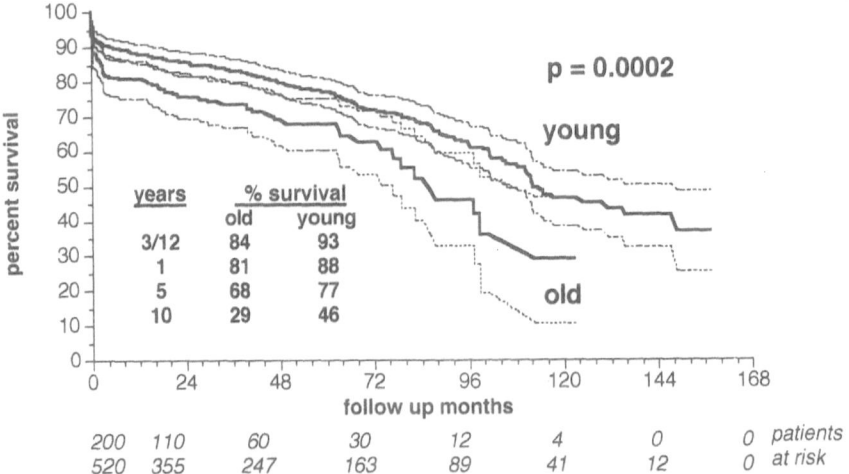

Figure 4.1. Kaplan-Meier survival of the old ($\geq$ 70 years) and young ($<$ 70 years) patients after valve surgery combined with CABG
(patients at risk – upper row: old patients, lower row: young patients).

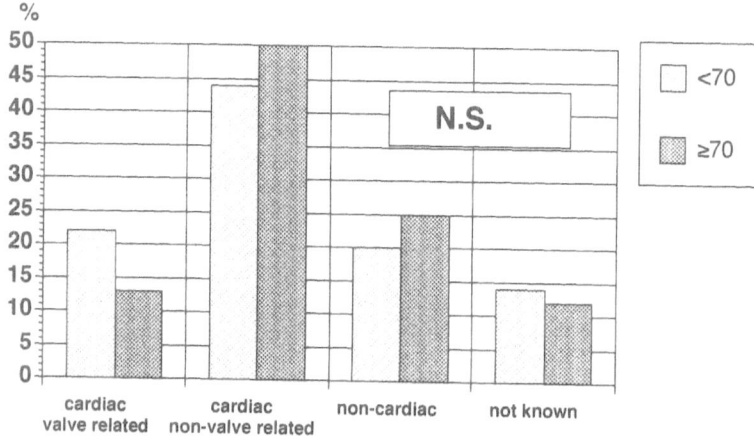

Figure 4.2. Mode of death during the follow-up (n = 221 deaths; mean follow up: 47.7 ± 39.8 months).

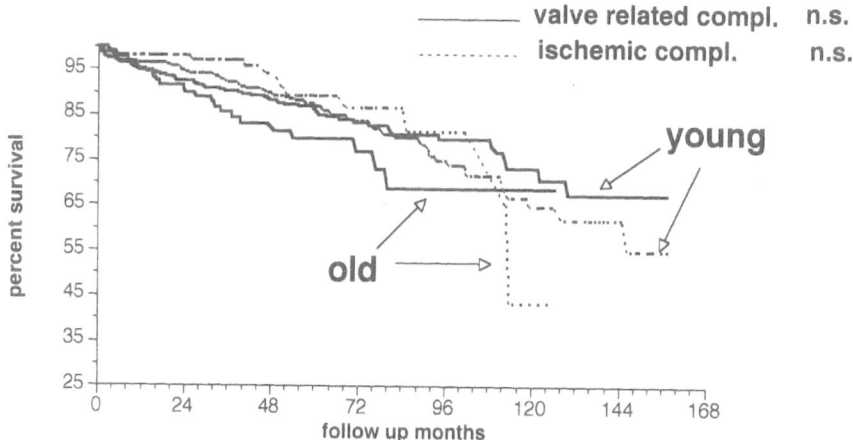

Figure 4.3. Freedom of valve-related and ischemic complications of old (≥ 70 years) and young (< 70 years) patients after valve surgery combined with CABG.

(including death at any time during follow-up) was 76%, 51% and 12% in the elderly, and 83%, 59% and 26% in the young patients (Figure 4.4).

We observed significant improvements in the functional state of the patients after the mean follow-up of 47.7 ± 39.8 months. Of the hospital survivors, 85% in the old group and 83% in the young group belonged to NYHA class I or II at the time of censoring (Figure 4.5). Although return to original occupation was uncommon even in the young group (8% versus 1% in old group), a vast majority of the elderly and the young performed regular household activities (Figure 4.6). The effect of the operation was qualified as positive by most of the patients, since 80% of the aged population and 81% of the young patients

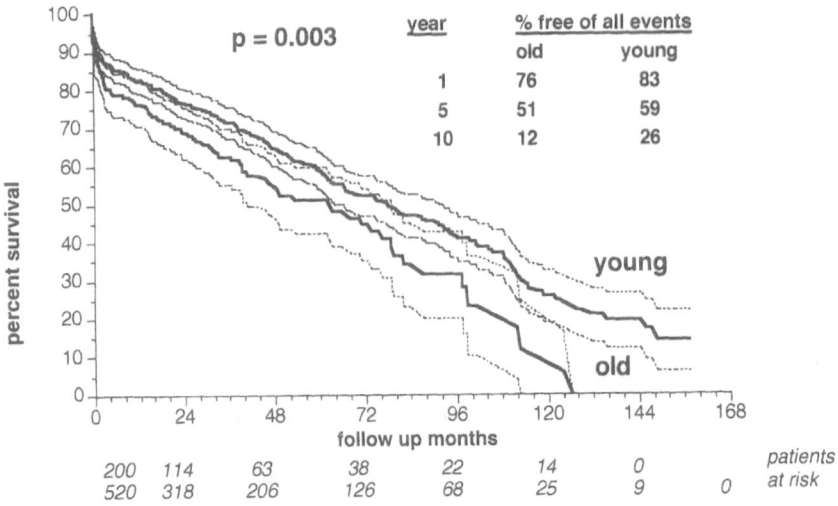

Figure 4.4. Freedom of all complications (death, valve-related and ischemic) of old (≥ 70 years) and young (< 70 years) patients after valve surgery combined with CABG (patients at risk – upper row: old patients, lower row: young patients).

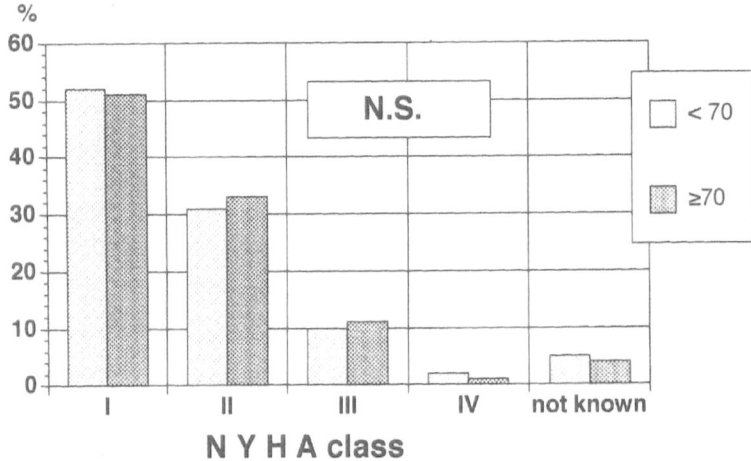

Figure 4.5. Functional class at follow-up (n = 519 survivors; mean follow-up: 47.7 ± 39.8 months). NYHA: New York Heart Association class.

considered their general condition to be better than preoperatively. Only 4% of long-term survivors in the old group and 5% in the young group experienced deterioration of their general condition following surgery (Figure 4.7).

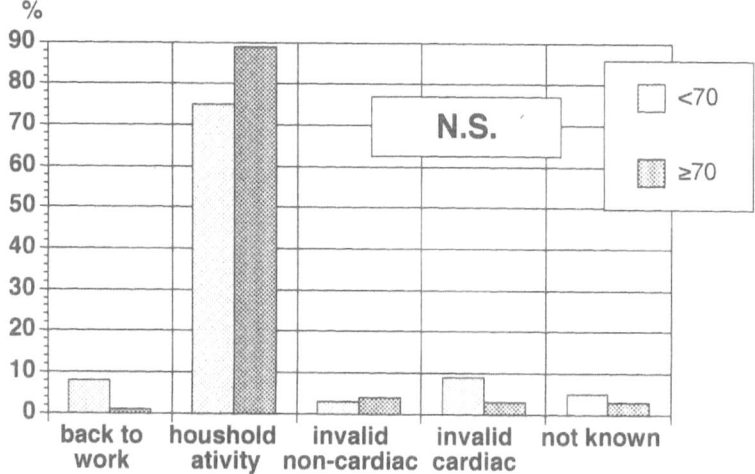

Figure 4.6. Activity at follow-up (n = 519 survivors; mean follow-up: 47.7 ± 39.8 months).

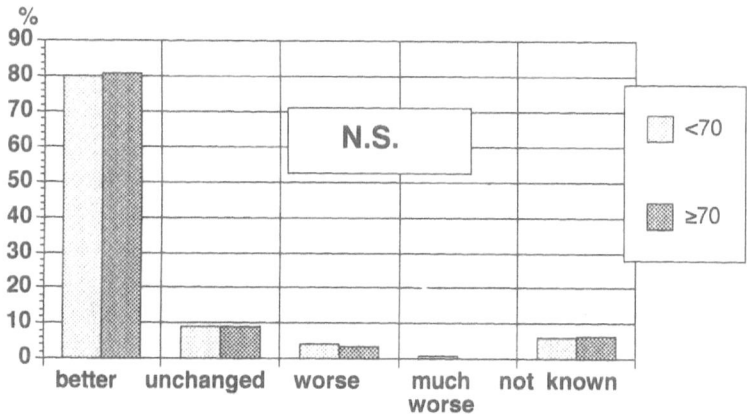

Figure 4.7. Patients' own judgement of general condition (n = 519 survivors; mean follow-up: 47.7 ± 39.8 months).

Discussion

Parallel with the physiological changes of the ageing organism, cardiovascular, respiratory, endocrine, renal and mental diseases are becoming more prevalent among the elderly [5]. Stenotic coronary artery disease occurs in approximately 60% of the aged population [6] and valve disease also becomes more frequent as senile valve tissue degeneration and arteriosclerosis progress.

Several studies have demonstrated that higher age (beyond 65 or above 70 years, or tested as a continuous variable) carries increased operative risk for isolated coronary or valve surgery, as well as combined valve+CABG surgery

[7–11]. This observation is well supported by our findings, which show a doubled hospital mortality for the elderly compared to the young patients. The ratio was similar in the subgroup of patients with AVR (11.9% versus 5.7%), but the difference was even more pronounced in the MVR group (13.6% versus 5.2%). Elderly patients having MtpVR fared slightly better than those younger, but this was probably due to chance alone, since the number of patients in this category was very small.

The early mortality rate for elderly patients undergoing combined AVR+CABG operations is reported to be 8–14%; this is consistently higher than that of isolated AVR, which runs around 3–8% [10, 12–14]. On the other hand, concomitant CABG surgery does not increase the risk among the younger population of AVR patients [15]. The considerably pronounced risk of combined MVR surgery is confirmed by Davis *et al.* [14], Fremes *et al.* [10] and Christakis *et al.* [16], who described 19–50% mortality, depending on the preoperative functional class, left ventricular function and urgency of the operation. Those undergoing emergency operation with severely depressed ventricular function fall into the highest risk category [16]. In our series, hospital mortality for MVR was also higher but only a mild difference could be registered between the AVR and MVR group.

Post-operative cardiac and general complications were more common in the old group due to higher incidence of low cardiac output syndrome, respiratory and renal insufficiency. Preoperatively, elderly patients had more extensive coronary artery disease and a larger percentage belonged to NYHA class III or needed emergency operations. These factors probably led to an advanced stage of myocardial damage which, in many of them, could be only partially restored by the operation and eventually resulted in higher mortality and cardiac complications. The more frequent occurrences of emphysema and bronchiolar obstruction, as well as decline in capacity of the immune response (all of which are seen regularly in elderly patients) can be implicated in the accumulation of respiratory complications [5, 17]. The decrease in renal blood flow and glomerular filtration rate, and the diminished capacity of sodium and potassium excretion in old people contribute to the increased prevalence of renal complications [5].

Long-term prognosis for the elderly following combined valve and CABG surgery is only partially known. Lytle *et al.* [18] observed 63% and 35% survival at 5 and 10 years, respectively, in patients older than 70 years after AVR combined with CABG. Similar (60–75%) five-year survival was documented by Galloway *et al.* [12] and Bergus *et al.* [19] in a heterogeneous group of patients after isolated and combined valve replacement. Data on late results after MVR+CABG in old patients are even less frequently published. A recent report by Davis *et al.* [14] describes 5- and 7-year survival being 73 and 63% (without hospital mortality). Our data (with hospital mortality included) compare favourably with those mentioned above, and confirm that combined valve replacement surgery, either AVR or MVR, has similar prognoses in the elderly.

Selection of valve prosthesis is an important decision in valve replacement, which has a substantial influence on long-term prognosis of the patients. In our series, elderly patients received predominantly biological valves (82% of AVR and 54% of the MVR). Recent reports have presented evidence that performance of tissue valves is excellent in elderly patients for up to 10–12 years after implantation, with 90–97% freedom of structural valve degeneration at 10 years [20, 21]. Similar to these data, 97% and 93% of the old patients in our study were free of valve degeneration at 5 and 10 years, respectively.

Although the advantage of internal mammary artery over saphenous vein is well established concerning long-term survival after coronary surgery [7, 22], it still remains to be proven in the field of combined valve and coronary surgery. In a recent review, Mannion *et al.* [23] still doubted whether the internal mammary artery can provide adequate flow to hypertrophied left ventricles frequently seen in valve surgery. Some authors have advocated the application of mammaries also in combined surgery [11, 24], reporting its use in 30–40% of their patients, but many surgeons still continue to perform bypass surgery predominantly with veins in this setting [18, 19, 25, 26]. Gardner *et al.* [27] and Edwards *et al.* [28] have presented evidence that the application of mammary artery reduces early perioperative risk of isolated CABG surgery in general, and in different subgroups of patients, including the elderly. Although our previous studies did not show that mammary artery has a favourable effect on 3-month mortality after combined valve and coronary surgery in a mixed group of elderly and young patients (Flameng, unpubl. data), we progressively extended the use of mammaries in combined operations and, in the last year of this study period, 71% of the patients received at least one of this type of arterial conduit.

Most of the hospital survivors in the old and young group experienced spectacular improvement in their functional class and activity following surgery. This was paralleled by positive judgements of the effect of the operation by the elderly as well as the young patients. Over 80% of the long-term survivors considered their condition to be better at follow-up than prior to surgery. Returning to the original occupation part-time or full-time was uncommon even in the group of young patients, but this variable is of limited value in describing well-being of the patients after cardiac surgery, since it is mostly determined by indirectly health-related factors such as age, socio-economic status or insurance conditions and familial circumstances. Despite all this, close to 90% of the late survivors in the old group were regularly engaged in household activity. These data, combined with a moderate rate of late complications during the follow-up, verify that good quality of life can be maintained even in elderly patients after combined heart operations.

In conclusion we can state that performing the high risk procedure of combined valve and CABG surgery in elderly patients seems justified by substantial improvement in the general condition and functional capacity of long-term survivors. Mortality and morbidity of the old patients, beyond the third post-operative month, is not different from those observed in younger patients. Biological prosthesis can be safely recommended for valve replacement since valve failure due to structural degeneration is extremely rare even after 10 years. Use of mammary artery as a bypass conduit should be encouraged, although further studies are necessary to prove its advantages in the setting of combined valve and coronary surgery.

References

1. Chen CC, Masuda M, Szabo Z, et al. Nucleoside transport inhibition mediates lidoflazine-induced cardioprotection during intermittent aortic crossclamping. J Thorac Cardiovasc Surg 1992; 104: 1602–9.
2. Pinson CW, Cobanoglu A, Metzdorff MT, Grunkemeier GL, Kay PH, Starr A. Late surgical results for ischemic mitral regurgitation: role of wall motion and severity of regurgitation. J Thorac Cardiovasc Surg 1984; 88: 663–72.
3. Edmunds LH Jr, Clark RE, Cohn LH, Miller C, Weisel RD. Guidelines for reporting morbidity and mortality after cardiac valvular operations. Ann Thorac Surg 1988; 46: 257–9.
4. Armitage P, Berry G. Statistical methods in medical research, 2nd ed. London: Blackwell Scientific Publication, 1987.
5. Beernaerts A. Surgery in the aged: associated pathologies of aged people. Acta Chir Belg 1993; 93: 112–4.
6. Weisfeldt ML, Lakatta EG, Gerstenblith G. Aging and the heart. In: Braunwald E, editor. Heart disease: a textbook of cardiovascular medicine, 4th ed. London: WB Saunders, 1992: 1656–69.
7. Kirklin JW, Akins CW, Blackstone EH, et al. ACC/AHA Task force report: guidelines and indications for coronary artery bypass graft surgery. JACC 1991; 17: 543–89.
8. Sethi GK, Miller C, Souchek J, et al. Clinical, hemodynamic and angiographic predictors of operative mortality in patients undergoing single valve replacement (Veterans Administration Cooperative Study on valvular heart disease). J Thorac Cardiovasc Surg 1987; 93: 884–97.
9. Scott WC, Miller DC, Haverich A, et al. Operative risks of mitral valve replacement: discriminate analysis of 1329 procedures. Circulation 1985; 72(Suppl II): 108.
10. Fremes SE, Goldman BS, Ivanov J, Weisel RD, David TE, Salerno T. Valvular surgery in the elderly. Circulation 1989; 80(suppl I): 77–90.
11. Kirklin JK, Naftel DC, Blackstone EH, Kirklin JW, Browns RC. Risk factors for mortality after primary combined valvular and coronary artery surgery. Circulation 1989; 79(suppl I): 185–90.
12. Galloway AC, Colvin SB, Grossi EA, et al. Ten-year experience with aortic valve replacement in 482 patients 70 years of age or older: operative risk and long term results. Ann Thorac Surg 1990; 49: 84–93.
13. Aranki SF, Rizzo RJ, Couper GS, et al. Aortic valve replacement in the elderly, effect of gender and coronary artery disease on operative mortality. Circulation 1993; 88(2): 17–23.
14. Davis EA, Gardner TJ, Gillinov AM, et al. Valvular disease in the elderly: influence on surgical results. Ann Thorac Surg 1993; 55: 333–8.
15. Lytle BW. Impact of coronary artery disease on valvular heart surgery. Cardiol Clin 1991; 9: 301–14.
16. Christakis GT, Weisel RD, David TE, Salerno TA, Ivanov J. Predictors of operative survival after valve replacement. Circulation 1988; 78(suppl I): 25–34.
17. Kennes B. Immunodeficiency in aging. Acta Chir Belg 1993; 93: 115–8.
18. Lytle BW, Cosgrove DM, Gill CC, et al. Aortic valve replacement combined with myocardial revascularization: late results and determinants of risk for 471 in-hospital survivals. J Thorac Cardiovasc Surg 1988; 95: 402–14.
19. Bergus BO, Feng WC, Bert AA, Singh AK. Aortic valve replacement (AVR): influence of age on operative morbidity and mortality. Eur J Cardio Thorac Surg 1992; 6: 118–21.

20. Burdon TA, Miller CD, Oyer PE, et al. Durability of porcine valves at fifteen years in a representative North American patient population. J Thorac Cardiovasc Surg 1992; 103: 238–52.
21. Jamieson WRE, Burr LH, Munro AI, Miyagishima RT, Gerein AN. Cardiac valve replacement in the elderly: clinical performance of biological prosthesis. Ann Thorac Surg 1989; 48: 173–85.
22. Loop FD, Lytle BW, Cosgrove DM, et al. Influence of internal mammary artery graft on 10 year survival and other cardiac events. N Engl J Med 1986; 314: 1–6.
23. Mannion JD, Armenti FR, Edie RN. Cardiac surgery in the elderly patient. Cardiovasc Clin 1992; 22: 189–207.
24. Ashraf SS, Shaukat N, Odom N, Keenan D, Grotte G. Early and late results following combined valve and coronary bypass surgery and mitral valve replacement. Eur J Cardio Thorac Surg 1994; 8: 57–62.
25. Czer LSC, Gray RJ, DeRobertis MA, et al. Mitral valve replacement: impact of coronary artery disease and determinants of prognosis after revascularization. Circulation 1984; 70(suppl I): 198–207.
26. He GW, Hughes CF, McCaughan B, et al. Mitral valve replacement combined with coronary artery operation: determinants of early and late results. Ann Thorac Surg 1991; 51: 916–23.
27. Gardner TJ, Greene PS, Rykiel MF, et al. Routine use of the left internal mammary artery graft in the elderly. Ann Thorac Surg 1990; 49: 188–94.
28. Edwards FH, Clark RE, Schwartz M. Impact of internal mammary artery conduits on operative mortality in coronary revascularization. Ann Thorac Surg 1994; 57: 27–32.

5. Cardiac surgery in octogenarians: Perioperative results and clinical follow-up

FRANCIS FONTAN, ALAIN BECAT, GUY FERNANDEZ, NICOLAS SOURDILLE, PASCAL REYNAUD and PAUL MONTSERRAT

Introduction

Due to increased life expectancy, particularly in Western societies, the cardiac surgeon is confronted more and more often with decisions as to the indication or contraindication of an operation for increasingly older patients. Although advanced age is recognized as a risk factor for death, favourable results have been reported after CABG in patients over 75 and after aortic valve replacement in octogenarians [1–4].

However, most of the results reported are of studies which were begun some time ago. We thought there was a possibility that the progress made in cardiac surgery, in myocardial protection, in intensive care, and in perfusion methods might have a favourable effect on these results. This study was undertaken to see if, in the light of current practice and knowledge, this progress would affect the results of cardiac surgery in octogenarians, both immediately and in the medium term.

Patients and methods

Patients

Out of 3823 patients operated on under extracorporeal circulation at the Clinique Saint-Augustin between January 1, 1990, and December 31, 1993, a group of 180 patients – 102 male (56.7%) and 78 female (43.3%) – were aged 80 or above (mean: 82.6 years, range 80.0–91.2). They made up the basis of this retrospective study. Follow-up information was obtained in January and February 1994, through telephone contact with the family physician or cardiologist, or with the patients themselves when the patient's physician was not aware of the patient's condition. Follow-up information was complete; no patient was lost to follow-up. All patients were symptomatic and were predominantly in NYHA or CCVS functional class III or IV prior to operation. All patients underwent preoperative catheterization and coronarography,

P.J. Walter (ed.), Coronary Bypass Surgery in the Elderly, pp. 55–59.
© 1995 *Kluwer Academic Publishers, Dordrecht.*

including the two patients who underwent different types of surgery, one for left atrial myxoma and one for acute aortic dissection.

Surgical techniques

Patients were operated on through a median sternotomy. Extracorporeal circulation was established by insertion of an arterial cannula into the ascending aorta and a single venous cannula through the right atrial appendage. The patients in whom mitral valve surgery or surgery for left atrial myxoma was performed had two venous caval cannulae inserted through the right atrial appendage and the right atrium. The patient with acute aortic dissection had the arterial cannula inserted into the right external iliac artery. Various types of membrane or bubble oxygenators were used and pulsatile arterial inflow was used in all patients. The temperature of the perfusate during cardiopulmonary bypass (CPB) was 33 °C, except that the perfusion was kept normothermic until after completion of proximal anastomoses, the first step in the operation performed before aortic cross-clamping in the patients who had CABG. The temperature of the perfusate during CPB was 18 °C in the patient with acute aortic dissection. The left venticle was vented when required by a catheter introduced through the right superior pulmonary vein and advanced to the left atrium or the apex of the left ventricle. Cardioplegia was performed according to the surgeon's preference, either cold crystalloid cardioplegia alone or cold hyperkalemic-enriched blood cardioplegia. Warm and initially hyperkalemic-enriched, pressure-controlled aortic root reperfusion was used by one of the surgeons according to a protocol already described [5, 6]. CABG was performed in 102 patients. Seventy-six patients had valve replacement either alone (48 patients) or in combination with CABG.

Results

Hospital mortality was 10% (Table 5.1) due to cardiac cause in 9 patients, either from low cardiac output or perioperative myocardial infarction. Hospital morbidity showed 3 patients who required re-operation for post-operative bleeding and one for non-infected sternal dehiscence. Three patients had a cerebrovascular accident; two experienced full recovery, but hemiplegia persisted in one. One patient with post-operative A-V block required insertion of a permanent pacemaker. The mean post-operative hospital stay was 7.8 days (range 5–28 days).

Follow-up information was obtained on all 163 patients discharged alive from the hospital. The total length of follow-up was 2762 months, mean follow-up 18.9 months (range: 1–49 months). Twenty-five patients died during the follow-up period, 10 (5.6%) from cardiac cause and 15 (8.3%) from non-cardiac cause. Interestingly, most of the late cardiac deaths occurred during the first post-operative year.

Table 5.1. Hospital mortality

Mode of death	No. patients	%
Cardiac	9	50.0
Neurological	3	16.6
General failure	4	22.2
Renal failure	1	5.6
Internal bleeding	1	5.6
Total	18	100

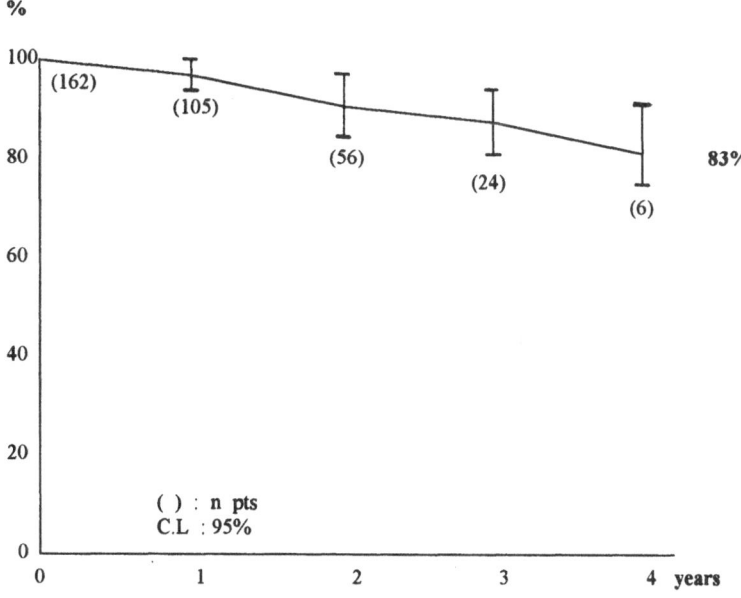

Figure 5.1. Actuarial curve of survival.

Cardiac-related morbidity was low among the surviving patients: 3 episodes of gastrointestinal bleeding in patients on anticoagulation therapy and one episode of transient ischemic attack. Among the 137 patients currently surviving, 96% were in NYHA or CCVS functional class I or II. Actuarial rate of survival was 83% at four years (Figure 5.1), whereas one-year survival from late cardiac death was 96% and at 3 years the figure was 93%.

Discussion

In France, the ageing of the population coupled with increased life expectancy has led to discussions concerning the operative risks of heart surgery for the growing number of patients over 80. The progress made in the last two decades (membrane oxygenators, pulsatile flow, refinements in perioperative myocardial protection management and in post-operative intensive care) has led surgeons to extend their operative indications to increasingly elderly patients. The results in terms of hospital mortality due to cardiac cause in our study (5%) are almost equal to those obtained in younger patients. The same goes for post-operative morbidity and the length of post-operative hospital stay. However, hospital mortality from non-cardiac causes (9 patients, 5%) in our study was significantly higher than in a younger population. This is not too surprising if one remembers that ageing leads to a decrease in a patient's resistance to invasive surgery, particularly when the technique of extracorporeal circulation is used. In addition, these patients are more likely to be prone to multiple organ failure, due simply to their age or to the consequences of their heart disease (especially if the latter has led them to show signs of cardiac failure), which weighs heavily in the post-operative period. Many studies have already shown that older age at operation is an incremental risk factor for death, both in early and late phases [7]. It would appear that, even today and despite the progress which has been made in cardiac surgery, this single factor, older age, has not yet been overcome, and indeed may never be.

The cardiac surgeon needs to very carefully weigh the operative risks for each individual patient, taking into consideration the state of the heart itself, the general state of the patient and the patient's overall resistance, so as to keep the incidence of hospital mortality from non-cardiac cause as low as possible. The decision is not a simple one nor is it currently subject to precise guidelines. It calls on the surgeon's clinical intuition.

The surgeon must also be particularly skilled in his operative procedure since there are additional procedural risk factors (risk factors of course existing whatever the age of the patient) for early death after the operation in older patients: longer global myocardial ischemic time, longer cardiopulmonary bypass time and revision for bleeding [8].

But the cardiologist and family physician must also be particularly vigilant in the preoperative monitoring of their patients for whom (unless there is a sudden and brutal onset of a coronary disease which until that point had remained silent) a deterioration in left ventricular performance is one of the most important incremental risk factors for early or late death after an operation [9]. Today, it would seem that a discussion about operative risks should take place before major left ventricular hypertrophy sets in, before the left ventricular ejection fraction suffers major impairment, and before manifestations of left ventricular failure appear. The medium-term results plead in favour of this argument, which also appears to be valid for younger populations. Life expectancy for operated patients then becomes the same as that for other population of the same age.

The quality of life of the great majority of these patients is, in general, excellent: they regain their autonomy and symptoms disappear or are greatly attenuated.

Conclusions

We believe that octogenarians can be operated on for cardiac disease and can hope for a significant improvement in their symptoms, and that for the great majority of patients, quality of life is vastly improved. The surgical team must do their utmost to reduce perioperative risk factors by carrying out the operation with maximum efficiency, skill and diligence, and by using the best myocardial protection possible. Even if operative contraindications which are cardiac in origin are difficult to determine for some patients, the operation must be envisioned before performance of the left ventricle is impaired and before the onset of left heart failure.

References

1. Horvath KA, DiSesa VJ, Peigh PS, et al. Favorable results of coronary artery bypass grafting in patients older than 75 years. J Thorac Cardiovasc Surg 1990; 99: 92–7.
2. Kirklin JW, et al. (ACC/AHA Joint Task Force Subcommittee on Coronary Artery Bypass Graft Surgery). Guidelines and indications for the coronary artery bypass graft operation. J Am Coll Cardiol 1991; 17: 543.
3. Utley JR, Leyland SA. Coronary artery bypass grafting in the octogenarian. J Thorac Cardiovasc Surg 1991; 101: 866.
4. Kleikamp G, Minami K, Breymann T, et al. Aortic valve replacement in octogenarians. J Heart Valve Dis 1992; 1: 196–200.
5. Fontan F, Madona F, Naftel DC, et al. Modifying myocardial management in cardiac surgery: a randomized trial. Eur J Cardiothorac Surg 1992; 6: 127–37.
6. Fontan F, Madona F, Naftel DC, et al. The effect of reperfusion pressure on early outcomes after coronary artery bypass grafting. J Thorac Cardiovasc Surg 1994; 107: 265–70.
7. Kirklin JW, Barratt-Boyes BG. Cardiac surgery, 2nd ed. New York: Churchill Livingstone, 1993: 316–7.
8. Logeais Y, Langanay T, Leguerrier A, et al. Etude des facteurs prédictifs du risque opératoire dans la chirurgie du rétrécissement aortique des patients âgés. Arch Mal Coeur 1994; 87: 201–9.
9. Kirklin JW, Barratt-Boyes BG. Cardiac surgery, 2nd ed. New York: Churchill Livinstone, 1993: 315.

6. Coronary artery bypass grafting and use of the LIMA in octogenarians

GIDEON SAHAR, EHUD RAANANI, ITZHAK HERTZ,
RON BRAUNER and BERNARDO A. VIDNE

Introduction

Improved medical care over the past few decades has increased life expectancy and, consequently, the number of aged persons in the general population has risen. For patients with coronary artery disease with ongoing ischemia despite maximal medical therapy, coronary artery bypass grafting (CABG) is still the only viable option. Recent reports [1–5] indicate that this intervention for select elderly individuals, who otherwise are in good physical and mental health, has substantially improved quality of life and led to decreased mortality and morbidity. We reviewed our results in a group of 52 consecutive octogenarian patients who underwent CABG or combined CABG and valve replacement in our institution. Among other variables analyzed in this study, special emphasis was given to the consequences of using the Lt. internal mammary artery (LIMA) as an arterial conduit for revascularization.

Patients and methods

Between January 1991 and October 1993, 2960 adult patients underwent CABG in our institution. Fifty-two of them (1.8%) were aged 80 years or older (mean age 82.1 years). Only 30% of this patient group were electively referred; 62% were urgent cases defined as unstable angina and treated by i.v. administration of nitroglycerin and heparin; four patients (8%) arrived in cardiogenic shock, requiring inotropic support (and in one case even mechanical assistance), and were operated upon on an emergency basis.

Medical reports were reviewed in detail to obtain relevant pre-operative data (Table 6.1). Lt. ventricular function data were obtained from cardiac catheterization or radionuclide study reports. Lt. ventricular ejection fraction (LVEF) was considered good or normal when it was greater than 50%, fair between 30–50%, and poor under 30%. Coronary artery disease was defined as significant when stenosis was greater than 70% of the arterial lumen.

Risk factors other than cardiac are listed in Table 6.1 and include renal

P.J. Walter (ed.), Coronary Bypass Surgery in the Elderly, pp. 61–68.
© 1995 *Kluwer Academic Publishers, Dordrecht.*

Table 6.1. Preoperative characteristics

Variable	No. of patients	Percent
Total of patients	52	100
Male	38	73
Female	14	27
Admission type:		
Emergent	4	8
Urgent	32	62
Elective	16	30
Unstable angina	43	84
Previous MI	21	40
Left main coronary artery disease	10	19
Previous CABG	0	0
Previous AVR	1	2
Ejection fraction:		
Good (> 50%)	27	52
Fair (30–50%)	21	40
Poor (< 30%)	4	8
Associated diseases:		
Diabetes mellitus	12	23
Hypertension	20	38
Peripheral vascular disease	7	13
COPD	4	8
Renal failure	4	8
Arrhythmia	7	13

failure, chronic obstructive lung disease, hypertension, diabetes mellitus and peripheral vascular disease.

All patients underwent standard cardiopulmonary bypass using a membrane oxygenator and moderate hypothermia (25–28 °C). Myocardial protection was achieved by introducing antegrade, cold crystalloid cardioplegia every 20–30 min and topical cooling of the heart.

All distal coronary anastomoses were accomplished first during a single cross-clamping period. Proximal anastomoses was done with partial clamping of the aorta on a beating heart.

Seven patients had concomitant coronary and aortic valve disease and underwent CABG+AVR. Distal vein graft anastomoses were done first. The valve was replaced later and the internal mammary artery (IMA) was anastomosed to the LAD in those cases when the LIMA was used as a conduit. In all cases (21 patients), the LIMA was used as a graft *in situ* for revascularizing the LAD.

Follow-up was performed for up to 34 months, and questions were addressed regarding patients' functional class (NYHA), residual or recurrent angina pectoris, performance of normal daily activities, use of medications, and rehospitalization for cardiac and non-cardiac reasons.

For statistical analysis, surgical mortality was defined as death within 30 days or during the same hospitalization.

Table 6.2. Operative data

	CABG (n = 45)		AVR + CABG (n = 7)		Total (n = 52)	
No. of grafts (mean ± SD)	27 ± 1.0		2 ± 0.9		2.6 ± 1.0	
	No.	%	No.	%	No.	%
LIMA	18/45	40	3/7	43	21/52	40
	Mean	Range	Mean	Range	Mean	Range
Cross-clamp (min)	43	22–75	86	70–97	50	22–97
CPB time (min)	88	40–143	124	107–149	92	40–149

Results

Preoperative data shown in Table 6.1 indicate that 84% (43 patients) had unstable angina, while 40% had at least one previous myocardial infarction. Significant stenosis of the Lt. main coronary artery was found in 19% of the patients. LV function was good in only 52% of patients, moderately impaired in 40%, and severely impaired in 4 patients. According to NYHA classification, 84% were defined as classes III or IV and, as indicated, they frequently had other systemic diseases as well.

The mean number of grafts performed in the CABG subgroup was 2.7 ± 1.0 compared to 2 ± 0.9 grafts in those patients who underwent CABG+AVR. In the first subgroup, mean ischemic time was 43 min and bypass time was 86 min, compared to 88 min and 124 min, respectively, in the second subgroup (Table 6.2).

The LIMA was used as a conduit in 40% of the patients, regardless of whether the operation was simple or combined.

Mortality and morbidity

One patient (2%) died on the second post-operative day. This patient was referred to the operating theater as an emergency, suffering from acute dissection of the Lt. main coronary artery following coronary angiography. He was in cardiogenic shock on arrival and was assisted by an intra-aortic balloon pump (IABP). The patient remained in a low output state after the operation and expired from multi-organ failure.

Ten patients had at least one major complication as listed in Table 6.3. Two patients with an extremely calcified aortic arch suffered permanent neurologic deficit post-surgery (4%). Several others had some degree of impaired renal function, which improved gradually, but one patient required dialysis for acute on chronic renal failure. Even though the IMA was used in 40% of the patients,

Table 6.3. Morbidity and mortality

	No. of patients	Percent
Early death	1	2
Patients with major complications	10	20
Reoperation for bleeding	1	2
Perioperative MI (ECG, enzymes)	1	2
Renal failure (peritoneal dialysis)	1	2
Respiratory failure (ventilation > 72 hours)	2	4
Neurological damage (permanent)	2	4
Sepsis	1	2
Sternal wound infection (muscle flap)	1	2
Leg incision infection	2	4
Permanent pacemaker (S.S.S.)	1	2
Post-operative hospitalization		
< 10 days	37	73
10–20 days	8	15
> 20 days	6	12

only one had severe sternal wound infection necessitating a muscle flap reconstruction. It is interesting to mention that in this specific patient, the IMA was not harvested and only vein grafts were used. Analysis of our data revealed that the use of the IMA was not associated with higher mortality or morbidity (Figure 6.1).

Cardiac arrhythmias occurred in 12 patients, mainly atrial fibrillation, which was controlled medically and converted to sinus rhythm before discharge. One

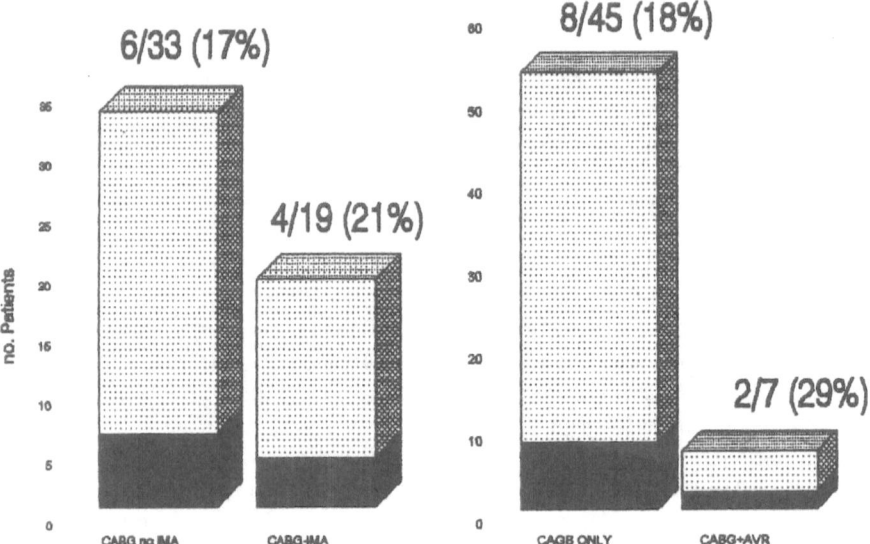

Figure 6.1. Occurrence of complications by type of operation.

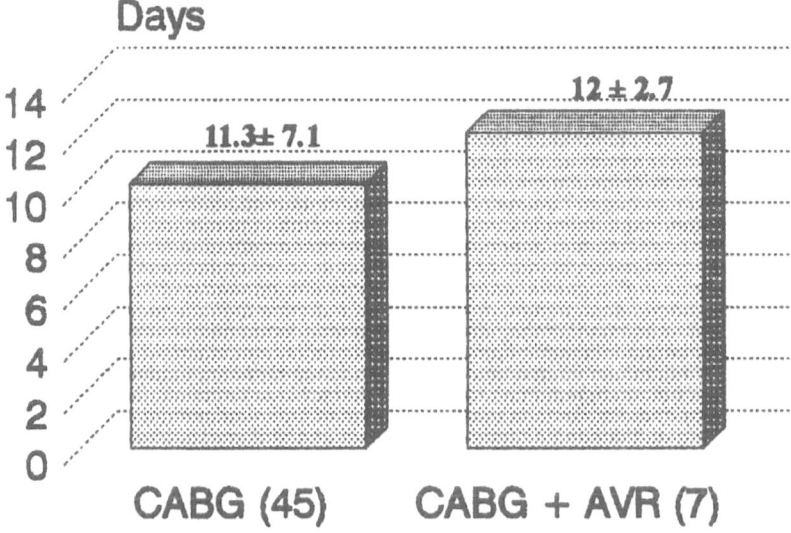

Figure 6.2. Mean hospital stay according to type of operation.

patient, with a sick sinus syndrome prior to surgery, required implantation of a permanent cardiac pacemaker.

The mean hospitalization stay, as illustrated in Figure 6.2, was 11.5 ± 7.3 days without any significant difference between the two subgroups (range 6–40 days).

Follow-up was performed for up to 34 months (mean 22 months). Two of the 51 surviving patients were lost to follow-up. Eight patients had to be rehospitalized during this period; two for cardiac and six for non-cardiac reasons. Only four patients (8%) still complained of either residual or recurrent angina pectoris.

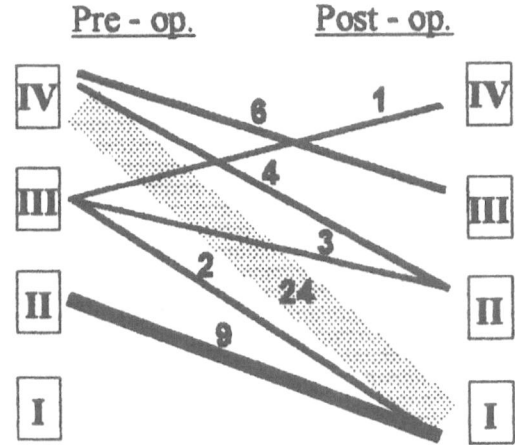

Figure 6.3. Post-operative change in NYHA functional class.

As mentioned previously, patients' functional state was assessed according to the NYHA classification and improved significantly from an average of 3.5 to 1.4 post-surgery (Figure 6.3). Eighty-four percent of the patients indicated improvement in their quality of life; six others (11.5%) did not notice any change, and one patient claimed that his condition had worsened. In addition to the subjective relief of symptoms, a significant reduction was noted in the consumption of medications, especially of anti-angina drugs and diuretics.

Discussion

Although significant advances have been made in the medical management of ischemic heart disease, it remains a predominant cause of mortality in developed countries. Increased life expectancy and subsequent aging of the world's population has prompted reviews of the results of revascularization in elderly patients [6–8].

In this study, as in others, the indications for coronary angiography were usually crescendo or post-infarction angina, resistant to maximal medical therapy. Analysis of the NYHA classification ratings indicate that most of the patients were in advanced stage (classes III–IV).

Open heart surgery in octogenarians is undoubtedly still considered very risky, and the literature is still lacking in solid data concerning surgical results in extremely aged patients. Recent studies suggest that with careful patient selection, CABG can be performed relatively safely, with mortality rates ranging from 0–3% for purely elective cases up to 35% for emergencies. The average mortality is 2–12% and it is only slightly higher than in younger patients with the same risk factors [1, 2, 4, 5]. Complications after cardiac surgery are reported to occur in 20–92% of patients [1, 2, 5, 9–11] but, on the whole, the experience of several institutions indicates that surgical intervention clearly provides improved survival compared with the continuation of medical therapy.

In this present study, the mortality rate was 2% in a group of 52 consecutive octogenarians during a mean follow-up period of 22 months. Serious complications occurred in 19% of the patients. The positive results can be attributed to several factors, among them patient selection made by the cardiologists even before considering angiography. As previously mentioned, most patients were not referred on an elective basis. Even so, surgeons should not consider patients suffering mental or physical instability as candidates, since this will hinder their ability to recover promptly from the operation. In this study, intra-operative management included meticulous surgical techniques and maintaining high perfusion pressures (80–90 mmHg), whilst making special efforts during the post-operative period towards early extubation, minimal sedation, early removal of chest tubes and catheters, and ambulation as soon as possible.

Previous studies have suggested some variables, such as emergency operation, impaired LV function, previous myocardial infarction and prolonged ischemic time (> 100 min), to be important risk factors. In our patients, one patient of the four who were referred as emergency cases died (25%).

Other risk factors did not seem to play significant statistical roles in mortality or morbidity rates. The reason might be related to good myocardial preservation and a relatively short cross-clamping time which minimized the impact of the risk factors.

The use of the IMA is of special interest and importance. This group of elderly and usually urgent patients is considered quite 'fragile' and most surgeons tend to perform the quickest operation possible. In this study, we noticed that although the use of the IMA is somewhat time-consuming, it has several advantages over the saphenous vein graft, since ischemic hearts tend to recover much better and faster (especially when the technique of first performing the distal anastomoses and later the proximals is used). Subsequently, the patient benefits from a good arterial conduit. The complication rate was certainly not higher when the IMA was used, and this fact encouraged us to increase the use of this artery from a rate of 23% of patients in 1991–92 to 58% in 1993 (Figure 6.4).

A subgroup of seven patients underwent combined surgery, CABG+AVR. One of them had severe LV dysfunction (LVEF, 30%). Ischemic time during their operations was almost double that of CABG alone. The IMA as a conduit was used in three patients (43%) and none of them died during follow-up. The complication rate was 29%. (These numbers, of course, are too small for statistical interpretation).

As listed in the table of complications, a cerebrovascular accident is one of the most serious events caused by manipulating an atheromatous aorta during surgery. This risk may be reduced by performing a trans-esophageal echo (TEE)

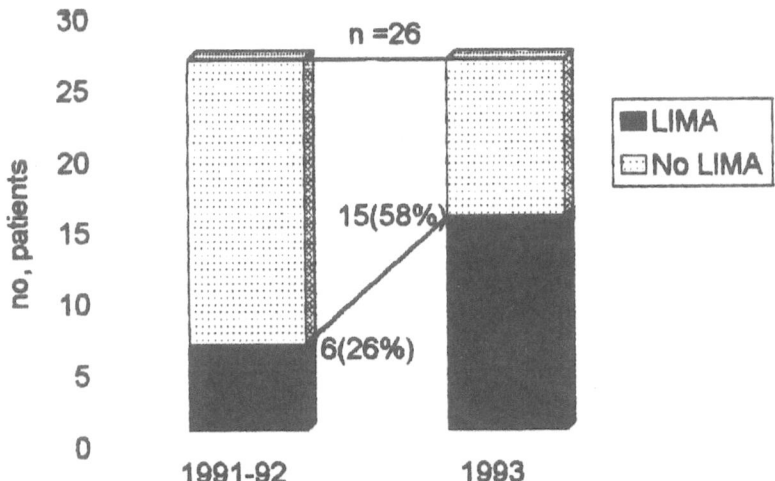

Figure 6.4. Increase in the use of LIMA – 1919–1993.

study during patient assessment, or even by using intraoperative echo which allows the surgeon to choose the right approach for each case.

We would conclude by suggesting that the positive results obtained by operation in this series, and additional data gathered on this complicated subject, may give rise to an increase in the total number of elderly patients referred for this kind of surgery. It is to be hoped that cardiologists, taking into account careful selection and correct perioperative management, will suggest CABG as a good alternative for treating coronary artery disease in octogenarians on an elective basis.

References

1. Ko W, Krieger KH, Lazenby WD, et al. Isolated coronary artery bypass grafting in one hundred consecutive octogenarian patients. J Thorac Cardiovasc Surg 1991; 102: 532–8.
2. Tsai T-P, Nessim S, Kass RM, et al. Morbidity and mortality after coronary artery bypass in octogenarians. Ann Thorac Surg 1991; 51: 983–6.
3. Horvath KA, DiSesa VJ, Peigh PS, et al. Favorable results of coronary artery bypass grafting in patients older than 75 years. J Thorac Cardiovasc Surg 1990; 99: 92–6.
4. Weintraub WS, Craver JM, Cohen CL, Jones EL, and Guyton RA. Influence of age on results of coronary artery surgery. Circulation 1991; 84(5 suppl II): 1226–35.
5. Glower DD, Christopher TD, Milano CA, et al. Performance status and outcome after coronary artery bypass grafting in persons aged 80 to 93 years. Am J Cardiol 1992; 70(6): 567–71.
6. Knapp WS, Douglas JS, Craver JM, et al. Efficacy of coronary artery bypass grafting in elderly patients with coronary artery disease. Am J Cardiol 1981; 47: 923–30.
7. Berry BE, Acree PW, Davis DL, Sheely CH, Cavin S. Coronary artery bypass operation in septuagenarians. Ann Thorac Surg 1981; 31: 310–3.
8. Stephenson LW, MacVaugh H, Edmunds LH. Surgery using cardiopulmonary bypass in the elderly. Circulation 1978; 58: 250–4.
9. Rich MW, Sandza JG, Kleiger RE, Connors JP. Cardiac operations in patients over 80 years of age. J Thorac Cardiovasc Surg 1985; 90: 56–60.
10. Edmunds LH Jr, Stephenson LW, Edie RN, Ratcliffe MB. Open-heart surgery in octogenarians. N Engl J Med 1988; 319: 131–6.
11. Tsai T-P, Matloff JM, Gray RJ, et al. Cardiac surgery in the octogenarian. J Thorac Cardiovasc Surg 1986; 91: 924–8.

PART THREE

Health care costs of elderly CABG patients

7. Age-specific costs of heart surgery and follow-up treatment in Germany

DETLEF CHRUSCZ and WOLFGANG KÖNIG

Introduction

More than 300,000 cardiac surgical interventions (diagnostic and therapeutic) took place in West Germany in 1992. Ten years before, the number of surgeries was about one sixth. The reason for this increase lies in the enormous increase in diagnostic and therapeutic possibilities in this field. Connected with this rise in numbers of operations is an expansion of the group of possible patients. Earlier, heart surgery was reserved for younger patients; today, the number of operations has increased in old and often more seriously ill patients.

The expansion of heart surgery to a growing number of patients implies rising costs for health insurance companies. Cost reductions could also exist because other treatments are no longer necessary, but there is little evidence for such an argument. Further, the growing number of heart surgeries leading to rising costs is only part of the story. In addition, operations on elderly patients may cause extra costs due to longer periods of convalescence after an operation. Due to the fact that there were no valid data available on age-specific costs of heart surgery in Germany, we have tried to estimate these costs.

Access to accurate data

Trying to ascertain the age-specific costs for coronary bypass surgery from routine health insurance data, one finds that age-specific data on surgical interventions are not available in Germany. One possibility for obtaining a rough overview of the development of bypass surgery is to look for diagnoses that are related to coronary bypass surgery in hospital cases, because health insurance firms are receiving an ICD-coded diagnosis at the patient's admission to the hospital.

An approximate analysis of the available, non-coded diagnoses makes it clear that most coronary bypass surgery is coded as ischemic heart disease. After the ICD-9 3-digit code, the following diagnosis codes are seen as causes for subsequent coronary bypass surgery: 410 (acute myocardial infarction), 413

71

P.J. Walter (ed.), Coronary Bypass Surgery in the Elderly, pp. 71–76.
© 1995 *Kluwer Academic Publishers, Dordrecht.*

(angina pectoris), 414 (other forms of chronic ischemic heart disease) and 444 (arterial embolism and thrombosis). On the one hand, this shows that it is impossible to classify bypass surgery as only one of the above-mentioned diagnoses and, on the other, it shows that diagnosis groups are too general to gain much evidence for coronary bypass surgery.

The exclusive transmission of diagnosis leads to a lack of information for health insurance companies. In the future, a remedy for this problem is expected with a revised version of the health reform law. When this comes into effect, hospitals will have to report, in addition to the diagnosis, the 5-digit ICPM code (International Classification of Procedures in Medicine) for their operations and other procedures. Only then will it be possible to directly determine the age-specific frequencies and costs of coronary bypass surgery [1]. As long as this law is not in effect, an analysis of coronary bypass surgery based on health insurance data is impossible.

A data source used for this analysis which provides some information on bypass surgery is the survey of the Hospital Committee of AGLMB and the Society for Thoracic-, Heart- and Vascular Surgery [2]. This survey provided data on the number of executed heart surgeries with a heart-lung machine, roughly differentiated by operations and age.

Development of coronary heart disease

Since the 1970s, coronary heart disease mortality has been declining in West Germany, as it has in most other Western and Northern European countries. The decline in mortality not only affects patients aged 50–65, but older patients as well. Life expectancy at birth increased between the mid-seventies and the end of the eighties by 4.3 years for males and females. Almost 0.9 years of this increase are related to the decline in cardiovascular mortality beyond the age of 60 years. In women, an even more dramatic decline of cardiovascular mortality is responsible for an increased life expectancy of more than 1.3 years in this age group. At the same time, a rise in cardiovascular morbidity during old age indicates an increase of interventions, as is supported by the rising number of heart surgeries in the past.

Heart surgery in Germany

In West Germany, the total number of heart operations with a heart-lung machine rose between 1978 and 1992 from 8,365 to 45,178 (see Figure 7.1). Comparing this number to the population, this means an increase from 136 to 701 heart surgeries per million residents. The development of the forms of surgery were also quite different. In 1978, only 3,042 coronary heart surgeries were carried out. This number increased tenfold to 31,338 in 1992. The number of heart-valve surgeries tripled, while the surgeries of congenital heart defects

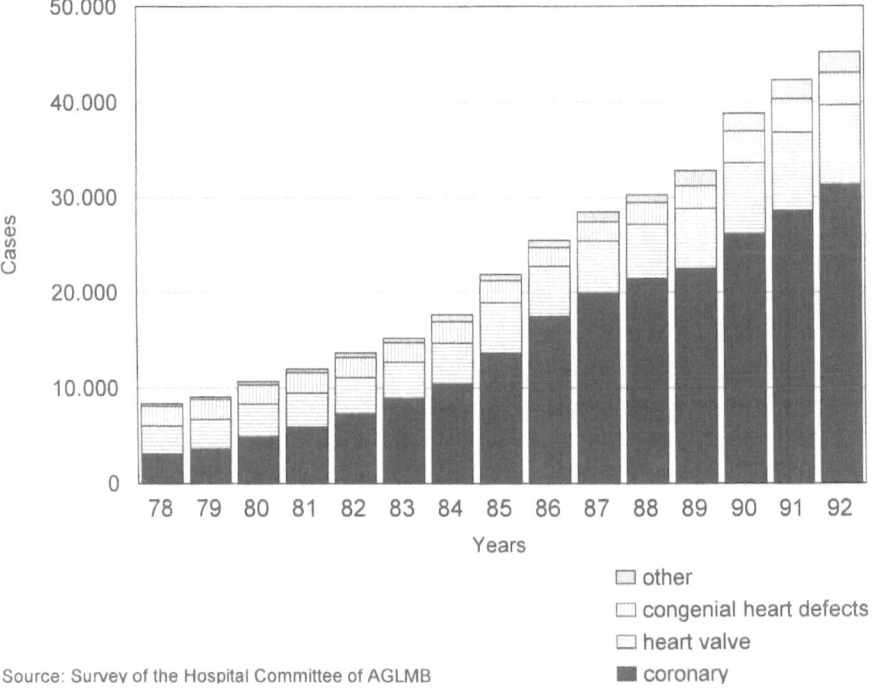

Figure 7.1. Open heart surgery in West Germany

only increased by 1.5 times. In 1992 the proportion of coronary heart surgery to total heart surgery with support of the heart-lung machine was about 70 percent.

The less invasive angioplasty technique (percutaneus transluminal coronary angioplasty – PTCA) replaced open heart surgery only to a certain extent. Earlier expectations that PTCA would be promoted as a less straining technique and the demand for coronary surgery would decrease did not materialize. In 1978, only 3% of the invasive treated coronary patients got a PTCA, but 97% received coronary surgery. For the first time, in 1987, more PTCAs were carried out than coronary surgery. In 1992, the number of PTCAs amounted to around 51,000, compared to 31,338 coronary surgeries.

The age distribution of operated heart patients shows that 37% of all heart surgeries took place between the ages of 60 to 70 years (see Table 7.1). At the same time, the proportion of surgeries carried out on patients beyond the age of 60 years has been increasing. More than half of all heart surgeries were performed on patients older than 60 years.

Table 7.1. Heart surgery and ischemic heart disease in West Germany in 1992

Age groups	Heart surgery with heart-lung machine[a]	Ischemic heart disease (ICD 410-414)[b]	
	Cases per 100,000 population	Cases per 100,000 population	Days per case
30–39	9.66	118.52	9.86
40–49	39.12	571.23	10.43
50–59	130.80	1498.15	11.77
60–69	254.13	2503.04	14.86
70–79	194.64	3017.52	17.47
80+	26.41	2834.71	17.88
All Ages	109.13	1757.20	14.65

[a] Survey of the Hospital Committee of AGLMB.
[b] Company health insurance funds.

Costs of heart surgery

The costs of heart surgery with heart-lung machine support in Germany comprise the general hospital allowance per day, plus a special charge for the surgery. In three cases, hospitals and health insurance companies have agreed upon a lump sum per case. In these centers, the lump sum varies between 20,500 and 22,900 DM. The lump sum is independent of the patient's duration of stay.

In most cases, the costs of heart surgery consist of two components: the special charge and a general hospital allowance per day. The special charge, as with lump sum cases, is independent of the length of hospitalisation. Special charges are arranged for heart surgery with heart-lung machine support, for heart surgery without the heart-lung machine, PTCA, and cardiac catheterisation. A more distinct differentiation, for instance, for coronary bypass surgery is not available. The special charges for a heart surgery with support of a heart-lung machine are between 13,800 DM and 23,800 DM. The general hospital allowance per day varies between 310 DM and 580 DM [3]. The average costs for heart surgery with a heart-lung machine and a ten-day period of hospitalisation reached 23,400 DM in 1992. The total expenses arising from the general hospital allowance per day are dependent upon the patient's period of hospitalisation. This is also age-dependent because the average duration of hospitalisation is longer for older aged patients due to generally longer convalescence periods.

Age-specific cost evaluation

An exclusive analysis of coronary bypass surgery is not possible with the information provided by the company health insurance funds. Available data from the statistics of types of sickness at least provide information on the age-specific incidence and age-specific period of hospitalisation of ischemic heart disease (see Table 7.1). Age becomes a cost factor if the age-specific period of hospitalisation is combined with the general hospital allowance per day. By comparing the general hospital allowance per day with the special charges for heart surgery with heart-lung machine, the combination of age-specific incidence rates of heart surgery, and the age-specific duration of hospitalisation from ischemic heart diseases, we can estimate the age-specific costs of heart surgery. In a similar way, the costs of rehabilitation clinic stays can also be estimated.

Considering an average general hospital per day allowance of 490 DM and an average special operation charge of 19,200 DM, a heart surgery with an average 14.7-day period of hospitalisation would cost 26,414 DM. The expenses for a subsequent stay at a rehabilitation clinic, for a regular 30-day stay, amount to 6,000 DM (average charge per day 200 DM). These 30 days of rehabilitation are an official regulation independent from the state of convalescence.

Costs for heart surgery increase with age (see Table 7.2), but the maximal difference amounts to less than 5,000 DM. At a total expense of 444 million DM, the age group 60 to 69 is causing much higher costs than other age groups. They are next followed by the 50–59 age group, with 294 million DM, and then by the 70–79 group with 231 million DM in 1992. The total costs for heart surgery with heart-lung machine support and the period of hospitalisation amount annually to 1.17 billion DM. Including the costs for a 30-day stay at a rehabilitation clinic, these expenses amount to 1.44 billion DM. This is approximately 2% of the national budget for hospital expenses of statutory health insurance programs.

Table 7.2. Costs of heart surgery in West Germany in 1992

Age groups	Costs (in DM)	
	Per case	Total
0–19	23,319	65,993,902
20–29	23,051	13,323,766
30–39	24,066	23,632,945
40–49	24,349	79,157,997
50–59	25,006	294,625,976
60–69	26,521	444,432,603
70–79	27,797	230,933,761
80+	28,000	19,292,242
All Ages	26,414	1,171,393,192

Conclusions

Based solely on demographic developments in the near future, the number of heart surgeries will probably increase. Using the population projection of the Federal Statistics Office, the population will decrease generally in Germany. But this development does not take place with the same intensity in all age groups. While the population of youth and adults is declining by about 18 million, the number of the elderly will increase by the year 2030 by 8 million [4]. This means that the number of people with the highest probability for heart surgery increases. If, contrary to the assumption of the Federal Statistics Office, that life expectancy rises only through the year 2000, a stronger increase in the elderly could be expected.

To summarize the findings on the age-specific costs of heart surgery in Germany: due to the German system of reimbursement, the average costs per heart surgery of younger patients are only slightly lower than the corresponding costs for older patients. The longer duration of hospitalisation of older people only causes a small difference in costs per case, compared to younger people. The increase in absolute cost totals arising from heart surgery in older patients is due to an increase in medical options for treatment that has made heart surgery possible at older ages. In addition to the expenses of heart surgery, there are other central criteria which need to be recognized in this discussion. These are the well-being of the patient, efficiency of the therapy and quality assurance [5, 6].

References

1. Von Bremen KP. Verschlüsselung der Diagnosen und Operationen in der Sozialen Krankenversicherung. Die Ersatzkasse 1993; 10; 341-6.
2. Bruckenberger E. Situation der Herzchirugie 1992 in Deutschland: Fünfter Bericht des Krankenhausausschusses. Hannover: Arbeitsgemeinschaft der Leitenden Medizinalbeamten, 1993.
3. Graeve G. Zugelassene Krankenhäuser: Betriebsstrukturen und Vergütungsregelungen. Düsseldorf: Deutscher Krankenhausverlag, 1994.
4. Sommer B. Entwicklung der Bevölkerung bis zum Jahr 2030: Ergebnis der siebten koordinierten Bevölkerungsvorausberechnung. Wirtschaft und Statistik 1992; 4: 217-22.
5. Stuck E, De Vivie ER, Hehrlein F et al. Multicentric quality assurance in cardiac surgery. Thorac Cardiovasc Surg 1990; 38: 123-34.
6. Bauer U. Qualitätssicherung in der herzchirugischen Versorgung. Die Betriebskrankenkasse 1991: 691-7.

PART FOUR

Clinical, economical and ethical controversies

8. Opportunities to improve the cost-effectiveness of CABG surgery

WILLIAM B. STASON

Introduction

Health care reform is generating an enormous amount of debate in the United States. Opinions vary widely, and the end results remain unclear. However, directions will, almost certainly, include:
- some form of universal coverage for a defined package of services to which all citizens will be entitled; and
- emphasis on increasing the cost-effectiveness of health care through a combination of incentives to control costs and increase the benefits of services that are provided.

To these ends, relevant costs will be those perceived by the payer (insurer, government, employer, or the individual) and relevant benefits will represent a balance between medical outcomes and effects on the quality of life. Quality of life is especially important to the elderly in whom the ability to pursue valued activities and freedom from discomfort may be valued far more than a few additional weeks or months of life.

Coronary artery bypass surgery (CABG) has been well demonstrated to increase both the length and quality of life in selected subgroups of patients. Though expensive, it may also be cost effective if it is applied:
- to patients who are most likely to benefit;
- by competent surgical teams; and
- in well-organized, well-staffed, efficient hospitals.

Bypass surgery has been found to be more cost effective than treatment of mild or moderate hypertension for left main disease and 3-vessel disease, about equally cost effective for 2-vessel disease, and much less cost effective for single-vessel disease [1]. Cost-effectiveness estimates for patients with extensive disease were driven primarily by improved survival benefits after surgery and, for 2-vessel disease, by whether the left anterior descending vessel was involved and by the severity of angina in patients on medical treatment. Surgical results in this study were obtained from surgical programs participating in controlled clinical trials during the late 1970s and early 1980s. If anything, current comparisons should favor bypass surgery even more, given the continued decline in operative

79

P.J. Walter (ed.), Coronary Bypass Surgery in the Elderly, pp. 79–89.
© 1995 Kluwer Academic Publishers, Dordrecht.

mortality rates and increasing use of expensive medications to treat hypertension, such as ACE inhibitors and calcium channel blockers.

The objectives of the present paper are to extend this cost-effectiveness perspective by:

1. summarizing current trends in bypass surgery in the Medicare program for elderly Americans;
2. discussing lessons being learned from the Medicare Heart Bypass Center Demonstration that offer insights into opportunities to improve the cost-effectiveness of surgery; and
3. by underscoring the importance of patient-centered care in enhancing both the quality and cost-effectiveness of health care.

Trends in bypass surgery under the Medicare program

Trends in bypass surgery performed on Medicare beneficiaries are summarized in Table 8.1. Results are based on an analysis of Medicare claims data for calendar years 1990 through 1992 [2].

During this period, the number of bypass operations performed on Medicare beneficiaries increased slightly more than 5% per year to a total of about 150,000 operations. By 1992, Medicare beneficiaries, most of whom are 65 years of age or older, accounted for approximately half of all bypass procedures performed in 880 cardiac surgery programs in the United States. Medicare cases averaged 170 operations per program in 1992 (equivalent to a total volume of about 340 cases). Many cardiac surgical programs are quite small, however, as indicated by the fact that those in the lower decile performed 36 or fewer Medicare operations per year.

The mean length of stay for bypass surgery in Medicare patients in 1992 was 13.5 days, and the mean cost for hospital care was about $25,000. Charges for physican services add another $5,000–$8,000 to total costs. Lengths of stay varied widely among hospitals and, on average, fell about 10 percent between 1990 and 1992. The cost of care in major teaching hospitals was 50% greater than in non-teaching hospitals ($33,000 vs. $22,000). The fact that hospital costs continued to increase between 1990 and 1992 despite shorter lengths of stay may reflect greater intensity of care or the failure of Medicare's Prospective Payment System reimbursement rates to reflect systematic changes in length of stay.

Hospital mortality for bypass surgery fell from 6.5% to 5.3% between 1990 and 1992. Case-mix adjusted mortality undoubtedly fell even more in view of the trend toward operating on 'sicker' patients during this period. Mortality varied 4.5-fold among hospitals, ranging from 2.1–9.0% between top and bottom deciles. No obvious differences in mortality were found between teaching and non-teaching hospitals, even though there is some evidence that teaching hospitals attract a more severely ill case-mix.

Table 8.1. Trends in coronary artery bypass surgery in the U.S. Medicare program: 1990–1992

	1990	1992	Percent change
Bypass procedures	129,270	150,027	+ 16.1
Cardiac surgical programs	833	880	+ 5.6
Medicare bypass procedures/program			
Mean	155	170	+ 9.7
Top 10%	333	363	+ 9.0
Bottom 10%	34	36	+ 5.8
DRG[a]			
106	62,892	85,443	+ 35.9
107	46,806	60,175	+ 28.6
108	19,572	4,409	− 77.5
Length of stay (days)			
Mean	15.0	13.5	− 10.0
Top 10%	18.5	16.2	− 12.4
Bottom 10%	11.6	10.5	− 9.4
Expenditures for hospital care			
National	$23,258	$24,928	+ 7.2
Major teaching	$29,818	$32,916	+ 10.4
Non-teaching	$20,620	$21,837	+5.9
Hospital mortality rate (%)			
Mean	6.5	5.3	− 18.5
Top 10%	11.2	9.0	− 19.6
Bottom 10%	2.5	2.1	− 16.0
Major teaching	6.8	5.8	− 14.7
Non-teaching	6.6	5.1	− 22.7

[a] More restrictive classification rules were adopted for DRG 108 in 1991.

Medicare Heart Bypass Center Demonstration

Overall results in the Medicare program provide the backdrop for the Medicare Heart Bypass Center Demonstration. This project began in 1991 with the primary purpose of examining the effects of paying hospitals a negotiated 'fixed global price' for all hospital and physician services connected with the admission during which bypass surgery is performed. Only patients who received bypass surgery as their only major surgical procedure, with or without coronary angiography on the same admission, were enrolled (DRGs 106 and 107, respectively). Patients who underwent concurrent valve replacement or other vascular procedures were therefore excluded.

Objectives are to determine the effects of the demonstration on the total costs of surgery, clinical outcomes, the appropriateness of clinical decisions, and on the ability of a designated Medicare Heart Bypass Center to increase its market share in its community.

Over 200 hospitals indicated an interest in the demonstration; 42 were asked to submit proposals; 27 completed proposals; and 7 were selected to participate based on price, extent of experience in open heart surgery, prior performance, and geographic distribution. Selected hospitals all have relatively high volume programs. Participants are:
- Boston University Medical Center, Boston, MA
- Methodist Hospital of Indiana, Indianapolis, IN
- Catherine McAuley Health System, Ann Arbor, MI
- Saint Joseph's Hospital, Atlanta, GA
- St. Luke's Episcopal Hospital, Houston TX
- St. Vincent Hospital, Portland, OR
- The Ohio State University Hospitals, Columbus, OH

Four hospitals began to enroll patients in mid-1991 and 3 others (St. Luke's, St. Vincent, and Methodist) began in mid-1993.

Opportunities to improve the cost-effectiveness of bypass surgery

The cost-effectiveness of bypass surgery is measured by the relationships between the costs and health benefits of surgery compared to other treatments for coronary artery disease (for example, angioplasty or medications); bypass surgery in one hospital compared to another hospital; or bypass surgery compared to treatments for other diseases such as hypertension or cancer.

The cost-effectiveness of bypass surgery can be improved by reducing costs, increasing benefits, or a combination. Near-term opportunities to reduce costs focus on hospital and physician charges. This is the approach being taken in the Medicare demonstration. Costs directly related to the surgical episode, however, tell only part of the story. This is especially true if initial cost savings are overshadowed by the subsequent costs of treatment for cardiovascular complications (for example, acute myocardial infarction), complications of surgery, or the need for repeat cardiovascular procedures. Comparisons between surgical programs and between angioplasty and bypass surgery need to take these subsequent costs into account. Surgical programs with higher rates of treatment failures or late complications will be more expensive in the long run. Similarly, angioplasty is less expensive initially but may be equally or more costly than bypass surgery in the long run if treatment failures or reocclusions necessitate repeat angioplasty or later surgery.

One opportunity for increasing the benefits of bypass surgery is through greater emphasis on selecting patients for bypass surgery in whom the potential benefits clearly exceed the risks. Several studies have raised important questions about the appropriateness of bypass surgery that is being done in the United States. At the extremes, a study in the mid-1980s found that 44% of patients in three western states received surgery for reasons that were felt to be questionable or frankly inappropriate indications [3]. A more recent study in

New York State identified only 9% such patients [4]. We can't be sure which findings are the more representative, but, almost certainly, there is room for further improvement.

Benefits can also be increased by improving the performance of surgical teams and their supporting hospital staffs. It is difficult to envision a surgical progam that cannot be improved.

Finally, considerable emphasis has been placed on the volume–quality relationship for cardiac surgery [5–16]. The evidence is complex, but a reasonable conclusion is that both hospital volume and surgeon volume are important considerations, other factors being equal. Actual performance of a program, however, is by far the best guide.

Findings from the Medicare Heart Bypass Center Demonstration

The Medicare Heart Bypass Demonstration Project exemplifies several opportunities to reduce costs or increase the benefits of bypass surgery. The results described are from an interim report [17].

Cost savings

The 'global rate' Medicare negotiated with the demonstration hospitals resulted in cost savings in the hospital portion of the bill ranging from 9% in the hospital with the lowest cost prior to the demonstration (from $21,600 to $19,600) to nearly 20% in the highest cost hospital (from $35,500 to $28,900). Reductions in physician fees were generally less, in part, because implementation of the resource-based relative value scale at about the same time had already reduced surgical fees. The Medicare Program estimates it has saved about $13 million on the first 2500 patients enrolled in the demonstration or about $5,100 per admission.

Participating hospitals have implemented some very creative cost-saving measures in response to these incentives.

– Lengths of stay have been shortened by as many as 5 days for DRG 106 and 2 days for DRG 107. DRG 106 offers more opportunity for shortening the length of stay because of efficiencies that can be gained through better coordination between the patient's prinicipal physician, the cardiac catheterization laboratory, and cardiac surgery during the pre-operative period.

– Same day surgery has been implemented for elective patients in several hospitals and appears to be well accepted by patients and physicians alike.

– Earlier extubation has reduced costs by shortening time in the surgical intensive care unit and by shortening overall length of stay. One hospital reports that the majority of patients can be extubated on the same day as surgery rather than waiting until the next morning.

– Several hospitals are exploring ways to reduce medication costs. For example, one hospital has saved $22,000 in a year by switching from brand name to generic protamine.

– Adherence to a *Critical Path* appears to be a particularly fruitful way to increase the efficiency of the care process. A *Critical Path* maps various aspects of pre- and post-operative care, including the monitoring of cardiac status, respiratory care, nutrition and hydration, physical activity, tests, teaching, and discharge planning, and specifies targets for each post-operative day. Content is discussed on a regular basis and revised as needed. Typically, willingness to modify traditional care patterns increases as evidence is obtained that patients can tolerate and accept an accelerated pace of care.

– Use of physician consultants such as infectious disease experts, nephrologists, and pulmonary specialists has been reduced by as much as 28% in one hospital.

– Finally, savings in administrative costs have resulted from reductions in the amount of paperwork required for billing. One bill covers all.

The universal feeling among participating hospitals is that cost savings have been achieved without any compromise in the quality of care and that patient satisfaction is as high or higher than previously. Patients are particularly happy about being protected from the traditional stream of bills from the hospital and physicians and about being protected against deductibles or co-payments.

Hospital mortality

One important measure of program effectiveness is hospital mortality. An overall, unadjusted, mortality rate of 4.2% in the first four demonstration sites compares favorably to the 5.3% figure for all Medicare patients. Both rates are for operations performed during 1992. Mortality is higher for DRG 106 than in DRG 107 (6.1% versus 2.9%) in part because DRG 106 includes more patients who are at higher risk because of unstable angina or a recent myocardial infarction.

Analysis of adjusted hospital mortality rates underscores the importance of taking case-mix into account. For example, one hospital had a significantly higher observed mortality rate (5.8% compared to 3.6% for the hospital with the lowest mortality rate). This finding was troublesome until case-mix adjustment revealed that the observed rate in this hospital was lower than the predicted rate. This hospital clearly operates on a more severely ill patient population. The converse was true for another hospital in which the observed mortality was higher than predicted.

Patient characteristics that were associated with hospital mortality are shown in Table 8.2. Pre-operative use of an intra-aortic balloon pump (IABP) conveys a 6-fold increase in the risk of surgery. Procedures performed on an emergent basis, a previous bypass operation, older age, the presence of congestive heart failure or chronic renal disease (marked by a serum creatinine of greater than 2 mg %), and procedures in patients with unstable angina or following an acute myocardial infarction were associated with with 2- to 4-fold higher risks of

Table 8.2. Patient risk factors for hospital mortality in Medicare Heart Bypass Center Demonstration participants

Univariate Risks

Risk Factor	Risk Ratio
Preoperative use of an IABP	6.4
Emergent bypass	3.8
Previous bypass	3.1
Chronic renal disease (serum Cr > 2 mg %)	2.8
Congestive heart failure	2.5
Age 80 or greater	2.3
Age 73–79	1.7
Acute myocardial infarction or unstable angina	2.0
Diabetes on treatment	1.6
Female gender	1.5
Black race	1.4
Left ventricular ejection fraction < 35%	1.4
Left main coronary artery stenosis (50% or greater)	1.3

Multiple Logistic Regression (N = 1951)

Risk Factor	Coefficient
Intercept	.000
Emergent bypass	.000
Previous bypass	.000
Pre-operative use of an IABP	.000
Congestive heart failure	.009
Diabetes on treatment	.018
Chronic renal disease	.014
Age 73–79	.040
Age 80 or greater	.008
Female gender	.096

hospital mortality. Female gender, black race, being on treatment for diabetes mellitus, a reduced left ventricular ejection fraction (< 35%), and the presence of stenosis of the left main coronary artery conveyed lesser degrees of increased risk.

Many of the same variables were independently associated with hospital mortality in a multiple logistic analysis. Emergent CABG, previous CABG, and pre-operative use of an IABP were the strongest predictors. Neither the presence of acute myocardial infarction or unstable angina, nor a left ventricular ejection fraction of less than 35% was significantly associated with mortality after controlling for the other variables. The effects of gender disappeared if height was added to the analysis.

The results of these analyses closely parallel other reports [16, 18–22]. The major difference is that each of these other studies identified left ventricular ejection fraction as an independent predictor of hospital mortality, while our study did not. The inclusion of a clinical diagnosis of congestive heart failure in our regression model may in part explain this finding. The relatively small univariate risk ratio of ejection fraction ($RR = 1.4$) makes it unlikely, however, that this is the only explanation.

Use of mortality data to improve the cost-effectiveness of bypass surgery

The potential values of mortality data such as these are at least three-fold. First, the relationships between patient characteristics and mortality can be used pre-operatively to better inform discussions with patients about the risks and benefits of surgery and improve case selection. Second, a hospital that monitors similar clinical information can use it to identify problem areas and improve performance. Regular feedback of program-wide and physician-specific severity-adjusted outcomes can serve as powerful stimuli to greater self-examination and efforts to improve performance. Third, public release of results will help the public become more discriminating consumers of the health care. Challenges are to ensure that the information released is accurate and that it is presented in a fashion that permits valid interpretation. Public release of program-specific data is just beginning in the United States but, almost certainly, will become the standard in the not far distant future.

Patient-centered care

The importance of patient perceptions is becoming ever clearer, both as a measure of the quality of care and the very practical matter of economic survival for hospitals in an increasingly competitive health care marketplace [23–25]. The finding that patient ratings of quality are associated with the financial strength of a hospital should provide strong incentives to health care executives [24]. Sensitivity to individual needs and preferences, effective coordination and convenience of services, clarity about who is responsible for care, and effective communication between patients and their physicians and nurses appear to be particularly important.

The usefulness of patient-centered information is exemplified in Figure 8.1 by data collected from 1,167 patients who received bypass surgery. These data are from a 68-hospital Patient Viewpoint database maintained by NCG Research, Nashville, TN. A questionnaire was sent to each patient following discharge in which he or she was asked to rate each dimension of care in terms of the performance of the hospital and the importance of that dimension to the quality of care. The importance of a dimension was derived by correlating the performance rating with the patient's expressed willingness to return, recommend the hospital to others, or 'brag' about the hospital stay. Findings are displayed as an importance-performance matrix in which the distance from

Open Heart & Cardiothoracic
DRGs 106, 107, 108
Importance/Performance Matrix

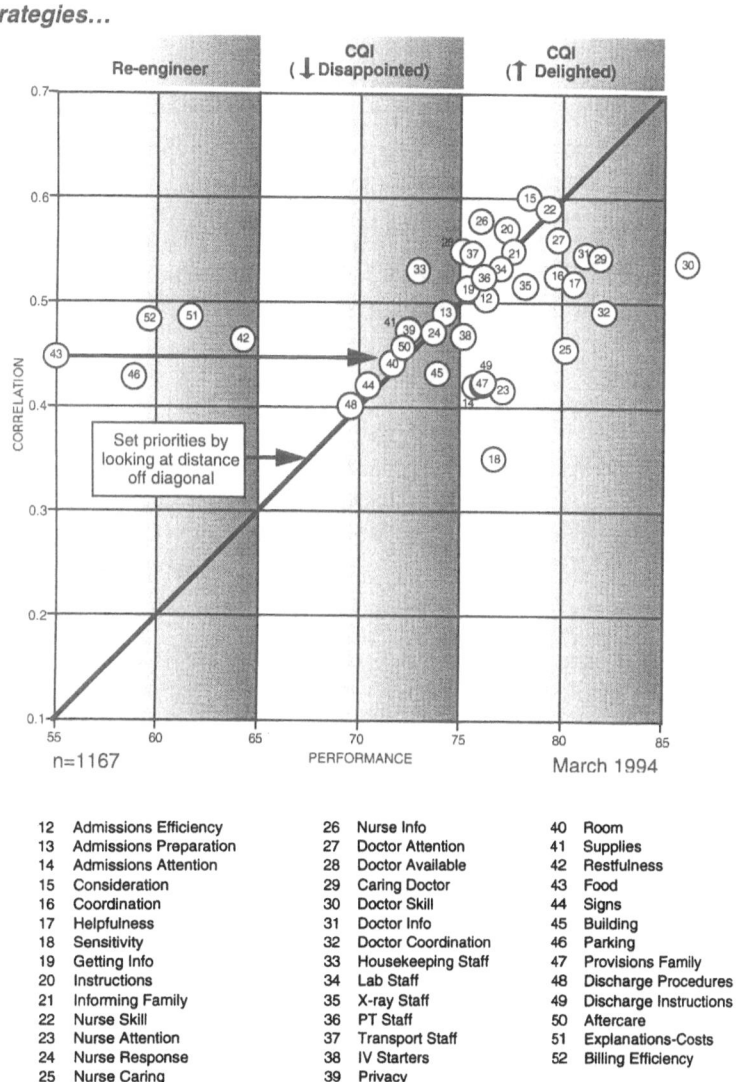

Based on data collected from 68 U.S. hospitals by NCG Research, Inc., Nashville, Tennessee.

Inpatient Viewpoint℠   NCG Research, Inc.

Figure 8.1. Importance-Performance Matrix for patients undergoing cardiovascular surgery. Each point represents a mean value for a particular attribute of inpatient care obtained from responses to a written post-discharge questionaire. Data were obtained by NCG Research Inc., Nashville, TN.

the diagonal represents the priority that should be given to a particular factor. Findings to the left of the diagonal, which represent areas of relatively low performance but high importance, are especially interesting. Examples are billing efficiency and explanation of costs, the patient's room and restfulness of the inpatient setting, and parking for visitors. Dramatic changes or 're-engineering' may be warranted to address these high importance-low performance areas. At the other extreme, areas of strong performance might justifiably be emphasized in promotional activities.

The bottom line is that the patient's perception of the quality of care one is receiving may not only influence near-term medical outcomes, but may also influence future decisions on where to seek health care.

Several of the Medicare Heart Bypass Demonstration hospitals are making concerted efforts to address patient issues and market their programs within their communities. Evidence of success is mixed; some hospitals appear to be increasing their market shares and others are not.

Conclusions and future analyses

In summary, the Medicare Heart Bypass Center Demonstration is achieving 9–20% cost savings in different hospitals and has created incentives for efficient care that may be saving even larger sums. Secondary effects on the costs of surgery reimbursed by other payers may ultimately be even more dramatic. At present, indications are that hospital mortality has been unaffected by the economic squeeze represented by the 'global price'.

Analyses in progress will extend findings on hospital mortality and also examine longer-term mortality, angina relief, factors that affect length of stay, re-admissions, and the appropriateness of decisions to perform bypass surgery.

Health care reform in the United States should take these lessons to 'heart' by:
- extending incentives created by global pricing to other procedures and to other conditions such as the management of acute myocardial infarction;
- taking steps to require all hospitals to maintain data systems that monitor case-mix adjusted performance; and
- seriously considering restrictions on low-volume cardiac surgical programs unless they can demonstrate they are cost competitive and are performing at least as well as higher volume programs in the same community.

References

1. Weinstein MC, Stason WB. Cost-effectiveness of interventions to prevent or treat coronary heart disease. Ann Rev Public Health 1985; 6: 41–63.
2. Dayoff D, Cromwell J. National and market area trends in Medicare heart bypass surgery. Report to the Health Care Financing Administration. Baltimore, M.D. under Contract No. 500–87–0029.

3. Winslow CM, Kosecoff JB, Chassin M, Kanouse DE, Brook RH. The appropriateness of performing coronary artery bypass surgery. JAMA 1988; 260: 505–9.
4. Leape LL, Hilborne LH, Park RE, et al. The appropriateness of use of coronary artery bypass graft surgery in New York State. JAMA 1993; 269: 753–60.
5. Luft HS, Bunker JP, Enthoven AS. Should operations be regionalized? The empirical relation between surgical volume and mortality. N Engl J Med 1979; 301: 1364–9.
6. Luft HS. The relation between surgical volume and mortality: an exploration of causal factors and alternative models. Med Care 1980; 18: 940–59.
7. Sloan F, Perrin J, Valvona J. In-hospital mortality of surgical patients: is there an empiric basis for standard setting? Surgery 1986; 99: 446–53.
8. Kelly JV, Hellinger FJ. Heart disease and hospital deaths: an empirical study. Health Services Research 1987; 22: 369–94.
9. Luft HS, Hunt SS, Maerki SC. The volume-outcome relationship: practice makes perfect or selective referral patterns? Health Services Research 1987; 22: 157–82.
10. Farley DE, Ozminkowski RJ. Volume-outcome relationships and inhospital mortality: the effect of changes in volume over time. Med Care 1992; 30: 77–94.
11. Showstack JA, Rosenfeld KE, Garnick DW, Luft HS, Schaffarzick RW, Fowles J. Association of volume with outcome of coronary artery bypass graft surgery: scheduled vs nonscheduled operations. JAMA 1987; 257: 785–9.
12. O'Connor GT, Plume SK, Olmstead EM, et al. A regional prospective study of in-hospital mortality associated with coronary artery bypass grafting, JAMA 1991; 266: 803–9.
13. Williams SV, Nash DB, Goldfarb N. Differences in mortality from coronary artery bypass graft surgery at five teaching hospitals. JAMA 1991; 266: 810–5.
14. Hannan EL, O'Donnell JF, Kilburn H Jr, et al. Investigation of the relationship between volume and mortality for surgical procedures performed in Neew York State hospitals. JAMA 1989; 262: 503–10.
15. Hannan EL, Kilburn H Jr, Bernard H, et al. Coronary artery bypass surgery: the relationship between in-hospital mortality rate and surgical volume after controlling for clinical risk factors. Med Care 1991; 29: 1094–107.
16. Hannan EL, Kilburn H Jr, Racz M, Shields E, Chassin MR. Improving the outcomes of coronary artery bypass surgery in New York State. JAMA 1994; 271: 761–6.
17. Cromwell J, Stason WB, Beaven M. Trends and differences in hospital mortality rates: an interim report on Medicare heart bypass centers. Report to the Health Care Financing Administration. Baltimore M.D. under Contract No. 500–87–0029, 1993.
18. Parsonnet V, Dean D, Bernstein AD. A method of uniform stratification of risk for evaluating the results of surgery in acquired heart disease. Circulation 1989; 79(suppl I): 3–12.
19. Hannan EL, Kilburn H Jr, O'Donnell JF, et al. Adult open heart surgery in New York State: an analysis of risk factors and hospital mortality rates. JAMA 1990; 264: 2768–74.
20. O'Connor GT, Plume SK, Olmstead BA, et al. Multivariate prediction of in-hospital mortality associated with coronary artery bypass graft surgery. Circulation 1992; 85: 2110–8.
21. Higgins TL, Estafanous FG, Loop FD, Beck GJ, Blum JM, Paranandi L. Stratification of morbidity and mortality outcome by preoperative risk factors in coronary artery bypass patients. A clinical severity score. JAMA 1992; 267: 2344–8.
22. Christakis GT, Ivanov J, Weisel RD, Birnbaum PL, David TE, Salerno TA and the cardiovascular surgeons of the University of Toronto. The changing pattern of coronary artery bypass surgery. Circulation 1989; 80(suppl I): 151–61.
23. Gerteis M, Edgman-Levitan S, Daley J, Delbanco TL, eds. Through the patient's eyes. San Francisco, CA: Jossey Bass Publishers, 1993.
24. Nelson EC, Rust RT, Zahorik A, Rose RL, Batalden P, Siemanski BA. Do patient perceptions of quality relate to hospital financial performance? J Health Care Marketing 1992; 12: 6–13.
25. Furse DH, Burcham MR, Rose RL, Oliver RW. Leverging the value of customer satisfaction information. Critical success factor in healthcare J Health Care Marketing 1994. In press.

9. Who gets bypass surgery – should the doctor, patient or computer decide?

JOHN KELLETT

Introduction

Seven years ago my father, then 74 years of age, developed angina. Many of my colleagues kindly offered him advice on his best treatment but, unfortunately, it was all conflicting! Subsequent to my father's successful management, I sought the opinion of 38 of my most experienced consultant physician colleagues (qualified for a mean of 23.1 ± 7.8 years) on the probable outcome of a 74 year old man (i.e. my father) who develops exercise-limiting angina and 3 mm ST deviation within four minutes of starting a Bruce protocol exercise test [1]. They estimated that such a patient treated medically had anything from a 5 to 75% chance of dying per year (mean $22.8 \pm 16.6\%$ per year). If the patient were to undergo coronary artery bypass surgery, their estimated chance of perioperative death ranged from 1 to 30% (mean $5.9 \pm 5.9\%$), and their estimated chance of major disabling stroke consequent to bypass surgery ranged from 0.1 to 20% (mean $4.1 \pm 4.2\%$). Life expectancy with medical treatment was estimated to range from 0 to 10 years (mean 4.8 ± 2.1 years); after bypass surgery life expectancy estimates ranged from 1 to 10 years (mean 5.9 ± 2.3 years). The number of years of life estimated to be gained from bypass ranged from -5 to 8 years (mean 1.1 ± 2.4 years). The old adage that doctors differ is true indeed!

Increasingly physicians are under pressure to consider myocardial revascularization without any explicit means of estimating the risks and likely benefits for the individual patient. It is my belief that this problem can be addressed by the use of 'decision analysis'. Many physicians may find this mathematical method of decision support, and especially the use of computers, a distasteful intrusion into their medical practice. However, decision analysis is NOT the same as an expert system using diagnostic or therapeutic algorithms. It can be applied to any problem that can be expressed as a choice between two or more strategies, all outcomes of which can be foreseen, and when the probabilities and utilities of these outcomes can be determined or estimated. For example, consider the choice between two strategies (Figure 9.1). Once the decision to chose between either of these strategies is made, the

P.J. Walter (ed.), Coronary Bypass Surgery in the Elderly, pp. 91–100.
© *1995 Kluwer Academic Publishers, Dordrecht.*

EXPECTED VALUE STRATEGY 1: (0.4*100)+(0.6*0) = 40

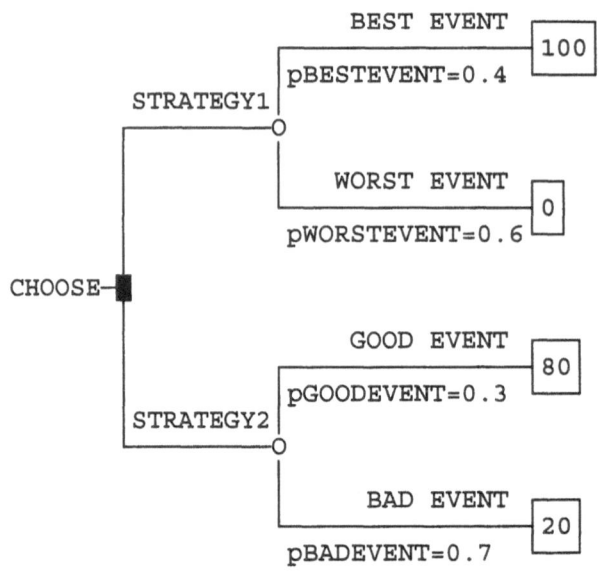

EXPECTED VALUE STRATEGY 2: (0.3*80)+(0.7*20) = 38

Figure 9.1. Example Decision tree that compares two different strategies: STRATEGY1 and STRATEGY2.

outcome is then beyond the control of the decision-maker and *entirely due to chance*. In the case of the first strategy (Strategy 1) there is a 0.4 chance of the best possible (BESTEVENT) outcome occurring. This outcome has arbitrarily been given a value (or utility) of 100. Unfortunately there remains a 0.6 chance of the worst possible outcome (WORSTEVENT) with a utility of 0. If Strategy 2 is chosen, there is a 0.3 chance of a good outcome (GOODEVENT) with a utility of 80, and a 0.7 chance of a bad outcome (BADEVENT) with a utility of 20. Which strategy should be chosen? The expected value of each strategy can be calculated by multiplying the probability of each outcome occurring by its utility. The sum of these products equals the expected value of each strategy. Strategy 1 therefore, has an expected value of $(0.4 \times 100) + (0.6 \times 0) = 40$. Strategy 2, on the other hand, has a lower expected value of $(0.3 \times 80) + (0.7 \times 20) = 38$. Strategy 1, therefore, is the *preferred* strategy.

Applying decision analysis to an individual patient

As decision analysis is a time-consuming process, it has usually only been used to draw up guidelines and/or strategies for the investigation and/or management of a patient population in general, providing only 'mean' expected outcomes for an overall patient population. In an attempt to apply decision analysis to the management of individual patients with coronary artery disease I have written a decision analysis of coronary artery disease management in a simple program called CABGTREE [2].

A simple decision tree maps out the outcomes of both medical and surgical treatment of coronary artery disease (Figure 9.2). The LONGTERM outcome of a medically treated patient depends on his (or her) age and the severity of coronary artery disease present. Although bypass surgery will benefit this outcome by decreasing coronary artery disease severity, it carries the risks of perioperative death (pDICABG) and major stroke (pCVA), especially in the elderly and/or those with extensive vascular disease. Life expectancy is calculated by a *Markov* simulation. In this process the probability of moving from the ALIVE to the DEAD state (pDIELONG) during a cycle of one year is estimated by adding the age-specific mortality rate and the disease-specific excess mortality rates relevant to the severity of coronary disease, either medically or surgically treated, plus the presence or absence of a major stroke. Life expectancy is the number of Markov cycles required for half a patient cohort to enter the DEAD state. The probability of death (pdiCABG) and major stroke (pCVA) associated with bypass surgery, and the excess mortality rates after surgery were obtained from a search of the MEDLINE literature. Since it has been shown to give an excellent estimate of survival [3], the standard treadmill exercise test was used to estimate the annual excess probability of death of a medically treated patient with coronary artery disease.

Life expectancy alone cannot fully express the 'utility' of a treatment option. For example, a year of life with severe angina or stroke will not be valued the same as a year of life without angina or stroke. Life expectancies, therefore, are modified to account for these 'quality adjustments'. The quality of life adjustments used assigned a value of zero to death, 0.5 to a year of life with a major stroke, and 1.0 to a year of life with either surgical or medical treatment. The utility of each outcome state, therefore, is its *Quality Adjusted Life Expectancy* (QALE) (i.e. the product of its quality of life adjustment and life expectancy), expressed in *quality adjusted life years* (QALYS).

Bypass surgery patients have a predictable return of angina, substantial late vein graft occlusion, and possibly increased progression of native coronary artery disease in grafted vessels [4]. Recent follow-up reports have shown a tendency for the mortality rates of bypass patients to approach that of comparable medically treated patients over time. This phenomenon may be less likely to occur in patients with internal mammary artery grafts. CABGTREE, therefore, assumed that there was progression back to pre-operative coronary artery disease severity and/or graft occlusion 10 years after bypass surgery. This

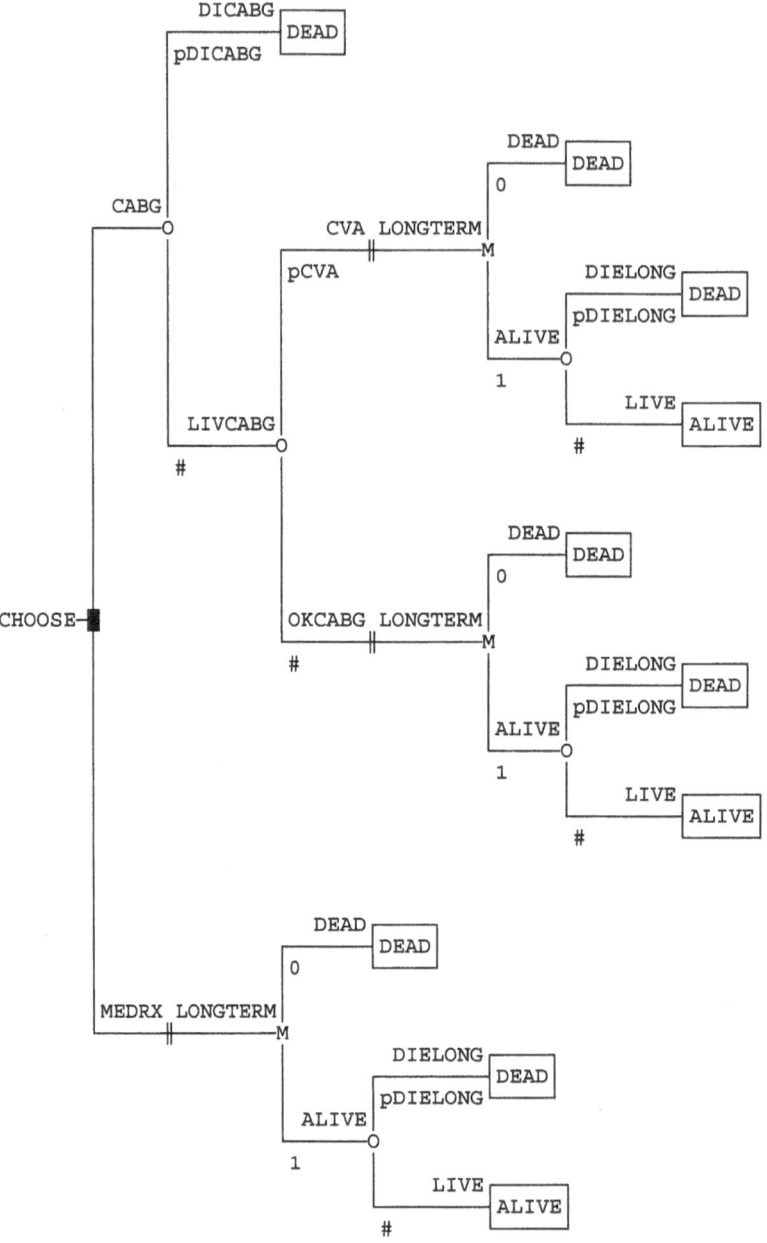

Figure 9.2. Decision tree for the treatment of coronary artery disease. CABG: coronary artery bypass graft, MEDRX: medical management, ■ : decision node, O: chance node, M: Markov node, DEAD and ALIVE represent terminal nodes, DICABG: perioperative death, LIVCABG: survival of surgery, CVA: perioperative major stroke, OKCABG: survival of surgery without major stroke, LONGTERM: life expectancy after surgical or medical treatment, DIELONG: death subsequent to treatment, pDICABG: probability of perioperative death, pCVA: probability of perioperative major stroke, pDIELONG: transitional probability (i.e. excess disease specific mortality rate plus age specific mortality rate) of each cycle of Markov process (probability of DEAD = 0 and ALIVE = 1 for initial cycle), # : residual probabilities.

scenario models the most probable natural history of saphenous vein graft [4] and fits in well with the most recent 10 to 20 year follow-up studies [5].

An example of CABGTREE use

A 74 year old man, with no significant past illnesses, presents with shoulder pain aggravated by exercise and relieved by rest. He develops 3.0 mm ST depression and disabling shoulder pain and chest tightness within four minutes on a Bruce protocol exercise test. CABGTREE shows that bypass surgery will, on the balance of probabilities, provide a benefit of 2.5 QALYS. The patient, however, is disturbed to find that, on average, he has a 6.1% risk of operative death and a 6.9% risk of perioperative major stroke. On reflection he considers these 'upfront' risks unacceptable, especially as he puts a low value on the possible 2.5 extra QALYS he might enjoy as an octogenarian. Moreover, the explicit demonstration of the risks and benefits of bypass surgery cause him to reconsider the severity of his symptoms, which he now realizes make very little impact on his quality of life. Medical treatment is therefore chosen, even though it is NOT mathematically 'preferred'.

What if CABGTREE'S structure or assumptions are incorrect?

'Sensitivity analyses' can be performed on a decision analysis model by varying one or more of the probabilities and/or utilities. If the recommended treatment changes as the probability of a chance event or utility of an outcome is varied, the decision is said to be sensitive to that parameter, and the recommended treatment changes at a certain 'threshold' probability or utility. If the preferred option, however, remains unchanged then that treatment strategy can be recommended with confidence. Sensitivity analyses allow the decision-maker to explore the interactions of various events by using the model to ask other questions: *what if* the patient were older? *what if* treatment were more effective? *what if* complications were more likely? etc. Any probability, utility or assumption in the model can be changed if the user wishes. Decision analysis forces doctors to appraise critically the information and beliefs upon which they base their decisions, and to recognize that they must often make decisions based on information which is deficient, defective and out-of-date. What alternative is there, however, to previously published reports, and/or documented clinical experience? Certainly an individual clinician's 'gut feeling' of what is likely to happen to his patients, would be an even more dubious basis for decision-making.

How does CABGTREE compare with a real doctor?

For many years I have worked as a summer locum internist at the Western Memorial Regional Hospital, Corner Brook, Newfoundland. Whilst there, I showed the CABGTREE program to Dr. Jamie Graham, the local consultant cardiologist. Referral for patients for coronary angiography from Corner Brook requires, in addition to the morbidity and risk associated with the procedure, a 700-km journey to the nearest tertiary care centre. Dr. Graham felt his referral decisions for angiography for possible bypass surgery were based on his clinical assessment of the likely risks and benefits after a standard exercise test. Happily, Dr. Graham's personal beliefs concerning the natural history of medically and surgically managed coronary artery disease were exactly captured and expressed by CABGTREE. I, therefore, decided to compare his decisions to refer patients for angiography with CABGTREE's recommendations.

Between March 1988 and July 1992 Dr. Graham performed 493 exercise tests. 190 patients were excluded because they had had prior angiography, suffered from bundle branch block, had associated valvular or congenital disease, cardiomyopathy or a previous angioplasty or bypass. The final study population was 303 patients, all of whom had a Bruce protocol exercise test performed.

Of the 303 patients studied, the 97 referred for angiography had more ST deviation during exercise, more angina, exercised for a shorter period of time, and were more likely to have had a prior myocardial infarction than the 206 patients not referred (Table 9.1). If medically managed, CABGTREE predicted the mean life expectancy of patients referred for angiography (13.6 ± 7.7 QALYs) to be significantly shorter ($p < 0.05$) than for those not referred (15.7 ± 8.0 QALYs). The mean life expectancy gain from bypass surgery was also predicted to be significantly greater ($p < 0.001$) in those referred (2.7 ± 1.9 QALYs) than in those not referred for angiography (1.0 ± 1.7 QALYs). *Despite these differences those referred for angiography may NOT come from a different population from those not referred.* One hundred and thirty seven of the patients

Table 9.1. Characteristics of patients referred and not referred for angiography

	Management strategy actually chosen		
	Not sent for angiography	Sent for angiography	p
Number	206	97	
Mean age	58.7 ± 10.4	56.4 ± 9.6	N.S.
Male	146 (70.9%)	72 (74.2%)	N.S.
ST deviation	1.7 ± 1.0	2.7 ± 1.4	< 0.001
Duration	6.9 ± 3.2	5.6 ± 3.1	< 0.001
Limiting angina	76 (36.9%)	52 (53.6%)	< 0.02
Prior MI	69 (33.5%)	58 (59.8%)	< 0.001
More than one exercise test	10 (4.8%)	8 (8.2%)	N.S.

Table 9.2. ST deviation during exercise testing by Quality adjusted life years (QALYs) predicted to be gained by patients referred and not referred for angiography – QALYs predicted to be gained from coronary artery bypass grafting (CABG) should angiography (angio) confirm patient suitable for bypass surgery

| QALYs predicted gained by CABG | Management strategy actually chosen | | | | |
| | Not sent for angiography | | Sent for angiography | | |
	n	ST deviation ± S.D. (mm)	n	ST deviation ± S.D.(mm)	p
≤ 4 to −5	1	1.0	–	–	
≤ 3 to −4	1	0.5	–	–	
≤ 2 to −3	1	2.0	–	–	
≤1 to −2	9	0.6 ± 0.2	1	0.5	
0 to −1	57	1.3 ± 0.5	8	1.6 ± 1.1	N.S.
> 0 to 1	46	1.6 ± 0.8	10	2.6 ± 1.8	N.S.
> 1 to 2	42	2.1 ± 1.1	23	2.8 ± 1.5	N.S.
> 2 to 3	18	1.9 ± 0.7	12	2.5 ± 1.2	N.S.
> 3 to 4	19	2.5 ± 1.4	15	2.5 ± 0.8	N.S.
> 4 to 5	8	2.6 ± 0.7	14	2.8 ± 1.0	N.S.
> 5 to 6	4	2.2 ± 0.6	12	3.6 ± 1.0	$p < 0.01$
> 6 to 7	–	–	2	3.7 ± 0.2	
Total	206	1.7 ± 1.0	92	2.7 ± 1.4	$p < 0.001$

not referred for angiography were predicted to benefit from bypass surgery, 93 gaining between 1.0 and 5.7 QALYs (Table 9.2).

There may be numerous factors that influence the decision to refer a patient for coronary angiography, such as patient life style, type of work, ability to articulate symptoms, addiction to tobacco, alcohol etc. Concomitant illness or other physical disabilities may make patients unsuitable for invasive investigations. Moreover, a patient's or a relative's body language may imply a desire for further investigation. Nevertheless, when deciding intuitively on referral for angiography for possible bypass surgery, a clinician must have some opinion as to the likely risks, benefits and costs. These opinions may be inconsistently applied by traditional, informal decision-making, with the result that some of the benefit that would result if the opinions were true, may be lost. The overall predicted life expectancy gain from Dr. Graham's intuitive decisions (i.e. by all patients combined, both referred and not referred for angiography) was 0.1 ± 2.5 QALYs per patient (Table 9.3). It would appear that the predicted life expectancy benefits from his appropriate referral decisions were very nearly cancelled out by his inappropriate ones. Had Dr. Graham's referral decision been solely directed by CABGTREE the overall gain per patient would have been 1.9 ±1.3 QALYs, and 128 extra patients (225 in total) would have been referred for angiography.

Table 9.3. Quality adjusted life years (QALYs) gained per patient by management intuitively chosen, and QALYs that would have been gained had the "preferred" management determined by decision analysis been chosen

Management strategy chosen	Management preferred by decision analysis		
	Bypass surgery predicted QALY gain	Medical management predicted QALY gain	Total QALYs gained per patient
QALYs gained per patient by management actually chosen			
Sent for angiography	3.0 ± 1.7 (n = 88)	−0.4 ± 0.5 (n = 9)	2.7 ± 1.9 (n = 97)
Not sent for angiography	−1.9 ± 1.4 (n = 137)	0.6 ± 0.7 (n = 69)	−1.0 ± 1.7 (n = 206)
Predicted life expectancy gained per patient by management chosen			0.1 ± 2.5 (n = 303)
QALYs gained had the preferred management been chosen			
Sent for angiography	3.0 ± 1.7 (n = 88)	0.4 ± 0.5 (n = 9)	
Not sent for angiography	1.9 ± 1.4 (n = 137)	0.6 ± 0.7 (n = 69)	
Predicted life expectancy gain per patient had the preferred management been chosen	2.3 ± 1.5 (n = 225)	0.6 ± 0.7 (n = 78)	1.9 ± 1.3 (n = 303)

'Quality of life' issues?

Assigning utilities to outcomes in any decision analysis is difficult, and patient preferences may differ markedly from those of their physicians. Several of Dr. Graham's patients did NOT accept his advice: 16 of the 97 patients he referred for angiography refused the procedure, despite having a predicted life expectancy gain from bypass surgery of 3.0 ± 1.7 QALYs (range 0.4 to 5.9). These patients might have changed their minds had they known their decision analysis results. Patients, however, may have quite perverse reasons for refusing angiography. One of Dr. Graham's patients with disabling angina, for example, turned down further investigation because he had excellent disability insurance. The prospect of bypass surgery possibly curing his angina and returning him to work, with a consequent loss of a monthly disability benefit did not appeal to him, nor did any anticipated gain in 'quality adjusted' life expectancy. Seemingly, a short life of idleness was preferable to a long life of honest toil! Restoration of a symptom-free state, therefore, has a surprisingly large variation in subjective value from patient to patient, and an inconsistent relationship to functional status. Surgical treatment for coronary artery disease may be associated with less angina, less limitation of activity, less need for drugs and increased survival compared with medical treatment. However, there is little evidence of a difference between medical and surgical therapy in other quality of life considerations such as return to work, and in the need for subsequent hospitalization. As many as one fifth of patients have stated that their global quality of life was no better or worse after surgery [6]. In actual practice, utilities have to be varied through a surprisingly large range before they alter the preferred decisions of CABGTREE. For example, the expected gain from bypass surgery for the average patient referred by Dr. Graham for angiography (56.4 years old with 2.7 mm ST deviation, no limiting angina and an exercise duration of 5.6 minutes) is increased from 1.99 QALYs to 2.04 QALYs when the quality adjustment of a major stroke is increased from 0.5 to 1.0, and decreased to 1.94 QALYs when stroke has a quality adjustment of zero (i.e. the same as death).

Future uses – audit and medico-legal issues

Provided it is based on the best information available at the time, and faithfully models the beliefs of the referring clinician, a decision analysis will always maximize the efficiency, and consistency of decision-making. The technique may, therefore, help audit management decisions more efficiently than more traditional methods and, in the event of limited resources, guide rationing. For example, if angiography had been 'rationed' by Dr. Graham to the 97 patients predicted by CABGTREE to gain the most from bypass surgery, then 3.9 ± 1.0 QALYs would have been gained per patient referred and 0.5 ± 1.1 QALYs would have been lost per patient not referred. The overall gain per patient (both referred and not referred combined) would have been 0.9 ± 2.3 QALYs, and the 'cut-off' predicted life expectancy gain required to justify referral for angiography would have been 2.3 QALYs.

Any doctor of a post-operative patient on a ventilator with a stroke would like to feel sure that, had the operation gone as planned, the patient would have been done a lot of good! Only by decision analysis can the original decision to operate be explicitly defended, even in the light of such a disastrous outcome. Decision analysis makes the best possible decision (in the light of the data currently available) time after time, with its risks and benefits clearly defined. Nevertheless, although decision analysis recommendations complement sound clinical judgement, they must never be a substitute for it.

Acknowledgements

I am especially grateful to Dr. Jamie Graham, Corner Brook, Newfoundland, Canada, for his honesty and bravery in allowing me to review his clinical decisions.

References

1. Kellett J. The management of coronary artery disease – a comparison of expert opinion and a decision analysis computer program. Irish J Med Sci 1993; 162(suppl 11): 3.
2. Kellett J. Bypass surgery or medical treatment for coronary artery disease – should decision analysis be used? Theor Surg 1992; 7: 223–5.
3. Mark DB, Shaw L, Harrell FE, et al. Prognostic value of a treadmill exercise score in outpatients with suspected coronary artery disease. N Engl J Med 1991; 325: 849–53.
4. Grondin CM, Campeau L, Thornton JC, Engle JC, Cross FS, Schreiber H. Coronary artery bypass grafting with saphenous vein. Circulation 1989; 79(6):124–9.
5. Muhlbaier LH, Pryor DB, Rankin JS, et al. Observational comparison of event-free survival with medical and surgical therapy in patients with coronary artery disease: 20 years of follow-up. Circulation 1992; 86(suppl II): 198–204.
6. Mayou R, Bryant B. Quality of life after coronary artery surgery. Q J Med 1987; 62: 239–48.

10. The economics of treatment choice
Making choices in coronary bypass surgery in the elderly

ALAN MAYNARD

Introduction

Resources always and everywhere are scarce and difficult choices about patient care are made each and every day in all health care systems. The policy issue is not whether resources are to be rationed but how, i.e. what criteria should be used to determine who will get treatment, who will be left in pain and discomfort, and who will be left to die humanely and with care from their nearest and dearest carers.

These life and death decisions are made every day in all health care systems where choice is made by clinicians often on the basis of poor scientific knowledge. The absence of a knowledge base to inform choices, and the variations in medical practice that result from uncertainty about the appropriateness of clinical practice are discussed in the first section.

Two alternative approaches to rationing health carer are explored in the second section: rationing by age and rationing in relation to the cost-QALY (quality-adjusted life year) characteristics of competing patient groups. Both these methods are criticised from methodological and empirical perspectives.

Finally it is argued that even if these methods were more robust and clinical and economic evaluation was not as deeply flawed as it is, the results of such work can only inform patient choices: final resource allocation or rationing choices will reflect not only the best scientific knowledge but also social values.

Inadequacies in the knowledge base

Ideally choices about treatment would be informed by knowledge about the value of what is given up by society in funding a procedure (i.e. its opportunity cost) and by knowledge about the value of what is gained from it (i.e. the value of enhancements in the length and quality of life), when the volume of activity is increased or decreased by a small amount (i.e. marginal cost and marginal value). In reality there are few cost data: most clinicians and managers do not know the value of the resources used to treat an elderly patient with angina.

101

P.J. Walter (ed.), Coronary Bypass Surgery in the Elderly, pp. 101–109.
© 1995 *Kluwer Academic Publishers, Dordrecht.*

Some health care systems are developing pricing systems but prices usually bear little relation to costs: prices either reflect 'what the market will bear' or are the product of regulated pricing systems (e.g. diagnostic related groups or DRGs) which do not reflect the value of social opportunity costs.

Whilst the existing compartmentalised financial systems are inadequate as a source of data about the opportunity cost of medical interventions to society, they tend to produce more information than is available about outcomes. For centuries there has been advocacy of outcome measurement but little action. For instance, the physician of the English King George II argued in 1732:

> In order, therefore to procure this valuable collection, I humbly propose, first of all, that three or four persons should be employed in the hospitals (and that without any ways interfering with the gentlemen now concerned), to set down the cases of the patients there from day to day, candidly and judiciously, without any regard to private opinions or public systems, and at the year's end publish these facts just as they are, leaving every one to make the best use he can for himself.
>
> Francis Clifton [1]

and an American physician, Codman [2] was equally clear about the need to measure performance in 1913:

> We must formulate some method of hospital reporting showing as nearly as possible what are the results of the treatment obtained at different institutions. This report must be made out and published by each hospital in a uniform manner, so that comparison will be possible. With such a report as a starting point, those interested can begin to ask questions as to management and efficiency.
>
> E.A. Codman [2]

Despite this powerful rhetoric over the centuries it is only now that outcome measurement is becoming a serious endeavour for most trialists. Many of the clinical trials in recent decades measured limited endpoints and only now is it generally accepted that these must be supplemented with data about survival duration and quality of life improvements.

However, with and without such data, many clinical trials are inadequately designed, poorly reported and refereed imperfectly. Altman [3] has argued that the motive for most clinical trials is not the development of knowledge but the enhancement of curriculum vitae and job advancement. Bailer [4] argued that there are more quacks (charlatans) in statistics than there are in medicine! This is a bold and disturbing assertion which when considered in the light of evidence about 'data torture' in some areas of medicine (e.g. Gotzsche [5] and Rochan *et al.* [6]) must make everyone cautious about the results of trials and anxious to evaluate evaluations carefully [7].

The ignorance about costs and effectiveness that permeates all areas of medicine produces uncertainty about the appropriateness of practices and much

Table 10.1. Magnitude of systematic variation (in ascending order) for selected causes of admission among 30 hospital market areas in Maine: 1980–82

Variation	Medical	Surgical
Low: 1.5-fold range		Inguinal hernia repair Hip repair
Moderate: 2.5-fold range	Acute myocardial infarction Gastrointestinal haemorrhage Cerebrovascular accident	Appendectomy Major bowel surgery Cholecystectomy
High: 3.5-fold range	Respiratory neoplasms Cardiac arrhythmias Angina pectoris Psychosis Depressive neurosis Medical back problems Digestive malignancy Adult diabetes	Hysterectomy Major cardiovascular operations Lens operations Major joint operations Anal operations Back and neck operations
Very high: 8.5+-fold range	Adult bronchioloitis Chest pain Transient ischemic attacks Minor skin disorders Chronic obstructive lung disease Hypertension Atherosclerosis Chemotherapy	Knee operations Transuretheral operations Extraocular operations Breast biopsy Dilation and curettage Tonsillectomy Tubal interruption

Source: Wennberg, McPherson and Caper [10].

variation in clinical behaviour. This has been well documented by Wennberg in the United States (e.g., Wennberg [8] and McPherson in the United Kingdom [9]). An example of these variations is shown in Table 10.1.

Whilst clinical and economic evaluation is poor and the knowledge base deeply flawed, some have argued that practice standards can be derived which can be used to make meaningful comments about the appropriateness of practice. For instance, an American study of the appropriateness of CABG procedures in 3 randomly chosen hospitals in the west of the United States in 1979–82 concluded that 56% of them were performed for appropriate reasons, 30% for equivocal reasons and 14% for inappropriate reasons. The percentage judged appropriate varied from 38–78% across the 3 hospitals [11].

The use of a 'conservative' U.K. panel and a more 'liberal' U.S. panel of experts concluded that the use of angiography and coronary artery by-pass procedures were not always appropriate in the Trent region of the U.K.-N.H.S.:

> Our study shows that inappropriate care, even in the face of waiting lists, is a significant problem in Trent. In particular, by the standards of the U.K. panel, one half of coronary angiographs were performed for equivocal or

inappropriate reasons, and two fifths of CABGs were performed for similar reasons. Even by the more liberal U.S. criteria, the ratings were 29% equivocal or inappropriate for coronary angiography and 33% equivocal or inappropriate for CABG.

Bernstein, Kosecoff, Gray, Hampton and Brook Study [12]

However, as the American physician Feinstein [13] has remarked: 'The agreement of experts has been the traditional source of all the errors through medical history', and the use of such approaches must remain contentious. The majority of health care interventions remain unevaluated from a cost-effectiveness perspective and medical practice is generally not knowledge-based but opinion-based.

Rationing health care

Introduction. Access to health care can be determined (or rationed) by the patient's willingness and ability to pay or by the patient's capacity to benefit per unit of expenditure. In principle it is the latter criterion (ability to benefit) which determines treatment availability in most Western health care systems. However, the operationalisation of this rule is difficult because of the poor knowledge base in medicine.

There is a widespread and continuing debate about the rationing of health care. The State Legislature in Oregon has a prioritised list of 745 treatment condition pairs which it proposed to use to define a basic package of health care for all low income groups (for a discussion see Strosberg [14]). The Dutch Government established a committee to define a basic package of health care benefits which was strong on logic but offered no prioritised listing of competing therapies [15].

Rationing by age. The American ethicist Daniel Calahan [16, 17] has argued that the fairest way to ration health care in the face of continually escalating demand was to adopt a flat age limit in the late 70s or early 80s and beyond which no high technology care would be available.

It was remarkable how little controversy Calahan's proposal provoked. As Levinsky [18] noted, if Calahan had proposed rationing on the basis of race or income, there would have been outrage. The absence of great rancour about rationing by age is indicative perhaps of a social recognition that age may be a relevant element in any rationing decision.

However, this approach is fraught with difficulty. Would the same cut off be used for women (who live longer) and men? Would the 'cut off' be defined for some technologies or all technologies? Would account be taken (how?) of the differences in the skills in surgeons and anaesthetists? Poor outcomes may be the product of poor health care rather than an absence in the elderly of ability to benefit (see e.g. Davenport [19]). The definition of the age cut off would be difficult in practice due to differential levels of capacity to benefit across age groups of particular ages.

Thus blind use of age as a rationing criterion could lead to the elderly being deprived of care, the provision of which is cost effective. Dudley and Burns [20] surveyed age-related treatment policies for the use of thrombolytic therapy and coronary care units (CCUs). They found that 20% of CCUs and 40% of consultants administering thrombolytic therapy had age-related treatment policies, despite some evidence that such interventions may be cost effective in elderly groups.

Rationing by ability to benefit. If resources are to be rationed by ability to benefit, it is necessary to measure benefit (health gains) and cost their incremental production. Researchers in the United States (e.g. Kaplan [21]), Canada (e.g. Goel and Detsky [22]) and the United Kingdom have used techniques centred on estimation of quality-adjusted life years (QALYs)*. Williams [23] used the Rosser-Kind Matrix and asked clinicians to plot patient progress through this matrix (before and after treatment). The duration of survival/quality of survival of each patient group could then be plotted (as in Figure 10.1).

This approach can be used to produce 'league tables' (e.g. Table 10.2), which rank procedures by the cost of producing one year of life of good quality (QALY). The implication of this ranking is that investment should be targeted

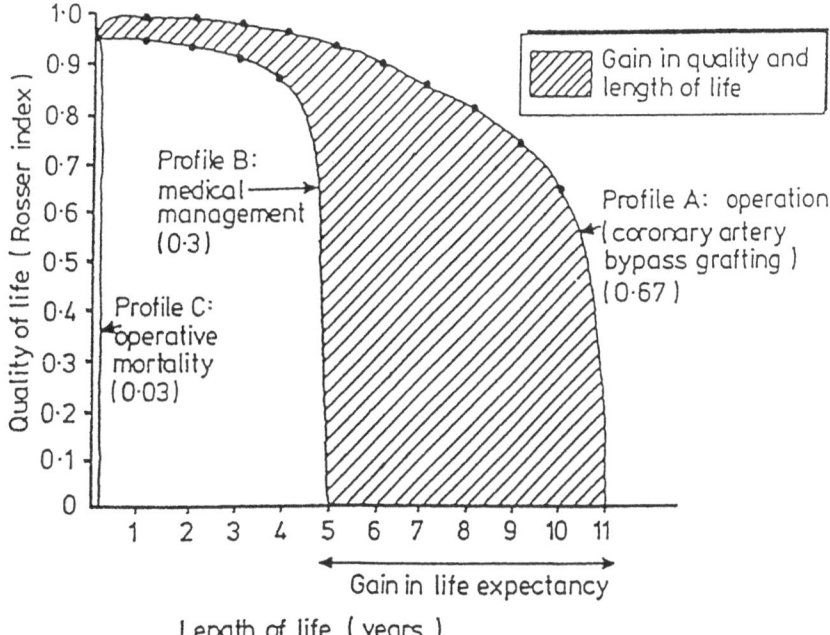

Figure 10.1. Expected value of quality and length of life gained for patients with severe angina.

* A QALY is one year of life of perfect quality.

Table 10.2. Quality-adjusted life year (QALY) of competing therapies: some tentative estimates

	Cost/QALY (£ August 1990)
Cholesterol testing and diet therapy only (all adults, aged 40–69)	220
Neurosurgical intervention for head injury	240
GP advice to stop smoking	270
Neurosurgical intervention for subarachnoid haemorrhage	490
Anti-hypertensive therapy to prevent stroke (ages 45–64)	940
Pacemaker implantation	1,100
Hip replacement	1,180
Valve replacement for aortic stenosis	1,140
Cholesterol testing and treatment	1,480
CABG[a] (left main vessel disease, severe angina)	2,090
Kidney transplant	4,710
Breast cancer screening	5,780
Heart transplantation	7,840
Cholesterol testing and treatment (incrementally) of all adults aged 25–39 years	14,150
Home haemodialysis	17,260
CABG[a] (1-vessel disease, moderate angina)	18,830
CAPD[b]	19,870
Hospital haemodialysis	21,970
Erythropoietin treatment for anaemia in dialysis patients (assuming a 10% reduction in mortality)	54,380
Neurosurgical intervention for malignant intracranial tumours	107,780
Erythropoietin treatment for anaemia in dialysis patients (assuming no increase in survival)	126,290

[a] CABG = coronary artery bypass graft.
[b] CAPD = continuous ambulatory peritoneal dialysis.
Source: Maynard [32].

on those procedures which produce QALYs at a low cost. CABG interventions (e.g. with LMV disease, severe angina) are seemingly quite cost effective (e.g. £2090 per year of good quality of life (or QALY)). CABG interventions for the elderly appear to have higher initial mortality rates (due to complicating factors such as hypertension, diabetes and renal failure) and then survival characteristics similar to young groups. The effective life of CABGs for these younger groups may often be only 10 years and thus the survival pay back period may not be greatly different from that of the elderly. Over time CABG surgery has become quicker e.g., in the first 12 years of some U.S. experience, times for the procedure fell by over 36%. These changes, because they reduce operative complications, may partly explain better outcomes in high volume institutions [24]. American data indicate that CABG costs across the age groups vary little (e.g. see Evans in this volume) and, thus, whilst better measurement of post-CABG quality of life (using, for instance the Short Form 36 (e.g. Brazier et al. [25]) and/or the Euroqol [26]) would be useful, a tentative conclusion may be that the cost-QALY characteristics of CABGs for appropriately selected elderly might not be significantly different from those of younger age groups. Outcomes for all groups may be improved by psychiatric screening and treatment as a routine part of the treatment package and such interventions may, due to reduced hospitalisation, be cost effective [27].

There are many technical problems with this approach. Are the reported QALY estimates marginal or average values? What are the confidence intervals for these point estimates? How robust is the Rosser-Kind index [28]? (Its values were based on only 70 non-randomly selected respondents and it appears to be difficult to replicate, i.e. how robust, valid and replicable is the Q in the QALY [29]? How robust are the clinical studies on which the LY in the QALY are based? These and other 'quality control' issues in the use of QALY estimates are often dealt with imperfectly [30].

Overview. Thus, because of the inadequacies in methods to measure cost, quality of life and survival duration, cost-QALY estimates are flawed and guestimates. The English Department of Health now has a list of nearly 500 cost-QALY estimates which it may publish to inform health care choices by purchasers. As better data appear for CABG procedures for the elderly, the tentative conclusion that they are relatively cost effective for appropriately selected patients will be confirmed or refuted. With the majority of CABGs being provided for the elderly and with treatment activity grouping most rapidly in this group, the monitoring of the cost effectiveness of these interventions is a priority [31].

Making choices

The method of clinical and economic evaluation are quite well defined (e.g. Sackett *et al.* [7] and Drummond *et al.* [33]). The practice of clinical evaluation is often poor (e.g. Bailar [4] and Altman [3]) and the practice of economic evaluation, which builds on this clinical deficits, can also be deficient (e.g. Freemantle and Maynard [34]). With clinical practice improving and technology developing, the cost effectiveness of therapies such as coronary bypass surgery for the elderly is constantly changing. The combined effects of poor evaluation and changing techniques means that decisions are often informed (or distorted) by biased results from past technologies.

If evaluative practices could be improved by creating greater openness and accountability which made practitioners more careful, more data would be made available to produce knowledge-based clinical practice and the degree of waste in health care practice could be reduced. However, progress in that direction will be achieved with difficulty and at great cost because existing institutions support behaviours which, if changed, would alter the distribution of job and incomes in ways which would engender great opposition to change.

As the evaluative sciences produce more information and practice becomes more knowledge-based, it will be important to recognise once again that decisions about who will live and who will die will be influenced by these results but not necessarily determined by them. Choices about the allocation of resources will be determined both by knowledge of which therapies are cost effective and by society's values. As Fuchs [35] argued:

> At the root of most of our major health problems are *value choices*. What kind of people are we? What kind of life do we want to lead? What kind of society do we want to build for our children and grandchildren? How much weight do we want to put on individual freedom? How much to equality? How much to material progress? How much to the realm of the spirit? How important is our own health to us? How important is our neighbour's health to us? The answers we give to these questions, as well as the guidance we get from economics, will and should shape health care policy.
>
> Fuchs [35]

References

1. Clifton, F. State of physick, ancient and modern briefly considered with a plan for the improvement of it. London: Bowyer, 1732.
2. Codman, E.A. The product of a hospital. Surgery, Gynaecology and Obstetrics, 1914. 18: 491–6.
3. Altman DG. The scandal for poor medical research. Brit Med J 1994; 308: 283–4.
4. Bailar JC. Bailar's laws of data analysis. Clin Pharmacol Ther 1976; 20:1: 113–9.
5. Gotzsche PC. Methodology and overt and hidden bias in reports of 196 double-blind trials of nonsteroidal anti-inflammatory drugs in rheumatoid arthritis. Controlled Clin Trials 1989; 10: 31–56.
6. Rochan PA, Gurwitz JH, Simms RW, et al. A study of manufacturer-supported trials of nonsteriodal anti-inflammatory drugs in the treatment of arthritis. Arch Intern Med 1994; 154: 157–63.
7. Sackett DL, Haynes BR, Guyatt GH, Tugwell P. Clinical epidemiology: as basic science for clinical medicine. Boston, Massachusetts: Little, Brown and Company, 1991.
8. Wennberg JE. Future directions for small area variations. Med Care 1993; 31(supp 5): 75–80.
9. McPherson K. Why do variations occur? In: Anderson TF and Mooney G, editors. The challenge of medical practice variations. London: Macmillan, 1989.
10. Wennberg JE, McPherson K, Caper P. Will payment based on diagnosis-related groups control hospital costs? N Engl J Med 1984; 311(5): 295–300.
11. Winslow CM, Kosecoff JB, Chassin M, Kanouse DE, Brook RE. The appropriateness of performing coronary artery by-pass surgery. JAMA 1988; 260:4: 505–9.
12. Bernstein SJ, Kosecoff J, Gray D, Hampton JR, Brook RH. The appropriateness of the use of cardiovascular procedures: British versus US perspectives. Intl J Tech Assess Health Care 1993; 9(1):3–10.
13. Feinstein A. Fraud, distortion, delusion and consensus: the problems of human and natural deception in epidemiology studies. Am J Med 1988; 84: 475–8.
14. Strosberg MA, Wiener JM, Baker R, Fein IA (editors). Rationing America's health care: the Oregon plan and beyond, Washington, DC: Brookings Institute, 1992.
15. Government Committee on Choice in Health Care. Choices in health care. Dunning Report. Rijswijk, The Netherlands: Ministry of Welfare, Health and Cultural Affairs, 1992.
16. Callahan D. Setting limits: medical goals in an aging society. New York: Simon Schuster, 1987.
17. Callahan D. What kind of life: the limits of medical progress. New York: Simon Schuster, 1990.

18. Levinsky MG. Age as a criterion of rationing care. N Engl and J Med 1990; 322(25): 1813–5.
19. Davenport HT. Anaesthetics and elderly patients. Brit Med J 1991; 303: 890–1.
20. Dudley NJ, Burns E. The influence of age on policies for admission and thrombolysis in coronary care units in the United Kingdom. Age Ageing 1992; 21: 95–8.
21. Kaplan R. A quality of life approach to health resource allocation. In: Strosberg MA, Wiener JM, Baker R, Fein IA, editors. Rationing America's health care: the Oregon plan and beyond. Washington DC: Brookings Institute, 1992.
22. Goel V, Detsky AS. A cost utility analysis of preoperative total parenteral nutrition. Intl J Assess Health Care 1989; 5: 183–95.
23. Williams A. Economics of coronary artery bypass grafting. Brit Med J 1985; 249: 326–9.
24. Cromwell J, Mitchell JB, Stason WB. Learning by doing in CABG. Med Care 1990; 1: 6–18.
25. Brazier JE, Harper R, Jones NMB, et al. Validating the SF-36 health survey questionnaire: new outcome measure for primary care. Brit Med J 1992; 305(684)6: 160–4.
26. EuroQol Group. Euroqol – a new facility for the measurement of health-related quality of life. Health Policy 1990; 16: 199–208.
27. Schindler BA, Shook J, Schwartz GM. Beneficial effects of psychiatric intervention on recovery after coronary artery by-pass surgery. Gen Hosp Psych 1989; 11(5): 358–64.
28. Rosser R, Kind P, Williams A. Valuation of quality of life. In: Jones-Lee MW, editor. The value of life and safety. Amsterdam: North Holland, 1982.
29. Carr-Hill RA, Morris J. Current practice in obtaining the 'Q' in QALYs: a cautionary note. Brit Med J 1991; 303: 699–701.
30. Drummond MF, Torrance G, Mason J. Cost effectiveness league tables: more harm than good? Soc Sci Med 1993; 37(1): 33–40.
31. Anderson GH, Lomas J. Monitoring the diffusion of technology: coronary artery bypass surgery in Ontario. Am J Public Health 1988; 78(3): 237.
32. Maynard A. The design of future cost-benefit studies. Am Heart J 1990; 3(2): 761–5.
33. Drummond MF, Stoddard GL, Torrance GW. Methods for the economic evaluation of health care programmes. Oxford: Oxford University Press, 1987.
34. Freemantle N, Maynard A. Something rotten in the state of clinical and economic evaluations? [editorial] Health Econ 1994; 3(2). In press.
35. Fuchs V. Rationing health care. N Engl J Med 1984; 311(24): 1572–3.

11. The role of age and life expectancy in prioritising health care

JOHN HARRIS

Introduction

I want to try to do two things. The first is sketch, in the broadest and most general terms, the moral principles that I believe should govern the allocation of resources in health care. The second is to say why the notorious QALY goes no way to respecting these principles nor indeed much else that is valuable or ought to be valued.

The equality principle

I shall not try to defend the equality principle today. That is a task for a book-length study. However, I shall assume that everyone here accepts that no allocation of public resources should discriminate unfairly between rival claimants or groups of claimants. This happens when each person's claim to the equal concern, respect and protection of the community, of the society in which they live, is not respected. This is the principle of equality: *that each person is entitled to the same concern, respect and protection of society as is accorded to any other person in the community.*

Even the principle architect of QALYs in the United Kingdom regards this as an important virtue of QALYs. Alan Williams has emphasised that a great virtue of QALYs is that they are consistent with equality because the involve the idea that 'one year of healthy life is of equal value no matter who gets it' and that each person's valuations 'have equal weight'.

The principle of equality involves the idea that people's lives and fundamental interests are of equal importance and that they must in consequence be given equal weight and be equally protected. This principle has powerful intellectual appeal and intuitive force. It is often enough to discredit a proposal or a theory simply to show that it violates this principle. When measures are said to be discriminatory or unfair it is this principle which is in play.

Recent philosophers of widely differing orientations and beliefs have given this principle a central role in their theories. Ronald Dworkin, Robert Nozick

111

P.J. Walter (ed.), Coronary Bypass Surgery in the Elderly, pp. 111–119.
© 1995 *Kluwer Academic Publishers, Dordrecht.*

and Jonathan Glover, for example, have all given it a central place,[1] although it is fair to say that they would all disagree as to just how it is to be interpreted.

If people's lives and fundamental interests are of equal value then it is unjust to treat people differently in ways which effectively accord different values to their lives or fundamental interests. Deliberately to give one person a better chance of remaining healthy and of having as long a life as possible than another is to value their life and their fundamental interest in health more than the person not so benefitted. It is to discriminate in their favour. Where literally all cannot be benefitted, equality requires that the method of selecting who will benefit and who will not is fair. This is why scarce resources which bear upon the value of life or the fundamental interests of persons, must be allocated justly.

No dogs in mangers

One method of allocation of a scarce resource which apparently satisfies the requirements of justice is of course not to allocate that resource to anyone! All are then treated equally, in the sense that they are all left equally without benefit of the resource in question.

Another superficially distinct but in fact morally similar procedure might be to go on redistributing resources until a distrubution was achieved which satisfies the 'envy test'. That is one in which no one envies anyone else's life chances as provided by those resources.[2]

This is often thought to be a viable application of the requirements of justice and indeed to constitute a just allocation of resources. The fallacy of such a supposition is easily illustrated. The principle of justice, and indeed the principle of equality, are *moral* principles. That is, they are principles with some moral content, principles that are designed to be more than impartial, that are designed among other things to respect and to do justice to persons. In some sense this must involve some benevolent attitude to persons which is often abbreviated as 'respect for persons'. Such an attitude to others is as different as it's possible to be from simply showing *an equality of lack of respect* or *an equal indifference to the fate of others*.

The failure to allocate resources that would save lives or protect individuals could not then be part of a claim to satisfy the requirements of equality because this principle has at its heart the claim that people's lives and fundamental interests *are of value, that they matter*. Anyone who denied life saving resources, or resources which would protect life and other fundamental interests, is not valuing the lives of those to whom she denies these protections. Although she is treating them all equally in the sense of treating them all *the same*, she is not treating them *as equals*, as people who matter and hence matter equally.[3] The alternative dog-in-the-manger approach treats all people as *equally unimportant* and hence as equally without value.

A parable

Jonathan Glover quoted this parable which derives from R. and V. Routley. It is quoted by Glover to illustrate the equal claims of future generations but it has lessons for our present concerns as well. We are asked to consider a bus journey:

> The bus carries both passengers and freight on its long journey. It is always crowded but passengers keep getting on and off, and the drivers change so that quite different people are on board at different stages of the journey. Early in the journey, a container of highly toxic and explosive gas is put aboard, destined for somewhere near the end of the route. The container is very thin, and the consignor knows it is unlikely to survive the journey intact. If it breaks, some of the passengers will probably be killed. Sending the container of gas on the bus seems an appalling act. The consignor might make various excuses. It is not *certain* the gas will escape. If it does, perhaps the bus will have crashed and killed everyone first. . . . He further tries to justify his act by pleading economic necessity: his business will crash unless he sends the container on the bus.

The point of the parable is of course that we are no more justified in killing future people than present people. However, its force would be not much diminished if we were told that the passengers were all young children or for that matter hospital patients or elderly people.

Glover ends his use of this parable by noting that 'people's moral claims are not diminished by when they live any more than by where they live And that is the equality principle'. Had his interest not primarily been in claims between generations he might have added that people's moral claims are not diminished by who they are, or how old they are, or by how rich or poor, powerful or weak they are or by the quality of their lives. The equality principle covers young and old, healthy and sick, weak and strong, regardless of race, creed, colour and gender quality of life or life expectancy.

Equal protection

Of the three elements into which the equality principle must be analyzed, (concern, respect and protection) perhaps the most important in the context of resource allocation is that of equal protection.

All governments and would-be governments boast the strongest commitment to national defence. The question that is seldom asked is what is national defence for, what justifies its prominent place in national priorities? The simplistic answer is of course that without national defence there might be no nation and hence no national priorities. But pressed further it is reasonable to ask what values and interests national defence subserves?

Arguably protecting citizens against threats to their lives, liberties and fundamental interests is the first priority for any state. This is the classic

Hobbesian argument for the obligation to obey the Sovereign. In 1651 Thomas Hobbes wrote:

> The obligation of subjects to the sovereign, is understood to last as long, and no longer, than the power lasteth, by which he is able to protect them.

On this view, any citizen's obligation to the State and to obey its laws is conditional upon the State for its part protecting that citizen against threats to her life and liberty. It was perhaps this interpretation of the purpose and rationale of national defence that best explains what might be offered as a justification for the Falklands war. In the Falklands it was not national integrity that was at stake but the protection of the lives and liberties of citizens.

With the spread of glasnost and the collapse of the strongest and most clearly perceived of possible threats to national integrity, most western states have re-examined their defence requirements but not reassessed the nature of their national defence needs. By that I mean they have not thought afresh about what is involved in meeting their obligations to defend and protect their citizens in the world that is emerging. To be sure they have all taken an opportunity to trim defence budgets traditionally conceived. What they have not done is thought about what should constitute 'national defence' in the next millennium.

If we go back to Hobbes and reflect on what citizens want and need in the way of protection I believe we will find that in most contemporary societies the most significant threats to life and liberty come not from the threat of armed aggression from without, but from absence of health care and other social welfare measures within. For most citizens threats to their lives and curtailment of liberty looms not in the form of soldiers with snow on their boots but from illness and accident. This is why it is arguable that the obligation to provide health care, and in particular life-saving health care, takes precedence over the obligation to provide defence forces against external (and often mythical) enemies.

There is a very good principle which states that real and present dangers should be met before future and speculative ones. This is why we are often willing to spend limitless amounts on rescue and less on longer term measures which would protect comparable numbers of lives. If a building collapses we don't tell those buried beneath or their relatives that the budget for digging survivors out has been exhausted and further rescue work must wait until the next financial year.

Another feature of the nation state's obligation to defend its citizens, which is often overlooked, is its egalitarian nature. Just as each citizen owes his or her obligation to obey the law regardless of such features as race, religion, gender or age, so the state must discharge its obligation of protection with the same impartiality. This seems unproblematic until we recall that recent developments in the allocation of health care resources are moving increasingly in the direction of valuing the lives of different groups of citizens at less than par.

One such development is the emergence of the QALY or quality adjusted life year. The essence of a QALY is that it takes a year of healthy life expectancy to be worth 1, but regards a year of unhealthy life expectancy as worth less than 1, the value varying with the quality of life. The inventors of QALYs believe that a beneficial health care activity is one that generates a positive amount of QALYs, and that an efficient health care activity is one where the cost per QALY is as low as it can be. A high priority activity is one where the cost-per-QALY is low and a low priority activity is one where the cost-per-QALY is high.

This is a powerful claim. It purports to provide three things: a measure of the benefit of health care, a measure of efficiency in health care, and a way of prioritizing the allocation of health care resources. It is this latter use which constitutes a threat to the principle that the lives of all citizens should be regarded as of equal value. This is because any principle which accords value not to people but to units of life-time, (life-years quality adjusted), must inevitably tend to favour younger, healthier people and others who will gain more quality adjusted lifetime if they are treated or rescued.

Two examples will illustrate this. Imagine twin sisters, one is disabled from birth with a painful condition that is untreatable and leaves her chair-bound and with a shorter life expectancy than her twin. The other is perfectly healthy. By the time they reach their twenties the disabled sister has, through much effort and resolution, carved out for herself a life she finds worthwhile despite its restricted nature and the pain she experiences. Both are then involved in a motor accident and require the same expensive treatment which will restore each to the condition she was in before. If resources are scarce QALYs dictate that the healthy sister get priority and this may mean that she will be the only one of the two to be treated. Having been born fortunate, her fortune will be rewarded by the QALY principle. Her sister, having once been unfortunate will have further misfortune heaped upon her.

Suppose next that a complete but expensive cure is found for a disabling and often terminal genetic condition which affects a minority ethnic group and usually strikes from age fifty onwards. Because of the late onset and the expense it is not very QALY efficient to treat, compared with rival claimants to resources. QALYs dictate that this group be left untreated.

Finally of course, QALYs must inevitably give a low priority to the care of the elderly.

The answer that is always given to the sort of argument I have set out here is that resources are scarce and that rationing is inevitable. This is of course true but misleading. If national health is, as I have suggested, not only a form of national defence but a form which has first claim on the national defence budget, then although resources will continue to be limited they will not be so scarce as we have been encouraged to accept. We should also remember that there are headings of public expenditure that are not limited in this way. We have not so far ever said that the criminal justice budget is limited and that no more murderers will be arrested nor given a fair trial because of the expense involved.

I believe, and I believe it is part of the political theory on which our particular democracy is founded, that each citizen has an equal claim to the protection of the state and, thus, upon the health resources of her own society. That no individual or group or type of individual should be regarded as having a more valuable life or a greater claim to lifesaving resources than any other. A society that says that particular citizens, whether individually identifiable in advance or not, will not be so protected has effectively declared such individuals to be outlaws – outside the protection of the state – and has forfeited its claim to their allegiance.

Conclusion

I have suggested that any principle of allocation of public resources for health care must obey the equality principle and that this is accepted by QALY defenders as well as being a crucial part of our public morality. We have seen that the QALY cannot hope to live up to any conception of justice based on the equality principle. We must now examine some of the other problems with the QALY.

What are QALYs?

Just to remind you – from the horses mouth:

> The essence of a QALY is that it takes a year of healthy life expectancy to be worth 1, but regards a year of unhealthy life expectancy as worth less than 1. Its precise value is lower the worse the quality of life of the unhealthy person. . . . If being dead is worth zero it is in principle possible for a QALY to be negative i.e. for the quality of someone's life to be judged worse than being dead.
>
> The general idea is that a beneficial health care activity is one that generates a positive amount of QALYs, and that an efficient health care activity is one where the cost per QALY is as low as it can be. A high priority . . . activity is one where the cost-per-QALY is low and a low priority activity is one where the cost-per-QALY is high.[4]

This is a powerful claim. It purports, as we have seen, to provide three things:
1. A measure of the benefit of health care,
2. a measure of efficiency in health care, and
3. a way of prioritizing the allocation of health care resources.

There is a benign and a vicious use for QALYs;

> *Benign: a patient choosing between rival therapies.*
> *Vicious: a mandarin choosing between rival claimants for therapy.*

We should note for the record that QALYS do not value people but simply units of lifetime. QALYS are ageist, they are sexist, they must value inconsequential gains in lifetime. QALYS favour cheaply and easily treated conditions. QALYS pre-empt economies of scale. QALYS violate the nation state's obligation to provide equal protection for all citizens and, hence, create outlaws. QALYS encourage the false belief that resources are critically scarce.

We have already examined some of these claims. For the remainder, I have only time to address two more now, and what better problem to examine in this context than discrimination against the old? The second issue is that of the quality adjustment part of the QALY's claim. For a substantiation of the other claims that I have made against QALYs, I must (regretfully) refer you to what I have written elsewhere.[5]

The anti-ageist argument

The anti-ageist argument which many criticisms of QALYs presuppose can be (and has been) stated thus:

> All of us who wish to go on living have something that each of us values equally although for each it is different in character, for some a much richer prize than for others, and we none of us know its true extent. This thing is of course 'the rest of our lives'. So long as we do not know the date of our deaths then for each of us the 'rest of our lives' is of indefinite duration. Whether we are 17 or 70, in perfect health or suffering from a terminal disease we each have the rest of our lives to lead. So long as we each fervently wish to live out the rest of our lives, however long that turns out to be, then if we do not deserve to die, we each suffer the same injustice if our wishes are deliberately frustrated and we are cut off prematurely.[6]

It is this outlook that explains why murder is always wrong and wrong to the same degree. When you rob someone of life you take from them not only all they have but all they will ever have, it is a difference in degree so radical that it makes for a difference in the quality of the act. However, the wrongness consists in taking from them something that they want. That is why voluntary euthanasia is not wrong and murder is.

Those who believe in discriminating in favour of the young or against the old must believe that, insofar as murder is an injustice, it is less of an injustice to murder the old than the young and, since they also believe that life years are a commodity like any other (specifically like money and time off),[7] it is clear that in robbing people of life you take less from them the less life expectancy they have.

The problem with anti-ageism

The main problem with the idea that I have called anti-ageism is that it leaves no room for exceptions at the extremes. So long as very old people wish to go on living even for a short time they, on this argument, have as large a claim on public resources to help them do so as does any other claimant. So that where, in extreme cases, a ninety-nine year old is in competition with a thirty-one year old for the only available ITU bed a coin should be tossed to see who gets it.

It is only if you are prepared to embrace this conclusion that you are truly anti-ageist.

Fairness & quality of life

The same ideas which underpin discrimination in favour of the young on the grounds of fairness would also entail trying to equalise quality as well as quantity of life. The argument here would be that resources required for survival should be distributed not only so as to favour the young but also so as to favour those whose quality of life has been relatively poor.

> Two patients ... both about 40 years old ... need a liver transplant but only one suitable liver is available. One of the patients [the first] has had a much worse life than the other. ... In this case it seems most fair to give the liver to the first person. This supports the life time view.[8]

Again, such a view has some appeal but it has two major problems, one practical and the other theoretical.

The practical problem is that we could never make decisions as to how to allocate lifesaving or indeed other scarce resources between people until we had their whole (and very complete and detailed) life history. Without it all sorts of injustices would be compounded. Better perhaps to treat each person as counting for one and none for more than one than even to embark on the massively invasive (of privacy) data collection which it would be necessary to hold and have instantly available on each and every citizen and which could never be complete, accurate or proof against abuse.

This incidentally is also the reason why it is wrong to discriminate against smokers, for example, in the provision of Coronary Artery Bypass Grafts.

The theoretical problem is that if it is right to attempt to even out quality of life as between people, then we should do so as a matter of public policy throughout society, not simply in the rare cases where resource allocation decisions in health care arise. This might have to include making sure that no one lived longer than the person who has the shortest lifespan and no one was happier than the most miserable.[9]

Equally, if fairness is the issue it is surely also unfair (even less fair?) to arrange things so that the burden of making society or the world a fairer place falls only on those who are in competition for lifesaving resources. If the bizarre claim that extra life years are not special is to be sustained, then those life years are not special *for anyone*, not even for those who do not need resources to keep them alive (and which of us does not?).

Of course those in favour of discriminating against the old can tough it out, they can embrace the problems I have here identified and say that is the price we pay for trying to be fair. Ultimately we will be comparing different moral priorities. However, there is much to be said for taking individual persons and their wishes and fundamental interests as what matters from the point of view of morality. This means that we must recognise that although their lives will all differ in length, happiness and success, in short in the degree to which their fundamental interests are satisfied, that people matter morally despite these differences, not because of them.

Notes

This paper draws on a number of my already published thoughts on justice, age and QALYs. Amoung sources used are my: More & Better Justice, in Sue Mendus and Martin Bell, editors, *Philosophy and Medical Welfare*, Cambridge: University Press, 1988: 75–97; Does Justice Require That We Be Ageist? Bioethics 1994; 8(1): 74–84; National Health = National Defence, Issues in Focus 1992; August: 38.

1. See Dworkin, *Taking Rights Seriously* London: Duckworth, 1977: 198; Robert Nozick *Anarchy State & Utopia*, Oxford: Blackwell, 1974: 33; and Jonathan Glover *What Sort of People Should There Be?* Harmondsworth: Penguin, 1984: 40–2.
2. See J. Harris, Does Justice Require That We Be Ageist? Bioethics 1994; 8(1).
3. See Ronald Dworkin's compelling elucidation of this distinction in Dworkin, Op. Cit., 1977: 227.
4. Alan Williams, The Value of QALYs, Health and Social Services Journal, July 1985.
5. See J. Harris, More & Better Justice, in Sue Mendus and Martin Bell, editors, *Philosophy and Medical Welfare*, Cambridge: University Press, 1988: 75–97; Rationing Life: Quality or Justice? In Mark Ockelton, editor, *Medicine, Ethics And Law*, Beiheft Nr. 32, ARSP, Steiner Verlag Wiesbaden GMBH, 1987: 104–12; EQALYty, in Peter Byrne, editor, *Health Rights & Resources*, King's Fund and Oxford University Press, 1988: 100–28; and QALYfying The Value of Life, Journal of Medical Ethics 1987; Sept: 117–23.
6. Harris, *The Value of Life,* **Routledge,** London, 1985, 1985: 89.
7. Kappel & Sandoe, QALYs: Age and Fairness, Bioethics 1992; 6(4): 314–5.
8. Ibid. pp 315–6.
9. This might of course be dysfunctional in terms of species survival but we will ignore this problem for obvious reasons.

12. When does the cost of living exceed the return on our investment?

The social and economic consequences of coronary bypass surgery in the elderly

ROGER W. EVANS

Introduction

Open heart surgery in the elderly has been the subject of numerous clinical reports, many describing the benefits patients derive [1–31]. Few of these reports have explicitly considered the cost associated with either coronary artery bypass surgery or cardiac valve replacement [10]. Nonetheless, this has not precluded expression of concern as to the financial implications of cardiac surgery in the elderly.

Increasingly, older people are being criticized for excess health care utilization and expenditures [32–49]. However, as in the general population, a small percentage of people are responsible for the majority of health care expenditures [50]. For example, in 1987, 30% of the U.S. population was responsible for 91% of all health care expenditures (see Table 12.1) [50]. Meanwhile, in 1990, about 4.8% (2.9 million) of all Medicare enrollees accounted for 64.4% of all Medicare payments [51]. This distribution of payments has remained stable during the past two decades.

While cost is an important consideration in treating the elderly patient, it should by no means be the only one. Quality of life is a critical issue we can no longer ignore [52]. In the case of complex surgery, there is always the fear that

Table 12.1. Distribution of health care expenditures for the U.S. population, 1987

Percent of U.S. population ranked by expenditures	Percent of total expenses
Top 1 percent	30
Top 2 percent	41
Top 5 percent	58
Top 10 percent	72
Top 30 percent	91
Top 50 percent	97
Bottom 50 percent	3

Source: [50].

P.J. Walter (ed.), Coronary Bypass Surgery in the Elderly, pp. 121–134.
© 1995 *Kluwer Academic Publishers, Dordrecht.*

Table 12.2. Age distribution of the United States' population: percent age 65 and over and age 80 and over

Year	Percent of population age	
	65 and over	80 and over
1960	9.2	1.4
1965	9.5	1.6
1970	9.8	1.8
1975	10.5	2.1
1980	11.3	2.3
1985	11.9	2.5
1990	12.6	2.8

Source: [55].

the patient may either die in the early post-operative period or endure long, debilitating, and dehumanizing stays in the intensive care unit [44]. Cost-effectiveness and cost-utility analysis requires that the cost, benefits and burdens of treatment be given careful consideration [53, 54]. In doing so, we are often forced to look beyond the individual patient in favor of a community or a social perspective. We can afford to do no less when we look at the demographics of developed countries.

As shown in Table 12.2, the population of the United States is aging [55]. In 1960, 9.2% of all persons were age 65 and over, compared with 12.6% in 1990. Since 1960, the percentage of the population age 80 and over has increased from 1.4% in 1960, to 2.8% in 1990. In 1900, a person 65 years of age could be expected to live an additional 11.9 years. By 1991, a 65 year-old was expected to live another 17.5 years (see Table 12.3) [55].

Personal health care expenditures have also increased substantially since

Table 12.3. Life expectancy at age 65 according to sex, United States 1900–91

Year	Remaining life expectancy (in years)		
	Both sexes	Male	Female
1900–1902	11.9	11.5	12.2
1950	13.9	12.8	15.0
1960	14.3	12.8	15.8
1970	15.2	13.1	17.0
1975	16.1	13.8	18.1
1980	16.4	14.1	18.3
1985	16.7	14.5	18.5
1990	17.2	15.1	18.9
1991	17.5	15.5	19.2

Source: page 44, [55].

Table 12.4. Per capita U.S. health care expenditures, 1929–92

Year	Per capita ($)
1929	26
1940	26
1950	70
1960	126
1965	175
1970	302
1975	536
1980	933
1985	1,496
1990	2,255
1992	3,160

Source: [56–58].

1950 (see Table 12.4) [56–58]. In 1950, the average per capita expenditure for health care was $70. By 1992 this amount had increased to $3,160 per person. The annual percentage change in personal health care expenditures has been the subject of extensive analysis. As shown in Table 12.5, at least three factors directly affect growth – prices, population, and intensity (defined as changes in the use of kinds of services and supplies) [55]. In 1990–91, 54% of the growth in personal health care expenditures was due to prices, 9% to population, and 37% to intensity. Clearly, medical technology, including open heart surgery, is of considerable significance. The interaction between age and technology has yet to be examined.

Table 12.6 summarizes, by age, the death rates for the three leading causes of death in the United States [55]. As shown, among persons age 65 and over, there were 9,386 deaths attributable to heart disease per 100,000 persons in 1991. As is

Table 12.5. Personal health care expenditures average annual percentage change

Year	Average annual percent change	Factors affecting growth (%)		
		Prices	Population	Intensity[a]
1960–61	11.3	31	27	42
1965–66	10.5	45	11	44
1970–71	9.9	65	11	24
1975–76	14.0	62	6	32
1980–81	16.2	70	6	24
1985–86	8.4	60	12	28
1990–91	11.6	54	9	37

[a] Intensity represents changes in use of kinds of services and supplies.
Source: page 163, [55].

Table 12.6. Death rates for three leading causes of death, according to age: United States, 1991

Age category	Deaths per 100,000		
	Heart	Malignant neoplasms	Cerebrovascular
All ages, age adjusted	146.1	132.6	26.5
All ages, crude	283.3	202.9	56.8
45–54 Years	118.7	154.1	16.7
55–64 Years	354.3	433.2	46.8
65–74 Years	850.5	855.0	139.0
75–84 Years	2,229.2	1,367.3	486.6
85 Years and over	6,306.5	1,716.6	1,525.9

Source: page 86, [55].

apparent, the death rate due to heart disease increases substantially as people age.

Not surprisingly, the number of coronary bypass operations performed per year has markedly increased since 1970, when 3,000 procedures were done. By 1989, over 360,000 procedures were performed (see Table 12.7). As shown in Table 12.8, the majority of these procedures were performed on males 65 years of age and older.

Despite concerns related to the cost of health care, and the inappropriate use of advanced medical technology, few reports have documented the cost of open

Table 12.7. Number of coronary artery bypass operations by year, 1970–89

Year	Number
1970	3,000
1975	57,000
1980	137,000
1985	230,000
1989	368,000

Table 12.8. Coronary artery bypass grafts in males age 45 and over: United States, 1980–91

Year	Number		Per 1,000 population	
	45–64 Years	65 and over	45–64 Years	65 and over
1980	72,000	27,000	3.4	2.6
1985	102,000	57,000	4.8	5.0
1990	132,000	137,000	5.9	10.6
1991	135,000	144,000	6.0	11.3

Source: page 129, [55].

heart surgery among the elderly [40]. In this report, I first examine the national experience with coronary bypass surgery in the elderly based on data for the Medicare program [51]. I then review the experience of the Mayo Clinic in 1992. My analysis will focus on unselected patients who were recorded as having undergone a coronary artery bypass graft, or had a cardiac valve replacement procedure. Some patients may have had both procedures.

Materials and methods

Often the concepts of *costs* and *charges* are used interchangeably [59–61]. Although the distinction between the two concepts is critical, true accounting cost data for any aspect of health care are rarely available. Instead, we often estimate costs based on billed charges. Alternatively, *expenditures* reflect the aggregate charges for the services received by patients with a common underlying problem. As a result, *cost of illness* studies frequently describe the level of expenditures incurred to treat a particular disease (e.g., cancer, heart disease). In such studies, the concept of cost is usually misleading.

Medicare Provider Analysis and Review (MEDPAR) data

Data on Medicare patients are accumulated annually by the Health Care Financing Administration (HCFA) and made available on a public use data tape referred to as the Medicare Provider Analysis and Review (MEDPAR) file [62]. The MEDPAR file for a given year contains one record for each Medicare-covered stay in a short-stay hospital for which the date of discharge occurred in that year. The MEDPAR file contains the Medicare identification number; dates of admission and discharge; up to 5 diagnoses including a principal diagnosis; and up to 3 procedures with the dates they were performed. The diagnoses and procedures are coded using ICD-9-CM.

Institutional Planning Data Base (IPDB)

The Institutional Planning Data Base is a repository for all data on billed charges associated with inpatient, emergency room and outpatient care at Mayo Clinic and its affiliated hospitals – St. Mary's Hospital and Rochester Methodist. Hospital Data are accumulated for all visits, examinations, tests and procedures. All charges for health services utilized by patients are aggregated according to major cost centers.

Results

The Medicare experience with coronary artery bypass surgery for 1983, 1985, and 1990 is summarized in Table 12.9. On the basis of their diagnosis-related

Table 12.9. Medicare short-stay hospital discharges for coronary artery bypass grafts (CABG), 1983–90

DRG	Description	Discharges (No.)			Average length of stay (days)			Average charge per discharge ($)		
		1983	1985	1990	1983	1985	1990	1983	1985	1990
106	CABG with cardiac catheterization	4,545	34,415	61,810	16.4	16.7	15.8	21,937	29,985	41,322
107	CABG without cardiac catheterization	50,340	33,755	46,765	15.5	16.0	12.3	20,960	22,063	33,394

DRG = diagnosis-related group.
Source: page 74, [63].

group (DRG), procedures requiring a cardiac catheterization are distinguished from those that do not [63]. As shown, there has been a remarkable growth in the number of CABGs performed on the Medicare patient population. In 1983, data on nearly 55,000 CABGs were included in the MEDPAR file. In 1990, data were available for 108,575 procedures. These figures may not include all patients who received a CABG. Some patients may have required medical care in addition to a CABG and, thus, their principal DRG may be different from DRG 106 or 107.

For both DRG 106 and 107, the average length of hospital stay has decreased, from 16.4 to 15.8 days for DRG 106 and from 15.5 to 12.3 days for DRG 107 [63]. Despite a reduced length of stay, the average charge per case has increased considerably. The average charge for DRG 106 increased from $21,937 in 1983 to $41,322 in 1990. While the increase is less substantial for DRG 107, it is still noteworthy, up from $20,960 in 1983 to $33,394 in 1990.

The data reported here understate the total cost of cardiac care. They are based on a single episode of care. As noted by Riley *et al.*, many Medicare patients are rehospitalized following a CABG or a percutaneous transluminal coronary angioplasty [62]. Table 12.10 presents the number of rehospitalizations for adverse events per 1,000 patients discharged alive. Adverse events have been classified into eight clinically coherent groups. The most common type of adverse event following CABG was 'other cardiac events'. Subsequent CABGs and PTCAs were rare, at 3 per 1,000 and 8 per 1,000, respectively. It should be noted that all rehospitalizations recorded here occurred within one year of surgery.

The Mayo Clinic experience with CABG in 1992 is summarized in Table 12.11. Procedures are distinguished according to the number of vessels involved

Table 12.10. Number of rehospitalizations for adverse events within one year of the procedure per 1,000 discharged alive, by adverse event group, for Medicare beneficiaries undergoing selected cardiac procedures, 1986–88

Adverse event group	Number of rehospitalizations for adverse events per 1,000 discharged alive	
	CABG	PTCA
Total	283	558
Subsequent CABG	3	61
Subsequent PTCA	8	140
Cardiac catheterization without revascularization	29	118
Angina, acute mycardial infarction, and other acute and subacute ischemic heart disease	50	129
Other cardiac events	130	81
Noncardiac vascular events	19	14
Infections	23	7
Other	22	10

Source: page 928, [62].

Table 12.11. Total charges per case and in-hospital mortality for coronary artery bypass grafts: Mayo Medical Center, 1992

| Number of vessels | Mean total charge per case $ | | | | | In-hospital mortality (%) | | | | |
	45–54 Years	55–59 Years	60–64 Years	65–74 Years	75+ Years	45–54 Years	55–59 Years	60–64 Years	65–74 Years	75+ Years
One	34,839	40,545	35,321	33,646	32,851	0.0	0.0	0.0	0.0	11.1
Two	38,369	41,926	34,941	35,179	38,115	5.6	0.0	0.0	0.8	10.2
Three	37,619	34,653	47,767	37,005	40,718	0.0	0.0	7.5	2.9	1.9
Four	37,251	35,066	37,135	41,750	43,293	0.0	0.0	0.0	7.7	1.4
Overall	37,357	38,577	40,591	36,592	39,283	2.0	0.0	3.1	4.2	6.8

Table 12.12. Total charges and in-hospital mortality for aortic and mitral valve replacement, 1992

Age group	Mean total charge ($)	In-hospital mortality (%)
45–54 Years	48,671	2.5
55–59 Years	53,009	2.9
60–64 Years	50,759	4.9
65–74 Years	47,022	6.3
75+	46,812	8.8
Overall	48,014	5.9

and the age of the patient. Data are provided on total charges per case and in-hospital mortality.

As shown, there is some variability according to the age of the patient and the number of vessels involved. However, the total charge per case does not necessarily increase with age. Meanwhile, in-hospital mortality among patients 75 years of age and older is actually higher for one- and two-vessel procedures. Finally, the overall results are revealing. The highest charge per case is for patients between 60 and 64 years. In-hospital mortality is highest among patients 75 years of age or older.

The data for aortic and mitral valve replacement are summarized in Table 12.12. Once again, the average charge per case is not as variable as one might expect, although in-hospital mortality does increase with age. Patients between the ages of 55 and 64 years incur the highest charges for their care.

Discussion

The data reported here are suggestive, not definitive. Charges do not reflect true accounting costs. Most hospitals are not reimbursed or paid on the basis of charges. For example, in the United States, the payment-to-cost ratio for Medicare patients is .91. For patients who are privately insured, the payment-to-cost ratio is 1.28. Nonetheless, in a single institutional setting, charges are a very worthy indicator of the relative differences in patient-related expenses.

Unfortunately, data such as those reported here inform the debate concerning health care and the elderly, but they do not resolve the dilemma. The underlying issues are far more complex. As noted previously, quality of life is an important consideration [52]. Equally critical, however, is the concept of productivity. Much of the debate today regarding the allocation of the health care dollar focuses on the general concept of a return on investment. Critics have essentially argued that the treatment of the elderly does not provide a reasonable return on investment. Younger people have more to contribute over a longer period of time than do the elderly. This is readily apparent from Table 12.13 wherein I have summarized mortality costs by age and sex for the United States in 1990. *Mortality cost* is defined as the value of lifetime earnings lost by

Table 12.13. Mortality costs by age and sex, 1990

Age	Mortality Cost Per Death ($)		
	Both sexes	Males	Females
15–24 Years	576,272	608,945	473,487
25–44 Years	588,325	646,637	447,826
45–64 Years	223,601	247,149	185,579
≥ 65 Years	19,520	20,005	19,092

Costs are discounted at 6% per year.
Source: page 100, [64].

persons who die prematurely [64]. The cost estimates presented here are based on the person's age, sex, life expectancy at the time of death, labor force participation rates, annual earnings, value of homemaking services, and a 6% discount rate by which to convert to present worth the potential aggregate earnings lost over the years.

As shown, the mortality cost is highest for males between the ages of 25 and 44 years [64]. Among females, the mortality cost is highest for persons 15 to 24 years. Clearly, as a person ages, their mortality cost decreases substantially. Overall, for persons 65 years of age and over, the mortality cost per death is $19,520. These data underscore the significance of productivity, but fail to take into account the fact that elderly persons have essentially made their contribution and are now taking advantage of the benefits for which they have paid. Of course, this assumes that the intergenerational transfer that has occurred is equitable.

The discussion of these data underscore the possibility of age becoming the basis for discrimination. Despite abundant evidence that elderly persons are highly diverse physiologically, psychologically, and socially, chronological age is a well-established focal point for discussions in the United States, regarding the allocation of health care resources [40]. For example, while the U.S. Congress, Office of Technology Assessment (OTA) recognizes that the elderly population is heterogeneous, it nonetheless legitimizes the usage of age 65 as an official marker [34]:

> Sixty-five, or any chronological age, is a poor indicator of biological function, physiological reserve, cognitive ability, or health care needs. The use of 65 is justified, however, by its prominence in available health and demographic statistics and its relevance to eligibility criteria in current Federal and State health care programs, especially Medicare.

Defining who is considered 'elderly' in relation to the use of advanced medical technology can be difficult [40]. The application of technology is a gradual process. Chronological age is often a consideration because of the ease with which it is determined, even though – according to many people – an individual's health status and probability of benefit are the real issues.

The correlation between chronological age and health status is often weak [40]. As this is recognized, the chronological limits placed on the use of new technology may be adjusted accordingly. For example, in 1967, only 7% of kidney dialysis patients in the United States were 55 years of age and over (see Table 12.14). In 1990, over 61% of all dialysis patients were 55 years of age and older. Moreover, in 1990, 14.1% of dialysis patients were 75 years of age or older. Obviously, the indications for treatment change over time, as has also been the case with open heart surgery.

The experience with cardiac surgery in the elderly is now extensive. The results are well known, but none of the randomized trials comparing coronary bypass surgery with medical therapy included patients over 80 years of age [44]. We know that both the morbidity and mortality associated with cardiac surgery increase with age. Data from the Coronary Artery Surgery Study revealed that the post-operative mortality rate at 30 days was almost three times higher among patients over 65 than those under 65 (5.2% versus 1.9%) [44]. Other studies have compared surgical results in patients over 70 years of age with those in patients under 70 and have revealed mortality ratios ranging from 3:1 to 4:1. Among patients over 80 years of age, the post-operative mortality rate at 30 days ranges from 9% to 29%. Elective operations for pure aortic stenosis are associated with the lowest mortality in this group. The mortality rates for emergency operations and combined procedures involving both coronary artery bypass surgery and valve replacement have been much higher.

Operative risk is not the only issue. Older patients often have a much longer post-operative hospital course, remain dependent on the ventilator longer after surgery, and have more post-operative complications (particularly neurologic complications) than younger patients. At the same time, however, the survivors have as much symptomatic improvement as younger patients and have actuarial survival curves that are similar to those for their unaffected peers [44].

Table 12.14. Age distribution of kidney dialysis patients in the United States

Year	Percent of patients by age category	
	≥ 55 Years	≥ 75 Years
1967	7.0	N/A
1980	48.5	5.3
1983	53.6	7.8
1985	58.4	10.1
1987	60.7	12.0
1990	61.8	14.1

N/A = not available.
Source: [40].

In conclusion, different perspectives emerge from the same data. The clinical perspective tends to underscore the surgical benefits, downplay the costs, and ignore the productivity issue. A societal perspective downplays the surgical benefits, underscores the costs, and highlights the productivity issue. Furthermore, the societal perspective is based on a generalized cost-effectiveness criterion which we must agree is inherently discriminatory to elderly patients [65]. Thus, clinical benefits can come into conflict with social goals and economic objectives. Indeed, as I have already noted, the data presented here inform the debate, but they do not answer the question as to what is the comparative value of a human life. What we can say is that, in purely economic terms, the return on our investment is inadequate to justify cardiac surgery in the elderly. Of course, the same is true of convicted felons upon whom we now spend in excess of $40,000 annually, excluding the social costs associated with their crime.

References

1. Stephenson LW, McVaugh HM III, Edmunds LH Jr. Surgery using cardiopulmonary bypass in the elderly. Circulation 1978; 58: 250–4.
2. Berry BE, Acree PW, Davis DJ, et al. Coronary artery bypass operation in septuagenarians. Ann Thorac Surg 1981; 31: 310–3.
3. Gersh BJ, Kronmal RA, Frye RL, et al. Coronary arteriography and coronary artery bypass surgery: morbidity and mortality in patients age 65 years or older. A report from the Coronary Artery Surgery Study. Circulation 1983; 67: 483–91.
4. Faro RS, Golden MD, Javid H, et al. Coronary revascularization in septuagenarians. J Thorac Cardiovasc Surg 1983; 86: 616–20.
5. Crater JM, Goldstein J, Jones EL, et al. Clinical, hemodynamic, and operative descriptors affecting outcome of aortic valve replacement in elderly versus young patients. Ann Surg 1984; 199: 733–41.
6. Gersh BJ, Kronmal RA, Schaff HV, et al. Comparison of coronary artery bypass surgery and medical therapy in patients 65 years of age or older: a nonrandomized study from the Coronary Artery Surgery Study (CASS) Registry. N Engl J Med 1985; 313: 217–24.
7. Lubitz J, Riley G, Newton M. Outcomes of surgery among the Medicare aged: mortality after surgery. Health Care Financing Review 1985; 6(4): 103–15.
8. Tsai TP, Matloff JM, Chaux A, et al. Combined valve and coronary artery bypass procedures in septuagenarians and octogenarians: results in 120 patients. Ann Thorac Surg 1986; 42: 681–4.
9. Tsai TP, Matloff JM, Gray RJ, et al. Cardiac surgery in the octogenarian. J Thorac Cardiovasc Surg 1986; 91: 924–8.
10. Stason WB, Sanders CA, Smith HC. Cardiovascular care of the elderly: economic considerations. J Am Coll Cardiol 1987; 10: 18A–21A.
11. Dustan HP, Hamilton MP, McCullough L, Page LB. Sociopolitical and ethical considerations in the treatment of cardiovascular disease in the elderly. J Am Coll Cardiol 1987; 10: 14A–17A.
12. Dorros G, Lewin RF, Daly P, Assa J. Coronary artery bypass surgery in patients over age 70 years: report from the Milwaukee Cardiovascular Data Registry. Clin Cardiol 1987; 10: 377–82.
13. Naunheim KS, Kern MJ, McBride LR, et al. Coronary artery bypass surgery in patients aged 80 years or older. Am J Cardiol 1987; 59: 804–7.
14. Mullany CJ, Elveback LR, Frye RL, et al. Coronary artery disease and its management: influence on survival in patients undergoing aortic valve replacement. J Am Coll Cardiol 1987; 10: 66–72.

15. Blakeman BM, Pifarre R, Sullivan HJ, et al. Aortic valve replacement in patients 75 years old and older. Ann Thorac Surg 1987; 44: 637–9.
16. Loop FD, Lytle BW, Cosgrove DM, et al. Coronary artery bypass graft surgery in the elderly: indications and outcome. Cleve Clin J Med 1988; 55: 23–34.
17. Edmunds LH Jr, Stephenson LW, Edie RN, Ratcliffe MB. Open heart surgery in octogenarians. N Engl J Med 1988; 319: 131–6.
18. Bessone LN, Pupello DF, Hiro SP, et al. Surgical management of aortic valve disease in the elderly: a longitudinal analysis. Ann Thorac Surg 1988; 46: 264–9.
19. Jamieson WRE, Burr LH, Munro AI, et al. Cardiac valve replacement in the elderly: clinical performance of biological prostheses. Ann Thorac Surg 1989; 48: 173–85.
20. Fremes SE, Goldman BS, Ivanov J, et al. Vavular surgery in the elderly. Circulation 1989; 80(suppl I): 77–90.
21. Fiore AC, Naunheim KS, Barner HB, et al. Valve replacement in the octogenarian. Ann Thor Surg 1989; 48: 104–8.
22. Califf RM, Harrell FE Jr, Lee KL, ct al. The evolution of medical and surgical therapy for coronary artery disease: a 15-year perspective. JAMA 1989; 261: 2077–86.
23. Levinson JR, Atkins CW, Buckley MJ, et al. Octogenarians with aortic stenosis: outcome after aortic valve replacement. Circulation 1989; 80(suppl I): 49–56.
24. Horvath KA, DiSesa VJ, Peigh PS, et al. Favorable results of coronary artery bypass grafting in patients older than 75 years. J Thorac Cardiovasc Surg 1990; 99: 92–6.
25. Deleuze P, Loisance DY, Besnainou F, et al. Severe aortic stenosis in octogenarians: is operation an acceptable alternative? Ann Thorac Surg 1990; 50: 226–9.
26. Galloway AC, Colvin SB, Grossi EA, et al. Ten-year experience with aortic valve replacement in 482 patients 70 years of age or older: operative risk and long-term results. Ann Thorac Surg 1990; 49: 84–93.
27. Freeman WK, Schaff HV, O'Brian PC, et al. Cardiac surgery in the octogenarian: perioperative outcome and clinical followup. J Am Coll Cardiol 1991; 18: 29–35.
28. Culliford AT, Galloway AC, Colvin SB, et al. Aortic valve replacement for aortic stenosis in persons aged 80 years and over. Am J Cardiol 1991; 67: 1256–60.
29. Olsson M, Granstrom L, Lindblom D, et al. Aortic valve replacement in octogenarians with aortic stenosis: a case-control study. J Am Coll Cardiol 1992; 20: 1512–6.
30. Bernard Y, Etievent J, Mourand JL, et al. Long-term results of percutaneous aortic valvuloplasty compared with aortic valve replacement in patients more than 75 years old. J Am Coll Cardiol 1992; 20: 796–801.
31. Wong JB, Salem DN, Pauker SG. You're never too old. N Engl J Med 1993; 328: 971–5.
32. Evans RW. Health care technology and the inevitability of resource allocation and rationing decisions (First of two parts). JAMA 1983; 249: 2047–53.
33. Evans RW. Health care technology and the inevitability of resource allocation and rationing decisions (Second of two parts). JAMA 1983; 249: 2208–19.
34. Office of Technology Assessment. Life-sustaining technologies and the elderly. Report No. OTA-BA-306. Washington DC: US Government Printing Office, July 1987.
35. Callahan D. Setting limits: medical goals in an aging society. New York: Simon and Schuster, 1987.
36. Callahan D. Rationing medical progress: the way to affordable health care. N Engl J Med 1990; 322: 1810–3.
37. Coddington DC, Keen DJ, Moore KD, Clarke RL. The crisis in health care: costs, choices, and strategies. San Francisco, CA: Jossey-Bass, 1990.
38. Lamm RD. The brave new world of health care. Denver, CO: Center for Public Policy and Contemporary Issues, University of Denver, 1990.
39. Levinsky N. Age as a criterion for rationing health care. N Engl J Med 1990; 322: 1813–6.
40. Evans RW. Advanced medical technology and elderly people. In: Binstock RH, Post SG, editors. Too old for health care. Baltimore, MD: The John Hopkins University Press, 1991: 44–74.

41. Barry RL, Bradley GV, editors. Set no limits: a rebuttal to Daniel Callahan's proposal to limit health care for the elderly. Urbana, IL: University of Illinois Press, 1991.
42. Binstock RH, Post SG, editors. Too old for health care? Controversies in medicine, law, economics and ethics. Glenview, IL: Scott, Foresman and Co., 1991.
43. Evans RW. Rationale for rationing. Health Mngt Quart 1992; XIV(2): 14–7.
44. Thibault GE. Too old for what? N Engl J Med 1993; 328: 946–50.
45. Kamm FM. Morality, mortality: death and whom to save from it. New York: Oxford University Press, 1993.
46. Callahan D. The troubled dream of life: living with mortality. New York: Simon and Schuster, 1993.
47. Molloy W. Vital choices: life, death, and the health care crisis. New York: Viking, 1993.
48. British Medical Journal Publishing Group. Rationing in action. London: BMJ Publishing Group, 1993.
49. Abrams FR. The doctor with two heads: the patient versus the costs. N Engl J Med 1993; 328: 975–6.
50. Berk M, Monheit A. The concentration of health care expenditures: an update. Health Affairs 1992; 11(4): 145–9.
51. Helbing C. Medicare program expenditures. Health Care Financ Rev Ann Suppl 1992; 23–54.
52. Walter PJ, editor. Quality of life after open heart surgery. Dordrecht, The Netherlands: Kluwer Academic Publishers, 1992.
53. Robinson R. Economic evaluation and health care: cost-effectiveness analysis. BMJ 1993; 307(6907): 793–5.
54. Robinson R. Cost-utility analysis. BMJ 1993; 307: 859–62.
55. National Center for Health Statistics. Health, United States, 1992. DHHS Pub. No. (PHS) 93-1232. Hyattsville, MD: Public Health Service, August 1993.
56. Rublee DA, Schneider M. International health spending: comparisons with the OECD. Health Affairs 1991; 10(3): 187–98.
57. Schieber GJ, Poullier J-P, Greenwald LM. Health care systems in twenty-four countries. Health Affairs 1991; 10(3): 22–38.
58. Schieber GJ, Poullier J-P, Greenwald LM. Health spending, delivery, and outcomes in OECD countries. Health Affairs 1993; 12(2): 120–9.
59. Evans RW, Manninen DL, Dong FB. An economic analysis of heart-lung transplantation: costs, insurance coverage, and reimbursement. J Thorac Cardiovasc Surg 1993; 105: 972–8.
60. Evans RW. Social, economic, and insurance issues in heart transplantation. In: O'Connell JB, Kaye MP, editors. Intrathoracic transplantation 2000. Austin, TX: R.G. Landes Co., 1993: 1–17.
61. Finkler SA. The distinction between cost and charges. Ann Intern Med 1982; 96: 102–9.
62. Riley G, Lubitz J, Gornick M, et al. Medicare beneficiaries: adverse outcomes after hospitalization for eight procedures. Med Care 1993; 31: 921–49.
63. Helbing C. Hospital insurance short-stay hospital benefits. Health Care Financ Rev Ann Suppl 1992; 55–96.
64. U.S. Bureau of the Census. Statistical abstract of the United States: 1993. 113th ed. Washington, DC: US Bureau of the Census, 1993.
65. Avon J. Benefit and cost analysis on geriatric care: turning age discrimination into health policy. N Engl J Med 1984; 310: 1294–301.

PART FIVE

The heart of the matter: Health-related quality of life after CABG in the elderly

13. Coronary artery bypass surgery and health-related quality of life: Data from the National Health and Nutrition Examination Survey

PENNIFER ERICKSON

Introduction

Coronary artery bypass graft surgery is being performed with increasing frequency. Although fewer than 100,000 were done in 1980, the number of grafts performed in short-stay hospitals throughout the United States increased four-fold in the ensuing decade [1]. This rapid expansion suggests that not only is the procedure safer and more available but, also, that different types of patients are now being considered for surgery. One example of the expanding case mix is that the procedure is increasingly being performed among persons 65 years and older [2]. These older patients have been found to have the same functional and emotional benefits after undergoing coronary artery bypass surgery as do patients who are less than 65 years of age [3]. Walter and colleagues extended this analysis by examining persons 75 years and older; these researchers also found that age was not a significant factor in determining benefits gained from bypass surgery [4].

These studies, however, have been based on samples of patients in health care settings, thereby precluding long-term tracing of the pre-surgical quality of life experience of the patients. Examination of health status months or even years before coronary bypass surgery, if performed, might lead to a better understanding of the relationship between the quality of life benefits attributed to this type of surgery. Such an investigation might indicate whether or not persons with a higher health-related quality of life are selected to receive coronary artery bypass graft surgery.

In the United States, a longitudinal epidemiological study that has been underway since 1971 is available to examine issues of the relationship between health status, subsequent surgery, and age. The current analysis is based on data from a cohort of a representative sample of the general population that was interviewed in 1982–1984, the first wave of the National Health and Nutrition Examination Survey (NHANES I) Epidemiological Followup Study (NHEFS). NHEFS data are used to study whether or not quality of life differed for persons who did and did not have coronary artery bypass surgery during the following five years. In addition to personal risk factors such as age and gender, the

137

P.J. Walter (ed.), Coronary Bypass Surgery in the Elderly, pp. 137–144.
© 1995 *Kluwer Academic Publishers, Dordrecht.*

influence of social factors including marital status and educational level on the subsequent surgery status are examined.

Material and methods

Study population. The NHANES I Epidemiologic Followup Survey is a cohort study that is based on the initial sample drawn for the NHANES I, which was selected to be representative of the U.S. population in 1971–1975 [5, 6]. In the late 1970s it was decided to convert this cross-sectional survey into a longitudinal study. The first followup, which consisted of a household interview in 1982–1984, attempted to trace and reinterview the 14,407 NHANES I respondents or their proxies who were aged 25–74 years of age in 1971–1975; 93 percent were successfully located [7].

The second followup, conducted in 1986, was limited to the 3,980 persons who were at least 55 years of age at the time of NHANES I; the 3,814 persons or their proxies who were successfully traced participated in a telephone interview in 1986 [8]. An attempt was made to reinterview the complete, non-deceased cohort of 11,750 persons in 1987; 11,018 persons or their proxies participated in this 1987 followup. Essentially the same questionnaire was used for the 1986 and 1987 interviews [9]. This analysis of health-related quality of life and coronary artery bypass surgery uses information collected in the 1982–1984, 1986 and 1987 followup surveys.

Coronary artery bypass surgery. Data on coronary artery bypass surgery was first collected in 1986. Of the 3,814 respondents or their proxies who were interviewed in 1986, 70 persons responded affirmatively to the question, 'have you ever had coronary artery surgery?' This same question was asked in 1987 for persons who had not reported bypass surgery in 1986 and resulted in an additional 115 persons who reported having had bypass surgery. One person who reported having ever had bypass in 1986 also reported having had an additional heart bypass in the 1987 interview. The two followup surveys conducted in 1986 and 1987 resulted in a total of 185 persons who reported having ever had bypass surgery.

Given the relatively few bypass surgeries that were performed in the United States in the early 1980s, it is likely that very few, if any, persons who participated in the 1971–1975 National Health and Nutrition Examination Survey (NHANES I) would have had bypass surgery at the time of the 1982–1984 interview. Based on the assumption that all bypass surgeries reported in either 1986 or 1987 occurred after the 1982–84 interview, data from the 1982–1984 survey are used to investigate the relationship of health-related quality of life and subsequent coronary artery bypass graft surgery.

Health-related quality of life. Data from the 1982–1984 followup were used to develop a multi-dimensional measure of health-related quality of life that is based on the Health Utility Index (HUI) Mark I [10, 11]. The HUI combines information on four concepts of health-related quality of life, namely, physical function, role function, social and emotional function, and health problems, into a single score that ranges from − 0.21 to 1.00. Scores of less than 0 represent states of health that are considered to be worse than death. A score of 1.00 represents no dysfunction on any one of the four concepts included in the HUI; this state of no dysfunction is sometimes referred to as perfect, or optimal, health [12]. Each HUI score can be interpreted as the proportion of a year that a person spends, on average, in perfect health. For example, a person with an average score of 0.75 over a one-year period is said to experience three-fourths of a healthy life year.

To create a health-related quality of life score for each person who participated in the 1982–1984 NHANES I Epidemiologic Followup Study (NHEFS), previously used methods for modelling health status were applied [13, 14]. First, items in the NHEFS questionnaire were matched to function levels used in the Health Utility Index (HUI). Then, each survey participant was assigned to one function level within each of the four concepts assessed by the HUI. Function level scores for each concept were combined to form an overall score that reflected health-related quality of life; a score was calculated for each participant using standard scoring methods that have been developed for use with the Health Utility Index; these are subsequently referred to as NHEFS-HUI scores [15]. Valid health-related quality of life scores were available for 10,163 persons who were alive at the time of the 1982–1984 followup.

Covariates. In the analysis of the relationship between coronary artery bypass and health-related quality of life, the following covariates were considered: gender, age in years, marital status, years of school, family income, and presence or absence of heart disease. For this investigation, a person was considered as having heart disease if he or she reported having angina, a heart condition, a stroke, or a transient ischemic attack. Information on all covariates is based on information that was collected during the 1982–1984 interview.

NHANES I is based on a complex multi-stage sampling design such that probability of selection varies by age, sex, residence and income. To obtain estimates which are representative of the U.S. civilian non-institutionalized population, sample weights should be used. Since the purpose here is to study relationships in a large national sample which include sufficient numbers of important sociodemographic subgroups in the U.S. population, rather than to estimate parameters on a national basis, sample weights have not been used in these calculations.

Findings

Percent distributions of selected demographic characteristics are shown in Table 13.1 for persons with and without bypass as well as for the total cohort.

Table 13.1. Percent distributions of selected demographic characteristics based on 1982–84 interview by self-reported coronary artery bypass surgery status in 1986 or 1987

Characteristic	No bypass	Bypass	Total
Sample size	9,997	166	10,163
Gender			
Males	39.8	69.8	40.3
Females	60.2	30.2	59.7
Age			
<65 years	58.4	50.9	58.3
65–74 years	10.3	26.0	10.5
75+ years	31.4	23.1	31.3
Marital Status			
Currently married	67.6	78.3	67.8
Never married	5.1	1.2	5.0
Previously married	27.3	20.5	27.2
Years of school			
<12 years	22.8	20.5	22.7
12 years	38.5	35.5	36.5
12+ years	40.7	44.0	40.7
Income			
<$7,000	18.4	16.3	18.3
$ 7,000–19,999	31.1	37.9	31.2
$20,000–34,999	24.0	24.1	24.0
$35,000+	26.5	21.7	26.5

Although more than half of the cohort is female, males were about twice as likely as females to have bypass surgery within the following five years. Bypass patients were also slightly older than the total cohort; about 50% of the bypass patients were 65 years or older compared to about 40% of the persons who did not receive treatment with bypass surgery. A higher percent of bypass patients were currently married compared to the non-bypass patients, 78 and 68%, respectively. Comparisons between the bypass and non-bypass groups with regard to education and income indicate that bypass patients tend to have more education and lower family income; income status may be a reflection of the older age of this group.

Mean health-related quality of life scores in 1982–84 for persons who reported having had a coronary bypass graft by 1986 or 1987 are compared with those for all persons without bypass surgery, regardless of the presence of a heart condition in 1982–84, in Table 13.2. Among persons who did not have bypass surgery, the mean score for males was higher than for females, 0.79 and 0.74, respectively. Among persons who subsequently had bypass surgery, mean health-related quality of life scores for both males and females were lower than for those persons in the no bypass group. The difference in scores between males and females is greater for the bypass than the non-bypass group. In the non-bypass group, quality of life is 0.05 points higher for males than for females. When bypass is reported, the difference in health-related quality of life scores

Table 13.2. Mean health-related quality of life scores based on 1982–84 interview by self-reported coronary artery bypass surgery status in 1986 or 1987

Characteristic	No bypass	Bypass
Sample size	9,997	166
Overall mean	.76	.68
Gender		
Males	.79	.70
Females	.74	.61
Age		
<65 years	.80	.70
65–74 years	.72	.66
75+ years	.63	.65
Marital status		
Currently married	.79	.69
Not married	.70	.65
Education		
<12 years	.68	.62
12 years	.80	.72
12+ years	.82	.73
Heart Condition		
No	.79	.83
Yes	.59	.63

for males and females is 0.09, or approximately twice that observed in the non-bypass group.

Comparing the bypass and non-bypass groups by age indicates that the health-related quality of life scores are highest in both groups for persons in the youngest age group. Within each group defined by bypass status, mean health-related quality of life scores decline with increasing age. In the oldest group, however, the health-related quality of life scores are approximately the same for both the non-bypass and bypass groups.

Approximately 18% of the sample reported having heart disease in 1982–84. Persons who had bypass surgery had a higher quality of life score than did persons who had heart disease but did not have bypass surgery; the means were 0.63 and 0.59, respectively. Of the 166 persons who reported having a bypass surgery by 1987, 38 persons reported no history of heart disease in 1982–1984. These persons had an average quality of life score above that of the general population without heart disease; the means were 0.83 and 0.79, respectively.

Mean health-related quality of life scores are shown in Table 13.3 for persons who reported having heart disease in 1982–84. The scores are similar for the bypass and non-bypass group, except for persons 75 years and older and for persons who were either never married or previously married in 1982–84. For both groups, the bypass group had higher mean scores than did the non-bypass group.

Table 13.3. Mean health-related quality of life scores based on 1982–84 interview for persons with heart disease by self-reported coronary artery bypass status in 1986 or 1987

Characteristic	No bypass	Bypass
Sample size	1,669	128
Gender		
Males	.63	.67
Females	.57	.56
Age		
<65 years	.66	.64
65–74 years	.58	.61
75+ years	.53	.63
Marital status		
Currently married	.63	.64
Not married	.53	.59
Years of school		
<12 years	.53	.57
12 years	.66	.67
12+ years	.69	.70

Discussion

In this study, persons 75 years and older in 1982–84 and who subsequently had bypass surgery by 1987 were found to have a higher health-related quality of life in 1982–84, on average, than did persons with heart disease in the same age group who did not have bypass surgery within the same five-year period. This difference suggests that bypass surgery may be performed selectively among persons over 75 years of age, with relatively healthier persons in this age group being treated with bypass surgery. Persons 75 years and older in 1982–84 who subsequently had bypass surgery had the same health-related quality of life, on average, as did persons in the same age group in the general population. Persons 75 years and older with heart disease who had bypass surgery had about the same mean quality of life as did the general population. One possible explanation for this similarity in scores is that persons in this age group have many comorbid conditions which result in lower quality of life scores.

The relationship between health-related quality of life and age and gender that is observed among people with heart disease as well as the total NHEFS cohort are similar to those observed in the health status literature. In general, men are found to have a higher point-in-time health status, or health-related quality of life; on the other hand, men tend to have higher mortality rates. Declining scores with increasing age is another general pattern that is observed for health status as well as health-related quality of life scores, especially those that are based either explicitly or implicitly on physical and role function. That these commonly observed patterns are observed in this study supports the validity of the NHEFS-HUI score and the use of this measure for analysis of heart disease in comparison with the general population.

This descriptive investigation indicates that national cohort data provide novel information about relationships between health-related quality of life and bypass surgery. In addition to suggesting that persons with heart disease might differentially be chosen for receiving treatment with bypass surgery, the use of a generic health-related quality of life measure, such as the NHEFS-HUI, allows for the comparison of the health status of persons treated with coronary artery bypass graft with the status of persons with heart disease but treated with other than bypass surgery. Further, a generic health status measure allows for the comparison of the health status of persons with heart disease to that of the general population. Continued analysis of these data will allow for further understanding of the fundamental relationship of coronary artery bypass surgery and health-related quality of life as well as the relationship to other conditions and types of treatments.

References

1. Graves EJ. Detailed diagnoses and procedures, National Hospital Discharge Survey, 1990. Vital and health statistics, series 13, no. 113. Hyattsville, Maryland: National Center for Health Statistics, 1990.
2. Feinleib M, Havlik RJ, Gillum RF, Pokras R, McCarthy E, Moien M. Coronary heart disease and related procedures. Circulation 1989; 79: 113–8.
3. Guadagnoli E, Ayanian JZ, Cleary PD. Comparison of patient-reported outcomes after elective coronary artery bypass grafting in patients aged ≥ and ≤ 65 years. Am J Cardiology 1992; 70(1): 60–4.
4. Walter PJ, Mohan R, Cornelissen C. Health-related quality of life five years after coronary bypass surgery at age 75 or above: a research approach to item selection. In: Walter PJ, editor. Coronary bypass surgery in the elderly. Dordrecht, The Netherlands: Kluwer Academic Publishers, 1994: 195–210.
5. Miller HW. Plan and operation of the Health and Nutrition Examination Survey: United States 1971–1973. Vital and health statistics, series 1, no. 10a. Hyattsville, Maryland: National Center for Health Statistics, 1973.
6. Engle A, Murphy RS, Maurer K, Collins E. Plan and operation of the HANES I Augmentation Survey of Adults 25–74 Years: United States, 1974–1975. Vital and health statistics series 1, no. 10a. Hyattsville, Maryland: National Center for Health Statistics, 1978.
7. Cohen BB, Barbano HE, Cox CS, et al. Plan and operations of the NHANES I Epidemiologic Followup Study 1982–84. Vital and health statistics, series 1, no. 22. Washington, DC: US Government Printing Office, 1987.
8. Finucane FF, Fried VM, Madans JH, et al. Plan and operations of the NHANES I Epidemiologic Followup Study 1986. Vital and health statistics, series 1, no. 25. Washington, DC: US Government Printing Office, 1990.
9. Cox CS, Rothwell ST, Madans JH, et al. Plan and operations of the NHANES I Epidemiologic Followup Study 1982–84. Vital and health statistics, series 1, no. 27. Washington, DC: US Government Printing Office, 1992.
10. Drummond M, Stoddart G, Torrance GW. Methods for the economic evaluation of health care programmes. London: Oxford University Press, 1987: 112–48.

11. Torrance GW. Multiattribute utility theory as a method of measuring social preferences for health states in long-term care. In: Kane RL, Kane RA, editors. Values and long-term care. Lexington, Massachusetts: Lexington Books, 1982: 127–56.
12. Patrick DL, Erickson P. Health status and health policy: quality of life in health care evaluation and resource allocation. New York: Oxford University Press, 1993: 19–26.
13. Erickson P, Anderson JP, Kendall EA, Kaplan RM, Ganiats T. using retrospective data for measuring quality of life: National Health Interview Survey and the Quality of Well-Being Scale. Qual Life and Cardiovasc Care 1988; 4(4): 179–84.
14. Erickson P, Kendall EA, Anderson JP, Kaplan RM. Using composite health status measures to assess the nation's health. Med Care 1989; 27(3 suppl): 66–76.
15. Erickson P, Kendall EA, Odle MP, Torrance GW. Assessing health-related quality of life in the National Health and Nutrition Examination Survey. Hyattsville, Maryland: National Center for Health Statistics, 1994.

14. The selection of health-related quality of life measures for older adults with cardiovascular disease

SALLY A. SHUMAKER and ROGER ANDERSON

Introduction

It is now well recognized that the assessment of health-related quality of life (HRQL) provides critical information regarding the effects of various treatments, as well as the natural history of diseases, on patients' day-to-day lives [1, 2]. HRQL may be of particular importance among older patients where the primary goal of treatment focuses on regaining and maintaining independent status for as long as possible, a major component of HRQL. In relatively costly treatments such as coronary artery bypass graft (CABG) surgery, assumptions regarding the risks and benefits of this intervention for older adults could influence decisions regarding who is considered appropriate for treatment. Thus, it becomes even more important to demonstrate the efficacy of CABG surgery in the kind of broad terms encompassed by HRQL among older patients.

The question arises, however, as to whether or not one can validly assess HRQL in an older population [3]. That is, are the available instruments applicable to an older cohort? And, are there population and measurement issues specific to older patients that systematically interfere with the validity of the HRQL data obtained? After providing a brief definition of HRQL, we consider some of the factors that may influence the quality of HRQL and other types of self-report data in clinical research involving older populations.

Defining health-related quality of life

A number of definitions of HRQL have been put forward over the past several years [2, 4, 5]. Although there are some discrepancies among definitions, the overlap is far greater than the differences. For the purposes of this chapter we define HRQL as '. . . those attributes valued by patients, including: resultant comfort or sense of well-being; the extent to which they were able to maintain reasonable physical, emotional, and intellectual function; and the degree to which they retained their ability to participate in valued activities within the

145

P.J. Walter (ed.), Coronary Bypass Surgery in the Elderly, pp. 145–154.
© 1995 Kluwer Academic Publishers, Dordrecht.

family, in the workplace, and in the community' [6]. This definition underscores the broad, multi-dimensional nature of the concept HRQL, and reflects the individual's personal perceptions of his or her well-being and functioning. Dimensions commonly associated with HRQL, include, at a minimum, physical and social functioning, mental and psychological well-being, and overall life satisfaction. In addition, HRQL researchers often include measures of energy and vitality, intimacy, sleep disturbance, disease-specific symptoms and pain perceptions [7].

There is no question that the concepts contained in HRQL are as important to older patients as they are to the general population. As noted by Williams and others [8, 9], the primary goal of elderly persons in terms of life quality is that they 'maintain or regain as much personal independence as possible'. However, due to a variety of factors associated with aging (e.g., increases in co-morbid conditions) there may be measurement concerns specific to an older cohort that must be attended to in order to obtain valid and reliable HRQL data.

Measurement issues in older populations

A number of factors can influence the quality of data obtained from self-report measures like those used in HRQL assessments. Most of these factors are relevant to all populations, not simply older people. That is, most of the concerns that threaten the validity of data obtained from an older person can apply to data obtained from a younger person. The critical difference is that many of the factors that threaten data quality are more prevalent in older people. For example, losses in visual and auditory acuity, fatigue, and co-morbid conditions can influence the quality of self-reported data. Although these conditions occur at all ages, they are more common in the elderly.

Ageism

At a very basic level, when discussing measurement problems in older cohorts, one must consider the issue of ageism or prejudice based solely on age [10]. Certain assumptions are often made about all older people that can influence an investigator's willingness to assess HRQL. For example, a survey researcher noted that one should 'design and interview (for the elderly) in the expectation that respondents' comprehension and concentration will be low' [quoted in 10]. However, the elderly are a heterogenous group of individuals and among most older cohorts of respondents there will exist highly varied levels of understanding and ability. Cognitive decline is not an inevitable aspect of aging. Furthermore, older respondents are often cooperative and willing to give more time to clinical investigators than are younger respondents. However, if an investigator enters into HRQL data collection from the elderly with the assumption that the respondents have a limited ability to understand and concentrate, the types of questions posed and the breadth of the data covered will be pre-determined. Ultimately, such assumptions will influence the data obtained and become a 'self-fulfilling prophecy' in that the investigators have, *a priori*, presumed that older people are only capable of providing a limited range of information with respect to their HRQL.

Similarly, assumptions are made regarding what dimensions of HRQL are important to older people, and the range of experiences they are likely to report. For example, measures of intimacy and sexual functioning may be excluded from HRQL assessments in older patients as intimacy is assumed to be non-relevant or embarrassing to an older cohort. Also, measures of physical functioning may exclude the higher ranges of activity since older people are often perceived as a relatively inactive group. Thus, in addition to selecting measures to cover all of the major dimensions of HRQL that are of potential relevance to older people and that may be affected by cardiovascular disease (CVD), for example, or such treatments as CABG surgery, a critical factor is the sensitivity of the content of each measure to the ranges of patients' levels of functioning at study baseline, and to changes (i.e., responsiveness of the measure) during a study period.

With regard to sensitivity, an optimal instrument will produce scores which are spread across the full range of functioning or health state. Instruments with skewed distributions of scores, such as clusters of scores at the lower (floor) and upper (ceiling) levels of functioning, will not permit possibly clinically significant distinctions among low or high scorers, and will not be responsive to deterioration or improvement in functioning in persons at the scale's minimum or maximum, respectively [11, 12].

It is common knowledge in public health that heterogeneity in health status is actually larger, not smaller, in older adult populations than in younger adults. However, there may be some uncertainty over diversity in the health status among older adults with disease. As noted, common assumptions about aging and chronic diseases are that people with illness experience sharply reduced functional capacity, and that there is a high prevalence of multiple co-morbidity, frailty, and inactivity [13]. Among clinicians, these generalizations may be reinforced by referral and treatment patterns in acute care facilities which over-select persons with multiple co-morbidity who are sicker or more severely ill than the general population with the same conditions. A much higher level of functioning is typical in epidemiological research designs which recruit community-living study participants. Here, many of the severely disabled persons have been selected out of the sampling frame by the fact of their institutionalization. Efforts to recruit the more severely ill in clinical studies tend to exclude elders who are homebound, have difficulty with ambulation, or rely on skilled medical care [14]. Thus, the range in level of functioning sought in an HRQL measure for older adults with chronic disease may need to be broader, rather than narrower, than those used in general patient populations of younger adults.

From existing national survey data in the United States, the health characteristics of subpopulations of older adults may be variously defined in terms of general functional status and morbidity. These data can provide a useful referent when selecting an HRQL measure for patient samples. For example, we know that approximately 32% of community-dwelling persons in the United States who self-reported prevalent ischemic heart disease (IHD) also report being limited in major activities [15]. Viewed differently, the majority of persons with IHD (i.e., 68%) in this sampling frame reported no major functional disability. Co-morbidity is another characteristic which disadvantages older patient populations with respect to the assumed appropriate measures of HRQL. Although the prevalence of multiple morbidity does increase with age, nearly one-third of community-living older adults report only one prevalent chronic condition, such as CVD, and between one-half and two-thirds of older adults report having only two chronic conditions. Thus, in general, significant proportions of older adults with a chronic health condition do not have known multiple co-morbidities [15]. Finally, it is noteworthy that, in older adults, the variability in functional levels found across levels of social class is substantially larger than that obtained for other ages [15].

A final issue which underscores the need for HRQL measures with ample range of functioning levels with older populations is responsiveness to treatment. Epidemiological studies of elderly adults have been illuminating. Where it was previously assumed that functionally disabled persons are in continuously declining health, descriptive studies have documented that a sizeable proportion of disabled persons will in fact regain functioning in one or more areas of activity over time [13, 16]. For example, in the Longitudinal Study on Aging (LSOA), a descriptive study of older adults in the United States, 11% of older adults self-reporting arthritis who were living in the community at the time of the initial interview reported improvement in their functioning two years later (R.T. Anderson, pers. comm.). Similar results have been obtained in representative samples of United States older adults [13]. The likelihood of substantial gains in functioning in older adults with chronic diseases may be even greater in interventions like CABG surgery. Thus, in selecting HRQL instruments for older patients, investigators must attend to both the broad heterogeneity of older patients at baseline, and the potential for improvement in HRQL over time.

Methods to ensure that an appropriate measurement range is incorporated into an HRQL measure under consideration includes a careful review of the psychometric data available on the instrument in older adult samples. The validity of the measure, particularly an instrument's ability to discriminate among 'known groups' of patients that differ in level or type of disability or functional state, or its correspondence to a known criterion is helpful. The instrument's 'floor' and 'ceiling' should also be directly reviewed. For example, norms reported for the Medical Outcome Study (MOS) Short-form 36 (SF-36) scales (range 0–100) for patients with congestive heart failure [17] reveal that a significant proportion of patients obtain the maximum score (highest level of functioning) in the Social Functioning subscale (38%) and Role-Emotional functioning subscale (53%). Almost 44% and 20% of the patients score at the minimum level of Role-Physical and Role-Emotional functioning, respectively. In contrast, the Vitality, Mental Health and Physical Functioning subscales appear to produce a broad range of scores for this patient population, having only small floor and ceiling effects. In a situation such as this, the investigators may find it imperative to increase the maximum or minimum levels of role functioning assessed by supplementing the HRQL instrument with a disease- or condition-specific measure, or to select a different HRQL measure altogether. Interestingly, the ranges in the SF-36 subscales noted above appear limited for less severely ill patients as well [17, 18].

The above example underscores the care needed to ensure adequate measurement of functional status of severely ill adults of any age. The critical point is that older patients are a highly variable group with respect to all dimensions of HRQL, and to attenuate scale ranges or limit the HRQL dimensions assessed will decrease the quality of data obtained and the investigator's ability to detect important treatment or disease effects. Each study group, as well as the planned intervention and its effects, must be carefully considered.

Life satisfaction measures in older and older adults

Major theoretical models of HRQL [1, 6] emphasize both functional capacity and subjective appraisals of life satisfaction. In older adult patient populations, however, relatively high levels of life satisfaction have been obtained despite the existence of severe illness or functional limitations [19, 20]. These results suggest that global life satisfaction measures may be insensitive to clinically significant differences in health status among older patient groups. Research on theoretical models of life satisfaction supports the view that this is a complex phenomenon [21, 22] and appears to be a synthesis of experiences in various life domains including, health conditions, personality characteristics, life views, emotional status [20], feelings of usefulness [23], past aspirations and plans [22], cognitive skills [24], and financial situation [20, 22]. Different experiences and life domains are assigned different weights in life satisfaction across age, gender, and social class groups [22]. For example, the expectations and aspirations regarding physical functioning for older adults with functional disability may shift from vigorous physical and recreational activity, to achieving or maintaining independence in the community and social integration. Therefore, the impact of a given health condition on an individual's goals, aspirations, and sense of mastery or accomplishment may change markedly with age.

Despite the potential for substantial heterogeneity in determinants of life satisfaction across individuals and life stages, measures of subjective well-being remain important clinical research tools because they can directly assess whether the effects of an intervention or treatment can be interpreted more broadly in terms of enhancing one's lifestyle or success in an individual's attainment of goals. Ultimately, these are the outcomes that patients desire. Thus, assessing life satisfaction can supplement functional assessments by keeping the patient's perspective as the central focus of the study.

Since a disease or its treatment can effect lifestyle differently among individuals, optimizing HRQL may be best achieved with individualized therapy [25] based on a patient's needs or preferences. Domain-specific life satisfaction measures can provide valuable data on the various HRQL dimensions (e.g., financial, productivity) affected by a given health condition weighted by the importance of that dimension to the patient.

Ambiguity and sensitivity

Poor wording in questions, or response formats, can produce missing or inaccurate data. A failure to respond to a question may be attributed to lack of comprehension when, in fact, it may be due to a problem in the wording of the question [26]. This mis-attribution is more likely to occur with older than younger patients. That is, investigators may assume that when errors occur in interviews with older respondents, the errors are due to declines in cognitive functioning of the respondents rather than in problems in the design of the question. Yet in one series of studies on survey research methods with older respondents, investigators did not find support for this assumption [26]. Error rates were not correlated with age when 'factual survey questions' were used and data were checked against 'external records' [26]. As noted by these same investigators, however, there is evidence that subjective questions (such as those used in HRQL instruments) may be more susceptible to measurement error in older versus younger respondents and this age-related difference may be due, in part, to the fact that older respondents are more influenced than the young by the formatting and structure of questions [26].

Evidence regarding differences in data quality (missing or inaccurate data), response sets, and acquiescence across age groups remains open to question. Some studies have found that self-report data obtained from older adults had lower internal consistency and reliability [27, 28], a larger number of missing items [29], and more socially desirable responses [30]. However, these studies do not distinguish between the effects of aging, per se, and the effects of chronic diseases, the latter of which may differ substantially across participant age groups.

In a study of MOS patients [31], investigators found that after controlling for disease severity and cognitive impairment, high quality self-report data on health and functional status could be reliably collected in older adults. The investigators found good validity, and only small differences attributable to age in reliability, item acquiescence, and noncommittal or neutral responses for the scales tested. While their results indicate that missing data are more likely among older versus younger respondents, the proportion of persons with missing data was relatively small, and usually involved only a single item missing on one or more subscales [31, 32].

In summary, rigorous studies of HRQL measures in older adults support the premise that HRQL assessments which rely on clear, unambiguously worded questions, and do not pose excessive response burdens, are as feasible for older adults as they are for younger patient populations. As a general rule, patient populations with a high prevalence of co-morbid diseases or impairments, regardless of age, may require mixed modes of form administration (e.g., self- and interviewer-administered) and questionnaire formats (e.g., larger font size, non-scannable forms) to accommodate the wide range in health status likely to be encountered. In addition, it is critical that questions be thoroughly pre-tested with older cohorts to determine that respondents understand the intent of the questions.

The issue of question sensitivity is common when discussing older respondents. That is, there is a recurring theme in survey literature that older people are more sensitive to certain types of questions and more likely to become emotional or distressed when queried about certain aspects of their lives. However, hard data, comparing emotionality among older and younger respondents are not available [31]. As noted by Carp [10], the critical issue is to identify those questions or subscales that may be threatening or sensitive for any population and introduce them properly to the respondent either with written instructions or by an interviewer. Also, it should be recognized that the fact that a question creates an emotional response does not, primae facie, render it bad or good.

Position effects

Respondents are influenced by the position of scales within a group of instruments or the position of an item in a single, multi-item scale. When using multiple instruments, it is often recommended that the order of presentation be randomized for each respondent in order to reduce such position effects. For example, it is known that after completing a depression scale some individuals' moods may be altered and this mood change could influence their responses to subsequent scales and measures. However, it is not often practical to randomize instrument ordering, especially when studying HRQL in large, multi-site clinical trials or national surveys. Therefore, it is incumbent upon the investigators to keep this potential bias in mind and order measures accordingly.

Older people are no more or less sensitive to position effects than younger respondents [31]. However, investigators should be concerned about the effects of fatigue on scale order and whether or not a particular patient population is more or less likely to become fatigued during the assessment process. For example, sicker patients are more likely to become fatigued than well people. The critical issue is to be aware of the fact that there could be loss of data toward the end of a group of measures and, if this is acknowledged at study onset, than the investigators can either reduce the length of the measures for all potential respondents, or put those scales at the end of the group of measures that are least important to the overall investigation.

Gatekeepers

One of the most critical issues in data collection that occurs with most cohorts but is more common among the elderly and the very young are gatekeepers [10]. That is, the individuals who interfere with the collection of information from the target patient. Gatekeepers can be both formal (e.g., physicians and nurses in medical settings) and informal (e.g., the patients' spouses or friends and family). In most cases, these individuals have the patient's best interests in mind and consider the collection of data from the individual to be a threat to the patient's emotional and physical well-being. HRQL data are often perceived as particularly threatening by health providers and family members due to the personal nature of such data. Thus, it is important for the investigators to properly educate the 'gatekeepers' regarding the rationale behind the collection of HRQL information.

In addition to guarding against access to the patients, formal and informal gatekeepers may influence the responses given to the questions on surveys. This is a particular problem when the investigator relies on mail-out surveys since he or she has no control over who 'helps' the respondent. In in-person interviews conducted in a medical setting when, for example, the respondent's spouse is present, there is a strong and natural inclination for the spouse to assist and protect the patient. This is true across all ages, but more likely to occur with older patients where both patient and spouse are out of the work force, the spouse often accompanies the patient to office visits, and the couple have a long history with one another. This problem can sometimes be minimized by explaining to the patient and spouse that it is important that the information come just from the patient, or by actually interviewing the patient in a separate room.

Proxy or surrogate respondents

Sometimes it is not possible to collect data directly from the target person and the investigator must rely on responses given for the patient by a proxy. Though proxy data may be collected at any age, it is more often relied upon in older ages due to co-morbidities and the assumption that an older person will be too 'taxed' by interviewing him or her directly. Most often the proxy is a spouse or close family friend, though a proxy can be anyone familiar with the patient. Studies conducted that compare proxy data to respondent-derived data indicate a low correlation between the two data sources. There are many factors that could explain this low relationship, including the fact that proxies do not have direct access to the HRQL of patients unless these issues have been discussed between them. Further, the more subjective the data collected (for example, measures of mood and emotional well-being), the less likely it will be that a proxy will provide similar responses to those provided by the patient or target person. Finally, investigators should keep in mind that most proxies have a vested interest in the HRQL of the patient and may unknowingly distort the data provided to protect their own self-interests. Thus, regardless of the age of the respondent, one should not use proxy data unless absolutely necessary.

Summary

To summarize, there are a number of factors that influence the quality of data obtained when collecting HRQL information from an older cohort. Most of these concerns are relevant to all age groups and should be considered whenever one is constructing or using an HRQL instrument. However, it is true that several factors are more likely to occur in older patient cohorts and should be carefully assessed prior to embarking on a full scale study. At the same time, the investigators should be certain that they have not allowed unfounded assumptions about the elderly regarding such things as the importance of certain issues to older people, the capabilities of the population, or the range of potential responses to a given scale or dimension of HRQL, to inappropriately influence the investigator's choices of instruments or the HRQL dimensions addressed within a given study.

References

1. Shumaker SA, Anderson R, Czajkowski SM. Psychological models of quality of life. In: Spilker B, editor. Quality of life assessments in clinical trials. New York: Raven Press, 1990.
2. Patrick DL, Bergner M. Measurement of health status in the 1990s. Ann Rev Public Health 1990; 11: 165–83.
3. Andrews FM, Herzog AR. The quality of survey data as related to age of respondent. J Am Stat Assoc 1986, 81: 403–9.
4. Schron E, Shumaker SA. The integration of health quality of life in clinical research: experiences from cardiovascular clinical trials. Prog Cardiovasc Nurs 1992; 7: 21–8.
5. Croog SH. Current issues in conceptualizing and measuring quality of life. In: Furberg CD, Schuttinga JA, editors. Quality of life assessment: practice, problems, and promise. NIH Publication No. 93–3503. Washington DC: US Govt Printing Office.
6. Wenger N, Furberg CD. Cardiovascular disorders. In: Spilker B, editor. Quality of life assessments in clinical trials. New York: Raven Press, 1990.
7. Berzon R, Shumaker SA. A critical review of cross national health-related quality of life instruments. Qual Life Newsl 1992; 5: 1–2.
8. Williams TF. Geriatrics: a perspective on quality of life and care of older people. In: Spilker B, editor. Quality of life assessments in clinical trials. New York: Raven Press, 1990.
9. Fretwell MD. The frail elderly: creating standards of care. In: Spilker B, editor. Quality of life assessments in clinical trials. New York: Raven Press, 1990.
10. Carp FM. Maximizing data quality in community studies of older people. In: Lawton MP, Herzog AR, editors. Special research methods for gerontology. Amityville, NY: Baywood, 1989.
11. Wilkin D, Hallam L, Doggett MA. Measures of need and outcome for primary health care. New York: Oxford University Press, 1992.
12. Streiner DL, Norman GR. Health Measurement Scales – a practical guide to their development and use. New York: Oxford University Press, 1989.
13. Suzman RM, Harris T, Hadley EC, Kovar MG, Weindruch R. The robust oldest old: optimistic

perspectives for increasing healthy life expectancy. In: Suzman RM, Willis, Manton KG, editors. The oldest old. New York: Oxford University Press, 1992.

14. Tell GS, Fried LP, Hermanson B, Manolio TA, Newman AB, Borhani NO. Recruitment of adults 65 years and older as participants in the cardiovascular health study. AEP 1993; 3(4):358–66.

15. National Center for Health Statistics. National Health Interview Survey: supplement on aging (NHIS-SOA). Washington, DC: Department of Health and Human Services, 1984.

16. Suzman RM, Manton KG, Willis DP, editors. The oldest old. New York: Oxford University Press, 1992.

17. Ware Jr. JE, Snow KK, Kosinski M, Gandek B. SF-36 health survey manual and interpretation guide. Massachusetts, 1993.

18. Anderson RT, Aaronson NK, Wilkin D. Critical review of the international assessments of health-related quality of life. Quality Life Res 1993; 2: 369–95.

19. Sullivan JG, Higginbotham MB, Cobb FR. Exercise training in patients with severe left ventricular dysfunction. Circulation 1988; 78: 506–5.

20. Stolar GE, MacEntee MI, Hill P. Seniors' assessment of their health and life satisfaction: the case for contextual evaluation. Intern J Aging Hum Devel 1992; 35(4): 305–17.

21. Hornquist JO, Hansson B, Akerlind I, Larsson J. Severity of disease and quality of life: a comparison in patients with cancer and benign disease. Qual of Life Res 1992; 1(2): 135–41.

22. Krause N. Race differences in life satisfaction among aged men and women. J Geron 1993; 48(5): S235–44.

23. Krause N. Stressful events and life satisfaction among elderly men and women. J Geron 1991; 46(2): S84–92.

24. Gray GR, Ventis DG, Hayslip B Jr. Socio-cognitive skills as a determinant of life satisfaction in aged persons. Intern J Aging Hum Devel 1992; 35(3): 205–18.

25. Wenger NK. Quality of life: concept and approach to measurement. Adv Card 1986; 33: 122–30.

26. Herzog R, Rodgers WL. The use of survey methods in research on older Americans. In: Wallace R, editor. The epidemiologic study of the elderly. New York: Oxford University Press. In press.

27. Alwin DF, Krosnick J. Aging, cohorts, and the stability of sociopolitical orientations over the life span. Amer J Socio 1991; 97: 169–95.

28. Andrews FM, Herzog AR. The quality of survey data as related to age of respondent. J Amer Stat Assoc 1986; 81: 403–10.

29. Gergen KJ, Back KW. Communication in the interview and the disengaged respondent. Public Opinion Quart 1966; 30: 385–98.

30. Campbell A, Converse PE, Rodgers LR. The quality of American life. New York: Sage, 1976.

31. Sherbourne CD, Meredith LS. Quality of self-report data: a comparison of older and younger chronically ill patients. J Geron Soc Sci 1992; 47(4): S204–11.

32. McHorney CA, Ware Jr. JE, Lu JFR, Sherbourne CD. The MOS 36-item short-form health survey (SF-36): III. Tests of data quality, scaling assumptions, and reliability across diverse patient groups. Med Care 1994; 32(1): 40–62.

15. Survival and health-related quality of life of elderly patients undergoing cardiac surgery

NOREEN CAINE, SUSAN TAIT and JOHN WALLWORK

Introduction

With an increasing number of elderly patients being referred for cardiac surgery, it is important to assess outcome in terms of quality of life alongside the more traditional measures of survival and morbidity. This was recognised at Papworth Hospital in the mid-1980s when this project was planned; in 1985, 20% of all cardiac surgery patients at Papworth were in the 65 year and older age groups and by 1991 this had increased to 40%. The first step was to conduct a retrospective long-term survival analysis involving all cardiac surgery patients aged 65 and older who underwent surgery during the 12-year period from January 1973 to December 1984 [1]. This was followed by a prospective study of the health-related quality of life and resource use of all patients accepted onto the waiting list for cardiac surgery during the period July 1990 to December 1991.

Retrospective survival analysis

Using a simple questionnaire sent to patients' general practitioners, complete follow-up data was obtained for 471 of the 562 patients who underwent cardiac surgery at Papworth Hospital during the period from January 1973 to December 1984. Of the remaining 91 patients, 73 were not traced and 18 were known to have died but the date of death was not available. These 91 were therefore excluded from the survival analysis but were compared in terms of age, sex and type of operation with the patients who were traced, in order, for the 73, to assess whether they were less likely to have survived, or, for the 18, to assess whether they were less likely to have survived as long. Most of the patients received either valve surgery (62%) or coronary artery bypass grafting (CABG) (21%) which was introduced in this centre in the 65 years and older patients in 1977. Early mortality, defined as death within 30 days of operation, or death before leaving hospital, was 7.3% (41/562) in the whole group, 5% (19/349) in the valve patients and 0% (0/117) for the CABG group.

P.J. Walter (ed.), Coronary Bypass Surgery in the Elderly, pp. 155–166.

The survival rates for the 471 patients in whom follow-up data was complete were 88.0% at one year, 74.4% at five years and 46.5% at ten years. When analysed by age, comparing the 65–69 group with the 70 and older group, older age was shown to have a slightly adverse effect but there was no statistically significant difference between the two groups ($p = 0.1$). In a multifactorial analysis stratified by type of operation, the relative annual risk of death associated with being aged 70 or older, was 1.45. Indeed the type of operation was the only important factor in predicting survival ($p < 0.001$), as demonstrated in Figure 15.1.

The 73 patients who were not traced were found to be no different in age, sex and type of operation than the 471 who were traced, but a higher proportion of the 73 had been operated on before 1980. However, time of operation was not found to be an important factor in predicting survival. No differences were found between the 18 patients in whom the date of death was unknown and the 81 patients who died and for whom the time of death was known.

Perhaps the most significant finding in this study came from the comparison of the observed survival experience in the study population with the life expectancy of the general population in these age groups. For the 430 patients who survived to leave hospital, i.e. excluding the 41 early deaths, the observed survival rates were 96.3% at one year and 81.5% at five years. The corresponding expected rates in the general population, using 1988 mortality statistics for England and Wales [2], were 96.4% at one and 88.0% at five years. Thus, the survival experience of patients who survived the first month after surgery was very similar to that of people aged > 65 in the general population.

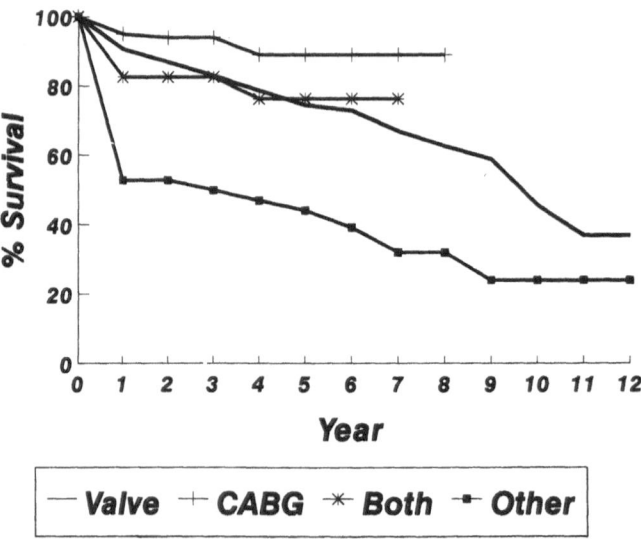

Figure 15.1. survival experience by type of operation (n = 471).

Prospective quality of life study

Having established that patients in the 65 years and older age groups could expect good outcome in terms of longevity, the next step was to establish the quality of the life experienced by these patients before and after surgery. By 1991, the proportion of cardiac surgery patients in these older age groups had risen to 40% of the total practice at Papworth hospital. The aims of the study were to determine the changes in health-related quality of life (HRQOL) experienced by elderly patients at intervals before and after cardiac surgery, and to identify the resource implications of an increasing number of operations being performed on elderly patients.

Study design

A prospective design was considered important in order to measure changes in quality of life both before and after surgery. Two comparison groups were included in the study design: just as in the survival analysis we sought to compare patient survival with life expectancy in the community, in the quality of life analysis we needed to compare outcome with the expected quality of life in the general population in these age groups. To this end, 150 randomly selected elderly people, matched for age, sex and location with the study population, were interviewed using the same health status questionnaires. The second comparison group was designed to test the assumption that the elderly use more hospital resources than younger patients during their admission for cardiac surgery. Resource use data was collected for a group of under 65 year old cardiac surgery patients, matched for type of operation and undergoing surgery during the study period.

The study population consisted of 154 patients aged 65 years and older accepted onto the cardiac surgery waiting list during the period July 1990–December 1991. Emergency cases not admitted from the waiting list were excluded from the study because of the need to establish baseline data in a pre-surgery interview.

The interviews were conducted by the same research assistant and took place in patients' homes at the time of acceptance onto the waiting list, at three monthly intervals pre-surgery and at three and twelve months after surgery. One interview, aimed mainly at testing cognitive function, took place in-hospital at seven days after surgery. The interview structure and content were tested and refined in a pilot study with a sample of 20 patients who had recently been accepted onto the cardiac surgery waiting list. The resulting interview had four main components:

The *Cardiac Surgery in the Elderly Questionnaire* (*CASE-Q*) is a combination of basic sociodemographic queries, medical and drug histories, an activities of daily living scale, symptom and activity Likert type scales, and queries regarding community health and social services resource use.

The *Nottingham Health Profile* (*NHP*) [3] is one of the most widely used measures of general health status in the UK. Part I consists of 38 questions in the six dimensions of physical mobility, energy, pain, sleep, social isolation and emotional reactions. A score from 0–100 can be calculated for each dimension, with a higher score indicating more extensive problems. In Part II of the NHP, patients are asked to indicate which areas of their daily lives are being affected by their current state of health.

The *Hospital Anxiety and Depression Scale* measures mood state and is a non somatic instrument in that none of its scale items refer to physical states which may confound with emotional health status [4].

A set of five *Cognitive Function tests*, selected to give an appropriate combination for measuring aspects of memory and concentration in this age group.

Statistical methods

For NHP Part I dimensions, mean scores are presented so that they can be compared with other published studies and with NHP norms [3], although it is recognised that the distributions are not Gaussian. Other data is presented as frequency distributions.

Since data is asymmetrical and discontinuous, non-parametric inference tests have been used: the Wilcoxon matched pairs signed rank test to compare NHP Part I scores before and after surgery and the McNemar test for Part II.

For the HAD responses, symptoms and mobility, where results are ordered categories (or Likert scales), for example, 'Never', 'Occasionally', 'Some of the time', 'Most of the time', 'Always', the data was dichotomised due to the small numbers in each of the cells. (HAD: scores 0–7 = 0, > 7 = 1; Symptoms: no symptoms = 0, symptoms = 1; Mobility: no restriction = 1, restrictions = 2). McNemar's test was used to compare frequencies before and after surgery for these measures.

Results

Of the 154 patients accepted for surgery during the study period, 2 patients did not wish to continue with the study after the initial interview, and 3 patients were withdrawn from surgery by their doctor. One patient refused surgery, 1 patient moved away from the area and 2 patients were dropped from the study because of language/compliance problems. After surgery a further 2 patients withdrew from the study and 1 patient was too ill to be interviewed at one year after surgery. There was 1 death prior to surgery and 11 deaths in the first year after surgery.

This resulted in 130 of the original 154 patients completing the study, from acceptance onto the waiting list to one year after surgery. The mean age of the 130 patients was 70 years, with a range of 65–82 years; 83 were male and 47 female and the average waiting time to surgery was 8 months (range 2–19 months). Most patients were suffering from ischaemic and/or valvular heart disease with 70 (54%) patients undergoing coronary artery bypass grafting, 44 (34%) valve surgery, 14 (11%) combined graft and valve surgery and 2 (1.5%) other surgery.

The quality of life analysis presented below is based on the same 130 patients who completed interviews both at acceptance to the waiting list and at one year after cardiac surgery, of whom 126 completed interviews at three months after surgery. The main focus of the analysis is the observed changes in general health status, mood state, symptom frequency and activity restrictions, comparing the baseline figures at acceptance for surgery with those at three and twelve months after surgery.

Nottingham health profile
The mean scores from Part I of the NHP at acceptance for surgery and at three and twelve months after surgery are given in Figure 15.2. These indicate improvements in health status in all six dimensions of the profile at three months after surgery. These differences were statistically significant at three months after surgery (p <0.05), with the improvements either maintained or further enhanced at one year. In Part II of the NHP, the areas of daily living in which most patients indicated a problem, pre-surgery, were in looking after the home, social life, hobbies and holidays (Figure 15.3). Again there were statistically significant improvements at three months after surgery, compared with pre-surgery, in all of the seven areas of daily living (p <0.05).

Anxiety and depression
In Figure 15.4, the proportion of patients whose scores on the Hospital Anxiety and Depression Scale indicated anxiety and depression levels above normal are given for time of acceptance for surgery and at three and twelve months after surgery. Pre-surgery, 52 (42%) patients had above normal anxiety levels,

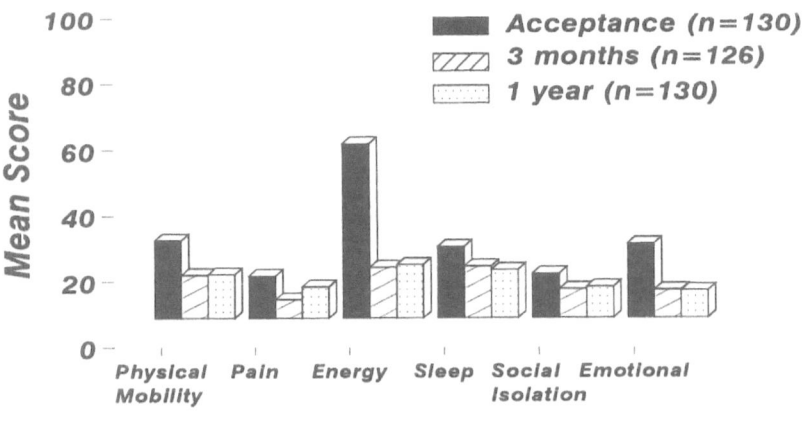

Figure 15.2. Nottingham Health Profile: Part I. Mean scores before and after cardiac surgery.

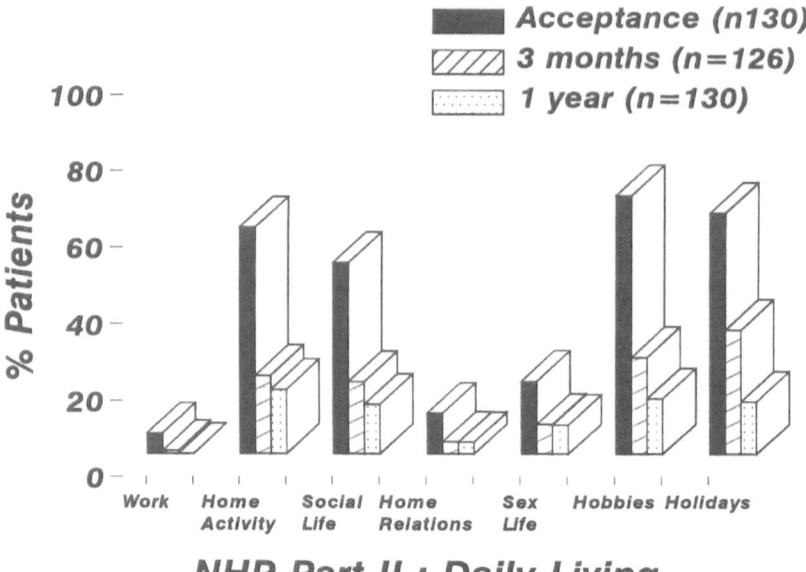

Figure 15.3. Nottingham Health Profile: Part II. Percent patients with problems related to health before and after cardiac surgery.

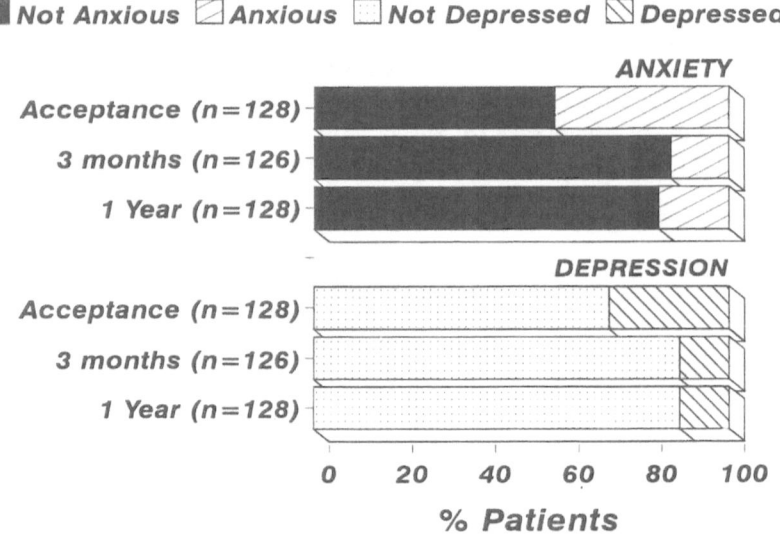

Figure 15.4. Hospital Anxiety & Depression Scale: Frequency of anxiety and depression before and after cardiac surgery.

reducing to 16 (13%) at three months and 22 (17%) at one year after surgery (*p* = 0.0000). Those with depression levels above normal were reduced from 38 patients (30%) pre-surgery to 15 (12%) at three months and one year (*p* = 0.0003). Furthermore there were no patients with above normal scores after surgery who had had normal scores pre-surgery.

Symptoms
Pre-surgery, 75% (97) of all patients, 93% (65) of CABG patients and 46% (20) of valve patients were experiencing chest pain. At three months after surgery these figures had reduced to 20% (25) of all patients, 18% (12) of CABG patients and 21% (9) of valve patients. At one year after surgery the patients saying they had experienced chest pain in the preceding month were 16% (21) of all patients, 16% (11) of CABG and 14% (6) of valve patients. The differences between the baseline measure and one year after surgery were statistically significant with a *p* value of <0.000 for both the whole group and the CABGs, and equal to 0.0013 for the valve group of patients. In Figure 15.5 the frequency of chest pain for all patients at time of acceptance on the waiting list and at three and twelve months after surgery are presented on a five-point Likert scale. Pre-surgery the frequency was distributed between 'occasionally', 'some of the time' and 'most of the time'. After surgery, all but 2% of the 20% of patients suffering chest pain were doing so 'occasionally'.

Breathlessness was experienced by 86% of all patients (112), 80% of CABG patients (56) and 91% of valve patients (40) pre-surgery. At three months after surgery these had reduced to 55% (69), 63% (42) and 40% (17), respectively. By one year after surgery, breathlessness was being experienced by 47% of all patients (61), 47% of CABG (33) and 48% of valve patients (21) (*p* values for

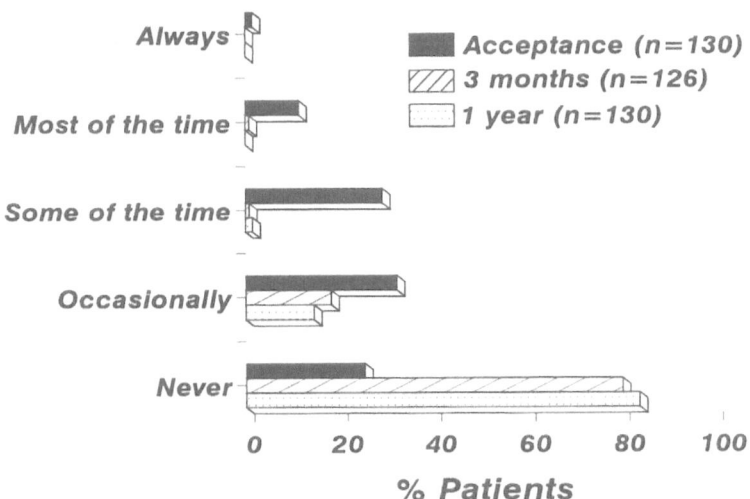

Figure 15.5. Frequency of chest pain before and after cardiac surgery.

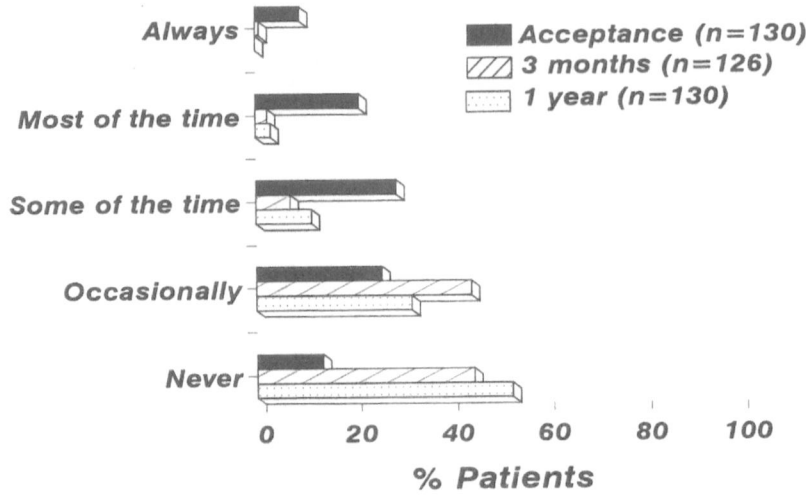

Figure 15.6. Frequency of breathlessness before and after cardiac surgery.

differences pre- and one year after surgery were <0.000 in all three groups). In Figure 15.6 the frequency of breathlessness for all patients at acceptance and at three and twelve months after surgery is presented. Pre-surgery, the frequency among those experiencing breathlessness was distributed across all levels, with 10% of patients saying the condition was constant. After surgery, as with chest pain, for the great majority of patients experiencing breathlessness it was 'occasionally' (90%), although for 7% of patients it was being experienced 'some of the time' and for 3% either 'most of the time' or 'always'.

An important aspect of symptom assessment and its affect on quality of life is a measure of the level of exertion at which symptoms become apparent to the patient. We did this by using a six-point Likert type scale, ranging from 'rest' to 'heavy lifting'. As can be seen in Table 15.1, the distribution on the exertion frequency scale did not change significantly after surgery for patients suffering from chest pain, with 79% of 97 patients saying they had chest pain either at 'rest' or 'walking slowly' pre-surgery, falling to 62% of the 21 patients who were still experiencing chest pain by one year after surgery ($p = 0.2891$). For patients suffering from breathlessness there was a greater improvement, from 70% of 112 patients complaining of breathlessness either at 'rest' or 'walking slowly', pre-surgery, to 28% of 61 patients at one year after surgery (p <0.000).

Mobility and activity restrictions
In order to establish the degree of independence being experienced in day to day mobility and activity, patients were asked to assess their own performance in the following terms: Can you perform this task 'yourself easily', 'yourself with difficulty', 'with help', 'not at all' or is this task never applicable to you? The choice of tasks was derived partly from an adaptation of the Townsend

Table 15.1. Levels of exertion at which patients experienced chest pain and breathlessness, comparing results pre cardiac surgery with those at three and twelve months after surgery

Exertion level	Chest pain						Breathlessness					
	Acceptance (n = 97)		3 months (n = 25)		1 year (n = 21)		Acceptance (n = 112)		3 months (n = 69)		1 year (n = 61)	
	No.	%	No.	%	No.	%	No.	%	No.	%	No.	%
Rest	52	(53.6)	12	(48.0)	11	(52.4)	36	(32.1)	14	(20.3)	10	(16.4)
Walking slowly	25	(25.8)	3	(12.0)	2	(9.5)	42	(37.5)	9	(13.0)	7	(11.5)
Working normally	14	(14.4)	3	(12.0)	6	(28.6)	22	(19.6)	15	(21.7)	19	(31.1)
Climbing stairs	3	(3.1)	2	(8.0)	1	(4.8)	7	(6.3)	10	(14.5)	9	(14.8)
Running	1	(1.0)	2	(8.0)	0	(0.0)	3	(2.7)	18	(26.1)	3	(4.9)
Heavy lifting	1	(1.0)	0	(0.0)	0	(0.0)	2	(1.8)	1	(1.4)	7	(11.5)
Not Applicable	1	(1.0)	3	(12.0)	1	(4.8)	0	(0.0)	2	(2.9)	6	(9.8)
Total	97	(99.9)	25	(100.0)	21	(100.0)	112	(100.0)	69	(99.9)	61	(100.0)

Table 15.2. Mobility and activity: comparison of the frequency with which patients could perform tasks 'yourself easily', pre-cardiac surgery and at one year after surgery

Mobility/activity	Acceptance on waiting list		1 Year after surgery		P Value
	No.	%	No.	%	
Getting out of bed	90	69.2	106	81.5	= 0.0101
Getting out of a chair	90	69.2	105	80.8	= 0.018
Walking downstairs	72	67.3	96	85.0	= 0.003
Walking upstairs	19	17.8	76	67.3	< 0.0001
Walking outside	28	21.5	91	70.0	< 0.0001
Dressing	92	70.8	117	90.0	< 0.0001
Toilet	96	73.8	118	90.8	= 0.0001
Washing	89	69.0	117	90.0	< 0.0001
Bathing	70	54.7	102	78.5	< 0.0001
Light housework	79	74.5	90	89.1	= 0.0005
Cooking	71	66.4	73	85.9	= 0.0001
Vacuuming	46	39.0	72	73.5	< 0.0001
Making beds	32	30.5	58	59.2	< 0.0001
Ironing	48	63.2	51	76.1	= 0.0074
Window cleaning	32	29.4	55	60.0	< 0.0001
Shopping	22	17.5	90	76.9	< 0.0001
Gardening	19	16.4	70	63.1	< 0.0001

Percentages are of those patients for whom the task was considered by them to be applicable to their daily lives.

Disability Scale [5, 6] similar to those of many other researchers [7] and partly from our own pilot study during which patients were asked to specify the activities of most relevance to their daily lives.

As can be seen in <Table 15.2, in all areas there were significant improvements in the number of patients who could perform these tasks with ease and without help, when comparing the results from the interviews at time of acceptance onto the waiting list and at one year after surgery. In mobility, the most striking improvements were in the number of patients who could walk upstairs, a change from 19 (18%) patients before surgery to 76 (67%) patients at one year after surgery (p <0.0001), and in those who could walk outside unaided, from 28 (22%) patients before, compared to 91 (70%) by one year (p <0.0001).

In several areas of activity, like dressing and washing, there was a modest 20% increase, from 70% to 90% of patients who could perform these functions with ease. In other areas there were more marked improvements: from 18% of patients being able to go shopping pre-surgery, compared to 77% who were able to do so unaided after surgery (p <0.0001). Similarly there was a change from 16% to 63% of patients who could manage the gardening (p <0.0001).

Early mortality and survival

Of the original 154 patients accepted for cardiac surgery during the study period, 1 died on the waiting list, 3 patients were withdrawn from surgery by their doctors, 1 refused surgery and 1 moved from the area. Of the remaining 148 patients who underwent surgery, 3 died in the first 30 days (2%), of whom 2 were CABG patients and 1 CABG + valve. A further 8 patients (5%) had died by one year after surgery.

The one year survival rates by type of surgery were 91% for CABG patients, 94% for valve patients and 92% for the combined operation.

Discussion

In many countries, perhaps particularly in the United States, it is now accepted that patients in older age groups should not be denied cardiac surgery on grounds of age alone [8]. The debate more recently has shifted from whether or not patients over a particular age should receive surgery, to the predictive value of a variety of risk factors which need to be taken into account when making decisions regarding older patients access to surgery [8–12]. It is clear from this study that the symptomatic benefit most patients derived from their surgery is enabling them to enjoy a greater independence in their day to day lives, compared to pre-surgery. However, we need a better understanding of the factors which are predictive of no or little improvement.

It is also becoming increasingly accepted that the outcome measures used to judge the benefits of cardiac surgery, in all age groups, should include a range of health-related quality of life assessments [13]. These should be used alongside rather than instead of the more traditional objective measures of early mortality, survival and morbidity, in order to provide the full picture from the patient's point of view. We would argue that it is important to include both generic and disease/age specific measures [13–15], and to conduct a prospective study, allowing 'real time' data collection and therefore proper analysis of any changes before and after surgery. Our study has demonstrated that it is feasible for elderly people, even those in some distress while waiting for surgery, to complete an interview lasting one to one and a half hours, which incorporates both generic and specific questionnaires and a range of cognitive function tests. A compliance rate in excess of 95% was achieved.

However, even when presented with evidence of acceptable risk and benefit, there are more subtle obstacles to access to health care for the elderly, which need to be recognised. We refer in particular to the length of waiting lists and the consequent longer waiting times involved for both investigation and surgery. In the U.K., general practitioners may refrain from referring elderly patients for cardiac surgery and indeed other forms of treatment, due to the likelihood that if they do refer, the waiting times would lengthen to such an extent that more and perhaps younger patients may die before they could be treated [16].

Informed by these debates, further analysis from our study will include assessments of the affect on both outcomes and resource use of a range of preoperative risk factors, including waiting times. Another important analysis will be the comparison of the health-related quality of life of the study population after surgery with that of the general population sample. The hypothesis to be tested is that the patients who survive cardiac surgery are returned to the kind of health related quality of life which might be expected for this age group. It is hoped that such analyses will contribute to a better informed and therefore a more explicit and rational decision making process; thus ensuring that the patients being selected for cardiac surgery will be those for whom there is the highest chance of benefit.

Acknowledgements

The retrospective survival analysis would not have been possible without the help of the general practitioners through whom we traced our cardiac surgery patients. In the prospective quality of life studies our thanks are due to the patients for taking part and to the British Heart Foundation for their financial support.

References

1. Livesey S, Caine N, Spiegelhalter DJ, English TAH, Wallwork J. Cardiac surgery for patients aged 65 years and older: a longterm survival analysis. Br Heart J 1988; 60: 480–4.
2. Office of Population Censuses and Surveys. Mortality statistics: review of the registrar general on deaths in England and Wales, series DH1, no. 13. London: HMSO, 1984.
3. Hunt SM, McEwan J, McKenna SP. Measuring health status. London: Croom Helm, 1986.
4. Zigmond AS, Snaith RP. The Hospital Anxiety & Depression Scale. Acta Psychiatr Scand 1983; 67: 361–70.
5. Townsend P. The last refuge. London: Routledge and Kegan Paul, 1962.
6. Townsend P. Poverty in the United Kingdom. Harmondsworth: Pelican, 1979.
7. Bowling A. Measuring health: a review of quality of life measurement scales. Milton Keynes: Open University Press, 1991.
8. Royal College of Physicians Working Group. Cardiological intervention in elderly patients. J R Coll Physicians London 1991; 25: 197–205.
9. Loop FD, Lytle BW, Cosgrove DM, et al. Coronary artery bypass graft surgery in the elderly: indications and outcome. Cleveland Clin J Med 1988; 55: 23–34.
10. Edmunds LH, Stephenson LW, Edie RN, Ratcliffe MB. Open-heart surgery in octogenarians. N Engl J Med 1988; 319: 131–6.
11. Elder AT, Cameron EWJ. Cardiac surgery in the elderly. Br Med J 1989; 299: 140–1.
12. Pifarré R. Open heart operations in the elderly: changing risk parameters. Ann Thoracic Sur 1993; 56: S71–3.
13. Mayou R, Bryant B. Quality of life in cardiovascular disease. Br Heart J 1993; 69: 460–6.
14. Fletcher AE, Gore SM, Jones DR, Fitzpatrick R, Spiegelhalter DJ, Cox DR. Quality of life measures in health care II: design, analysis and interpretation. Br Med J 1992; 305: 1145–8.
15. Cox DR, Fitzpatrick R, Fletcher AE, Gore SM, Janer DR, Spiegelhalter DJ. Quality of life assessment: can we keep it simple? J R Stat Soc 1992; 155: 353–93.
16. Le Fanu J. Never too old to be saved. The Times 1993; 27 April.

16. Health-related quality of life after coronary revascularization in older patients

PAUL D. CLEARY, EDWARD GUADAGNOLI and
JOHN Z. AYANIAN

Introduction

Clinicians and researchers increasingly are recognizing the limitations of using only measures of physiologic function and mortality as measures of the effectiveness of medical and surgical treatment. As a consequence, there is growing interest in the use of more comprehensive, patient-based measures of health-related quality of life (HRQL) to evaluate medical care. This is especially true with respect to the evaluation of cardiac surgery [1], partly because symptom relief and improvement in functioning are such central goals for the treatment of many patients. Recently, there has been a great deal of interest in assessing the relative effectiveness of coronary artery bypass grafting (CABG) and percutaneous transluminal coronary angioplasty (PTCA) in older, compared to younger, patients [2, 3]. In this chapter, we report data from two completed studies and describe a study currently being conducted that address this issue. These studies are: (a) a study of HRQL before and after treatment for six medical and surgical conditions, including CABG, in six academic medical centers in California and Massachusetts; (b) a study of HRQL before and after treatment for selected medical and surgical conditions, including CABG, at Brigham and Women's Hospital (BWH) in Boston; and (c) a study of HRQL in a probability sample of persons over the age of 65 who were hospitalized for a heart attack in New York or Texas. We refer to these studies as the Six Hospital Study, the BWH Study and the AMI PORT (Acute Myocardial Infarction Patient Outcome Research Team) Study, respectively.

One goal of this chapter is to review data from the first two studies showing that the HRQL scales used can differentiate among different medical and surgical treatments, in terms of their impact on HRQL. A second goal is to compare the impact of CABG in younger and older patients. A third goal is to summarize some of the difficulties of making inferences from observational studies of clinical populations and review one study design that we think has the potential of providing important new information in this area.

P.J. Walter (ed.), Coronary Bypass Surgery in the Elderly, pp. 167–177.
© 1995 *Kluwer Academic Publishers, Dordrecht.*

Health-related quality of life

There are several dimensions that capture most of the elements that individuals consider when they discuss quality of life [4–8]. These include disease-specific symptoms, general health perception, somatic discomfort, physical, social and role functioning, cognitive functioning, and psychological well-being [8–17]. In the studies reported herein we used measures that included a battery of generic subscales, the Functional Status Questionnaire (FSQ) [18] and condition-specific measures of angina, dyspnea, and cardiac capacity [19].

The six hospital study

The Six Hospital Study was an investigation of variations in case-mix, process of care, and outcomes in six acute care, university-affiliated, teaching hospitals in California and Massachusetts. The study was designed to investigate whether patients receiving different types of care varied with respect to the outcomes measured, controlling for case-mix. In this chapter, we report data from the eligible patients who had coronary artery bypass graft surgery (CABG), total hip replacement (THR), transurethral proctectomy (TURP), or cholecystectomy (CHOLE). These procedures were chosen because they are relatively common and it was possible to identify an initial inception cohort of patients through operating room logs and discharge abstracts, using clearly defined criteria.

To maximize the homogeneity of the patients to be studied, a set of inclusion and exclusion criteria were developed for each condition. These criteria have been reported in detail elsewhere [20]. In all cases patients were undergoing elective surgery, were older than 18 years of age, and were excluded if they had metastatic cancer, were receiving chemotherapy, had AIDS, or had received an organ transplant.

Study sites

The hospitals from which study subjects were selected are not-for-profit, university-affiliated, teaching hospitals. Hospitals were selected in this way to maximize homogeneity in the standards of care delivered. Three of the hospitals were located in California and three were located in Boston. They represent both small and large hospitals, with the number of yearly admissions during the period corresponding to this study ranging from about 1,200 per year to more than 42,000 per year.

Procedures

Data on case-mix and the process of care were abstracted from the medical records of each study patient. Questionnaires were sent to patients having a cholecystectomy or transurethral prostatectomy three months post-discharge. CABG patients received follow-up questionnaires six months post-discharge and total hip replacement patients were assessed one year after discharge. These times were suggested by our consults as the period during which we would be most likely to detect differences in outcome related to the process of care.

Chart reviews

We recorded information from patients' medical records about socio-demographic characteristics, characteristics of the admission, disease-specific severity measures, information about the surgical procedure, the occurrence of in-hospital complications, resource use, and co-morbidity.

Co-morbid conditions may have an impact on patients' disease management and outcomes during the months following hospitalization [21]. For example, the presence of insulin-dependent diabetes, mild renal failure, and angina in a patient undergoing cholecystectomy may have an impact on short-term function, symptoms, and rate of response to therapy. In order to control for differences in co-morbid conditions, we recorded information on co-morbidity from the medical record of each patient using the approach developed by Greenfield and colleagues [22, 23].

Outcome questionnaire

The outcome questionnaires included questions about sociodemographic characteristics, perceived general health, disability, use of health services, symptoms related to the primary condition, social support, social functioning, basic and intermediate activities of daily living (BADL and IADL), well-being, satisfaction with medical care and health, perceived change in health status, employment, and role functioning, as well as education and income. The questionnaire also asked about former daily activities, well-being, employment and role functioning. Among patients who agreed to participate in the study (approximately 91% of all selected patients), about 88% returned a usable questionnaire. The response rate was 81.3% for cholecystectomy patients, 88.6% for CABG patients, 93.7% for total hip replacement patients, and 91.1% for prostatectomy patients.

Analyses

Sample characteristics are described by presenting means and standard deviations. To simplify the analysis and presentation we rescaled each functional status measure so that it varied from 0 (worst functioning) to 100 (best functioning).

To assess the sensitivity of the different functional status scores over time, we calculated a paired-t statistic for the difference between the pre-surgical and post-discharge self-report of functioning. This measure provides an indication of the change in scores relative to the standard deviation of change scores [24, 25].

To compare the results of bypass surgery in different age groups we classified patients according to whether or not they were younger than 65 years of age. We compared mean outcome scores between these two groups of patients, statistically adjusting for gender, race, education level, marital status, severity of co-morbid conditions, American Society of Anesthesiology (ASA) classification, re-operation status, number of days intubated, pre-admission functional status, unstable angina on admission, symptomatic heart failure, insulin-dependent diabetes, prior AMI, major post-operative complications, and whether the patient had an internal mammary artery graft.

Results

Patients' average ages ranged from 46 to 69 years, the proportion male ranged from 26% to 100%; but only between 7% and 8% were not Caucasian for three of the conditions. Twenty-one percent of those having a cholecystectomy were non-white. The only group with any substantial limitation of basic activities of daily living was the group of patients having a total hip replacement.

The t-scores for most of the scales suggest significant improvements due to surgery for all patient groups (Table 16.1).

Table 16.1. T-scores of differences on functioning scales

	Condition			
Variable	CHOLE	THR	TURP	CABG
Basic activities of daily living	3.4	17.5	−0.7*	6.8
Intermediate activities of daily living	1.9*	18.1	−1.1*	12.3
Well-being	5.1	9.4	3.1	8.1
Work performance	1.7*	5.7	2.7	0.8*
House work	4.4	11.0	1.5*	2.8
Social activities	2.6	13.4	0.2*	7.4
Fatigue	3.6	10.6	−0.8*	8.0
Confusion	1.3*	2.0	0.15*	−1.2*

* Not significant

However, the patterns of changes clearly differentiate among the different conditions. These changes are consistent with clinical impressions of physicians caring for the different patient groups and the impact of the different procedures. Thus, these results have face validity and lend support to the use of these types of scales for evaluating the outcomes of CABG surgery.

CABG had a larger impact on BADL scores than cholecystectomy or prostatectomy and a smaller impact than total hip replacement, as expected. The patterns for the IADL scores were similar and the impact of CABG was much greater for IADL scores than for BADL scores, again an expected finding, considering the initial condition of CABG patients and the expected clinical changes in patients after CABG surgery.

For each of the scales analyzed, the t-scores were second highest for CABG patients, with a couple of notable exceptions. For all patients, the scale of confusion was the least likely to show any changes after surgery and with the exception of the work performance scores, the scales indicated the least change in TURP patients.

When we compared older to younger CABG patients, the older patients were significantly more likely than younger ones to have left main occlusion and were less likely to receive an internal mammary artery graft. The only other statistically significant difference was that older patients reported better pre-admission mental health than younger patients [2].

The improvements in functioning after CABG surgery were very similar in the two age groups. The proportion of patients reporting specific symptoms and the Specific Activity Schedule scores also did not vary significantly between the two age groups. None of the generic or condition-specific HRQL scores, except for mental health, were significantly different between the two age groups. A graph showing the changes between the pre- and post-surgical assessments of IADL scores for patients less than and older than 65 years of age is presented in Figure 16.1. The only significant difference between the two age groups was that older patients reported better mental health than younger ones. The results were comparable when we adjusted for potentially confounding factors [2].

INTERMEDIATE
ACTIVITIES OF DAILY LIVING

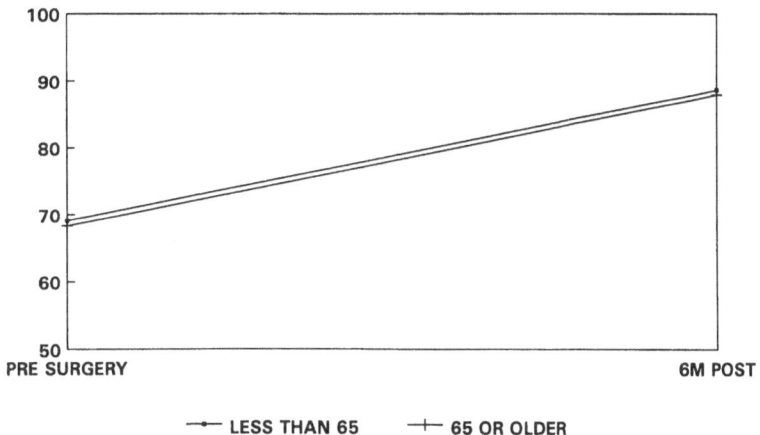

Figure 16.1. Changes in intermediate activities of daily living in Six Hospital Study.

Discussion

As might be expected, by far the greatest improvements in basic and intermediate activities of daily living occurred among patients having a total hip replacement, although CABG patients also showed large improvements in IADL scores. Interestingly, the only scale, aside from confusion, that showed no change for CABG patients was work performance. This is consistent with other findings in the literature [e.g. 26], although it is not fully understood why CABG surgery does not have a more beneficial impact on employment.

These data provide useful information about the level of functioning in a variety of domains prior and subsequent to surgery for patients of different ages. We think that the high compliance rates, internal consistency, construct validity, and sensitivity to changes argue for more widespread use of these types of scales when evaluating age-related differences in outcomes for medical interventions.

The BWH study

The BWH study was similar to the Six Hospital Study with respect to several of the conditions studied, the measures used and the analytic approach. One major difference concerned the nature of patients selected for study. The goal of the Six Hospital Study was to explain inter-institutional differences in process of care and outcomes and thus we tried to maximize the similarity of patients by using restrictive eligibility criteria. In the BWH study, on the other hand, we wanted to evaluate the performance of our measures and estimate the associations among them in more representative groups of patients.

A major purpose of the BWH Study was to select the most appropriate data elements for use in a routine information system for identifying patients at high risk of adverse outcomes. The conditions described here are CABG (n = 454), breast surgery (n = 375), cholecystectomy (n = 646), hysterectomy (n = 499), total hip replacement (n = 325), and total knee replacement (n = 341). In the BWH Study all outcome questionnaires were administered six months after discharge, rather than at varying times, as was the case in the Six Hospital Study [27, 28].

Analyses

To compare the improvement in health-related quality of life reported by patients treated for different conditions, we present the scores on the IADL scale prior, and subsequent, to treatment. To assess the relationship between patient age and changes in health-related quality of life, we grouped CABG patients into three age groups; under 60 years of age, between 60 and 69, and 70 years of age or older. The scales we examined were angina, IADL and a single question that asked patients to rate how much better or worse they felt, compared to the time prior to their surgery. To simplify the analysis and presentation of these data, we rescaled each change measure so that it varied from 0 (no change) to 100 (most change). The IADL scores, also, we scored so that they varied from 0 (worst functioning) to 100 (best functioning).

Results

The results on changes between pre- and post-surgical scores on the scale of limitations in Intermediate Activities of Daily Living are similar to those from the Six Hospital Study, in that the changes were a function of both the condition and dimension assessed. Also similar to the results of the Six-Hospital Study, when we compared the improvement of CABG in different aged groups of patients (less than 60 years of age, between 60 and 69 years of age, and 70 years of age or older), the improvement in health-related quality of life measures were as great, or greater, in the older patients, compared to the younger patients (Figure 16.2).

CHANGES IN QOL MEASURES

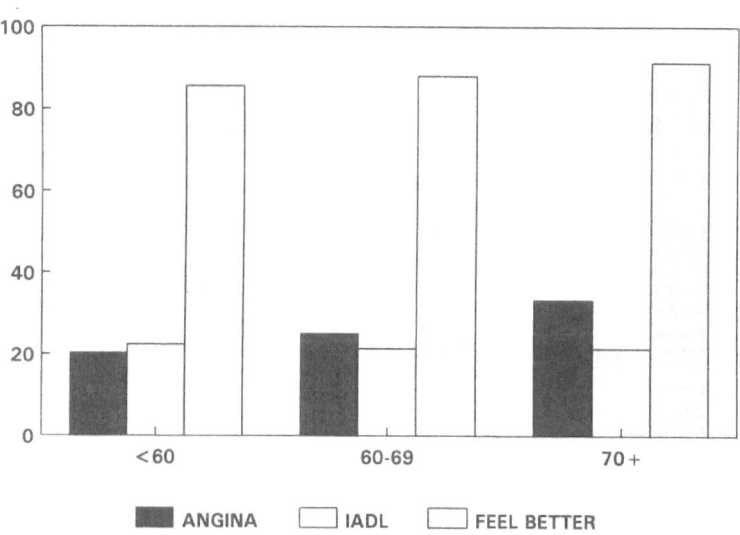

Figure 16.2. Changes in angina, instrumental activities of daily living and reports about feeling better in different age groups of patients in the BWH study.

Discussion

As was found in the Six Hospital Study, CABG patients showed less improvement in IADL scores than joint replacement patients, but substantially more than patients in the other conditions. Changes in IADL scores and condition-specific measures, such as angina and dyspnea, were analyzed; they were also consistent with the Six Hospital Study and previous studies in the literature, in that the improvements in older patients were as great as, or greater than, improvements in younger patients.

The AMI PORT study

One of the difficulties interpreting the data from these and other studies of age-related differences in outcomes is that often studies are not able to control adequately for age-related differences in case-selection. Even when detailed clinical data are collected, persons of different ages may differ on unmeasured characteristics that are strongly related to the outcomes of interest. One strategy for overcoming this problem is to examine populations in large geographic areas (e.g. states) that have different treatment patterns. In such a study it may be possible to estimate the incremental benefit or harm associated with more or less treatment in different age groups.

The purposes of the AMI PORT include examining regional variations in the way patients who have had an acute myocardial infarction (AMI) are treated, with an emphasis on cardiac catheterization and revascularization, the extent to which regional differences in clinical characteristics explain geographic differences in treatment patterns, and the outcomes associated with different treatment patterns. The AMI PORT Study collected data from a probability sample of persons in New York and Texas who had been hospitalized for an AMI between February 1, 1990 and May 31, 1990, who were discharged alive, and who were between the ages of 65 and 79.

To select the sample, we first obtained claims and administrative data from the Health Care Financing Administration (HCFA) on all Medicare enrollees who were residents of Texas or New York and who were hospitalized with a diagnosis of AMI. A total of 11,856 patients were coded as having an AMI during the study period and not in the previous year.

We excluded patients over the age of 79 because of the high mortality rate and low cardiac catheterization rates in those patients. We also excluded patients who were eligible for Medicare because they had end stage renal disease or because of disability, were referred for care from a hospital in which the admitting diagnosis was not an AMI, were treated in a non-acute care hospital, received care for their index admission in a hospital not in their home state, had non-continuous Medicare Part B enrollment, were discharged alive in less than five days, had a date of death prior to their recorded admission date, received their care in a Federal hospital, or were a member of an HMO. The rationale and application of these exclusion criteria have been described previously [29].

One of the eventual goals of our study is to compare the outcomes of patients who do and do not have a cardiac catheterization in the first 90 days after hospitalization, so we wanted approximately equal numbers of patients in each state who had and had not received a cardiac catheterization. Catheterization is a particularly important procedure because it is a necessary step prior to revascularization and catheterization rates may be a useful marker for more aggressive treatment styles. Thus, to draw our sample, we selected all patients who had received cardiac catheterization, about 40% of the non-catheterization patients in New York, and about 70% of the non-catheterization patients in Texas.

Using information from the HCFA 'Name and Address' file, we attempted to telephone all patients in this sample who were not known to be dead at the time of the follow-up study, approximately 18 to 24 months after the date of hospital discharge.

Patient interview

The interview asked patients about their race, education, marital status, whether they lived alone or with someone else, employment status, and family income. It also included ten scales to assess their current health or evaluation of their health. The general areas we assessed were general health perception, cardiac symptoms, pain, fatigue, functional status, emotional well-being, disability, and utilities for their current state of health. These data, which will be available this year, should be very valuable for estimating the relative benefit of different revascularization rates in clinically similar groups of older patients.

Conclusions

The majority of previous studies on age-related differences in outcomes among patients having coronary bypass graft surgery have found that older patients are more likely to be female, have unstable angina, have emergency surgery, and have more advanced coronary disease. Although operative mortality is significantly related to patient age, older patients often do as well or better than younger patients when the criterion is improvement in HRQL [3].

A major imitation of available studies is that it is difficult to adjust for possible case-mix differences other than age. Studies usually report basic clinical information for groups that are compared, but there are numerous factors that clinicians evaluate when making decisions about whether to perform cardiac surgery. Many of these variables are not recorded in medical records or are recorded inconsistently. To make inferences about the relative impact of revascularization, we have undertaken a large observational study in two regions of the United States in which the rates of revascularization differ dramatically but whose populations are not expected to differ. This research approach will allow us to assess the relative impact of higher rates of revascularization in different age groups, not confounded by regional differences in case-mix. We think this research approach will help elucidate some of the issues related to the potential benefits and risks of revascularization in different patient groups.

Acknowledgements

Work on this paper was supported by a grant from the Agency for Health Care Policy and Research (#HS06341) and the MacArthur Foundation Research Network on Successful Midlife Development. We thank Barbara J. McNeil, M.D., Ph.D. for her central role in the design and conduct of the three studies described here.

References

1. Walter PJ. Quality of life after open heart surgery. Boston: Kluwer Academic Publishers, 1992.
2. Guadagnoli E, Ayanian JZ, Cleary PD. Comparison of patient-reported outcomes after elective coronary artery bypass grafting in patients > 65 years of age to those <65 years of age. Am J Cardiol 1992; 70: 60–4.
3. Mohan R, Amsel BJ, Walter PJ. Coronary artery bypass grafting in the elderly – a review of studies of patients older than 64, 69, or 74 years. Cardiology 1992; 80: 215–25.
4. Andrews FM, Withey SB. Social indicators of well-being: Americans' perceptions of life quality. New York: Plenum, 1976.
5. Berg RL, Hallauer DS, Berk SN. Neglected aspects of the quality of life. Health Serv Res 1976; 11: 391–5.
6. Burt RS, Wiley JA, Minor MJ, Murray JR. Structure of well-being form, content, and stability over time. Sociol Meth Res 1978; 6: 365–407.
7. Flanagan JC. A research approach to improving our quality of life. Am Psychologist 1978; 33: 138–47.
8. Patrick DL, Erickson P. Assessing health-related quality of life for clinical decision making. In: Walker Sr, Rosser RM, editors. Quality of life: assessment and application. Lancaster, UK: MTP Press, 1988: 9.
9. Deyo RA. Measuring functional outcomes in therapeutic trials for chronic disease. Controlled Clin Trials 1984; 5: 223–40.
10. Feinstein AR, Josephy BR, Wells CK. Scientific and clinical problems in indexes of functional disability. Annals Intern Med 1986; 105: 413–20.
11. Jette AM. Health status indicators: their utility in chronic-disease evaluation research. J Chronic Dis 1980; 33: 567–79.
12. Jette AM. Concepts of health and methodological issues in functional assessment. In: Gresham G, Granger C, editors. Functional assessment in rehabilitation medicine. Baltimore: Williams and Wilkins, Inc., 1984.
13. Levine S. The changing terrains in medical sociology: emergent concern with quality of life. J Health Soc Beh 1987; 28: 1–6.
14. McDowell I, Newell C. Measuring health: a guide to rating scales and questionnaires. New York: Oxford University Press, 1987.
15. Sackett DL, Chambers LW, MacPherson AS, Goldsmith CH, Mcauley RG. The development and application of indices of health: general methods and a summary of results. Am J Public Health 1977; 67: 423–8.
16. Schipper H, Levitt M. Measuring quality of life: risks and benefits. Cancer Treatment Reports 1985; 69: 1115–23.
17. Ware JE. Standards for validating health measures: definition and content. J Chronic Dis 1987; 40: 473–80.
18. Jette AM, Davies AR, Cleary PD, et al. The functional status questionnaire: its reliability and validity when used in primary care. J Gen Intern Med 1986; 1: 143–9.
19. Cleary PD, Epstein AM, Oster G, et al. Health-related quality of life among patients undergoing percutaneous transluminal coronary angioplasty. Med Care 1991; 29: 939–50.

20. Cleary PD, Greenfield S, McNeil BJ. Assessing quality of life after surgery. Controlled Clin Trials 1991; 12: 189S–203S.
21. Kaplan MH, Feinstein AR. The importance of classifying initial co-morbidity in evaluating the outcome of diabetes mellitus. J Chron Dis 1974; 27: 387–404.
22. Greenfield S, Blanco DM, Elashoff RM, Ganz PA. Patterns of care related to age of breast cancer patients. JAMA 1987; 257: 2766–70.
23. Greenfield S, Aronow HU, Elashoff RM, Watanabe D. Flaws in mortality data: the hazards of ignoring comorbid disease. JAMA 1988; 260: 2253–5.
24. Guyatt G, Walter S, Norman G. Measuring change over time: assessing the usefulness of evaluative instruments. J Chron Dis 1987; 40: 171–8.
25. Liang MH, Larson MG, Cullen KE, Schwartz JA. Comparative measurement efficiency and sensitivity of five health status instruments for arthritis research. Arth Rheum 1985; 28: 542–7.
26. Smith HC, Frye Rl, Piehler JM. Does coronary bypass surgery have a favorable influence on the quality of life. Cardiovasc Clin 1983; 13: 253–64.
27. Katz JN, Wright EA, Guadagnoli E, Liang MH, Karlson EW, Cleary PD. Differences between men and women undergoing major orthopedic surgery for degenerative arthritis. J Gen Int Med 1994. In press.
28. Haas JS, Cleary PD, Guadagnoli E, Fanta C, Epstein AM. The impact of socioeconomic status on the intensity of ambulatory treatment and health outcomes after hospital discharge for adults with asthma. J Gen Int Med 1994. In press.
29. Udvarhelyi IS, Gatsonis C, Epstein A, et al. Acute myocardial infarction in the Medicare population. Process of care and clinical outcomes. JAMA 1992; 268: 2530–6.

17. Longitudinal health-related quality of life assessment in five years after coronary artery bypass surgery – does benefit continue with advancing age?

RAVINDER MOHAN, PAUL J. WALTER and ERIK VAN HOVE

Introduction

In 1987 we started a prospective study of quality of life after coronary artery bypass surgery. By that time, a certain relief from angina through operation had been well documented and randomized studies had additionally shown survival benefits of surgical over medical treatment. Reductions in drugs, care and sickness benefits were considered to neutralise the cost of the operation. However, other reports of post-operative symptoms and complications [1, 2], as well as problems in psychosocial [3, 4] and vocational [5] adjustment, cast a shadow on the usefulness of surgery. The requisite aim of the operation had broadened to improving quality of life. This investigation initially began by longitudinally studying the change in functional and psychosocial status in the first year after operation.

Another concern has gained overriding importance in the last few years. The mean patient age has increased everywhere, e.g., in Belgium from 48 years in 1972 to 64 years in 1990 [6]. Operations in older patients have a more complicated course and higher mortality, thus creating another incentive for refusing surgery. Since the closer one gets to retirement age, societal worth decreases in economic terms and, in very old patients, e.g., older than 75 or 80 years, it is further argued that the number of remaining years of life are neither enough, nor likely to be spent with a good enough quality of life to warrant an operation. In slightly younger patients, i.e. aged about 65 years (the mean CABG patient age today), the aim of the operation is as much for longer survival as for better quality of life. At that age, life expectancy, for instance, in Belgium, is 16.3 years and, by preventing imminent death, survival after operation may exceed 15–20 years and beyond. It is now believed that the operation also improves quality of life, supposedly, to an equally long time, but no study has yet investigated this beyond 1 year. Previous quality of life data cannot be extrapolated, as it was dominated by a return to employment, which loses meaning for older patients.

We therefore continued our longitudinal quality of life investigation until 5 years after operation and compared the results for patients younger and older

179

P.J. Walter (ed.), Coronary Bypass Surgery in the Elderly, pp. 179–194.
© 1995 *Kluwer Academic Publishers, Dordrecht.*

than 60 years of age. In this study we did not study very old patients, i.e. older than 80 years, as this group may have problems particular to such advanced age and because such patients constitute only 1% of current CABG patients. This investigation was therefore intended to study the longitudinal effect of increasing chronologic age in the usual CABG patient, averaging 60 years old. By newer concepts, it is now recommended to study 'Health-related quality of life' (HRQOL), a key basis of which is limitation in performance of social roles, which includes employment and household roles. In many patients of this age, a return to the last few years of employment continues to be an important concern.

Patients and methods

This study is a longitudinal follow-up of 271 patients who underwent isolated coronary artery bypass surgery at the University Hospital of Antwerp from 14 January 1987 to 11 November 1989. Criteria for inclusion in the study included elective operation, isolated coronary artery bypass surgery, willingness to be included in the study (i.e. answering questionnaires after the operation), patient appearance of being reasonably intelligent and able to understand what may be asked of him or her, and possibility of reading and understanding either Nederlands (Dutch) or German. These patients were studied in-hospital a few days before their operation and then by mail, using self-administered questionnaires which were filled in at home at 4 months, 1 year and 5 years after the operation. An attempt was made to maintain the longitudinal nature of the study by asking the same questions as those asked before the operation and at earlier follow-ups, but some changes were made at 5 years because of a better understanding of health-related quality of life measurements and because of previous follow-up responses of patients. At the last follow-up, at 5 years, of the total 271 patients, 14 were excluded, i.e. no questionnaires were sent to them at the 5-year follow-up because of one of the following reasons: (i) neither their address nor telephone number was available in hospital files or previous questionnaires completed until 1 year; (ii) they had indicated by the end of the first-year follow-up that they did not wish to continue to be a part of the study or they had failed to reply persistently despite reminders at earlier follow-ups; or (iii) their preoperative data itself was highly insufficient.

Thus, this study consisted of 257 patients who were questioned before operation and to whom questionnaires were sent at 5 years as well. They were divided almost equally into two groups according to age, with the dividing line kept at the mean age of 59 years for all patients: Group 1 – <60 yrs old, 'younger', n = 135, mean age 53.4 years at CABG; Group 2 – + 60 yrs old, 'older', n = 122, mean age 65.9 years at CABG. At the 5-year follow-up (mean follow-up of 58 months) they had mean ages of about 58 and 71 years, respectively, i.e. a difference of 13 years.

Item selection

Quality of life was assessed by a 5-component construct of physiological function, intellectual function, emotional state, performance of social roles and general satisfaction.

Physiological function
This includes the medical details and functional performance of activities. Medical details collected before operation included, among others: New York Heart Association (NYHA) classes for angina and for dyspnea, left ventricular ejection fraction, number of myocardial infarctions and duration of angina, medications used, severity of coronary disease and number and type of grafts placed, ventricular function on ventriculography, need for inotropes, perioperative myocardial infarction, need for hemodialysis, duration of mechanical ventilation, post-operative probable or definite confusion, days in intensive care, atrial or ventricular fibrillation, pain longer than 48 hours, duration of hospital stay and hospital mortality.

Angina. A *visual analogue scale* (a line 10 cm long) was employed for the patient to mark between 0 (minimum difficulty) and 100 mm (maximum difficulty), reflecting the extent of difficulty in 11 various exertions. The first question of this scale asked about difficulty with angina (chest pain). The scale was given before and at all follow-up times of 4, 12 and 58 months after the operation.

Thus, angina was rated longitudinally before operation and at 4 months, 1 year and 5 years after operation by a visual analogue scale. At the 5-year follow-up, angina was also measured on the *London School of Hygiene Questionnaire* [7].

Dyspnea. Before operation only: New York Heart Association Classes; at 5-year follow-up only: London School of Hygiene Questionnaire.
Functional performance of physical activities was measured by a visual analogue scale (0–100 mm) given preoperatively and at all follow-up times (including the follow-up at 5 years). Respondents were asked about perceived difficulties with angina (mentioned above), and with 10 different kind of exertions: bicycling, work, walking, fast walking, cold, climbing stairs, sexual activity, rest, light and heavy exertion. Patients could opt out of activities that were not applicable to them. From the number of activities reported with difficulties, a mean *difficulty index* could be calculated, giving a quantitative and precise longitudinal change in functional ability and disability (Figure 17.1).

Preoperatively, patients filled out the scale twice – their *experienced difficulties* status before operation, and their *expected difficulties* after. Other physical status questions were asked only at 5 years; these were self-designed questions on the occurrence of cardiac events (i.e. myocardial infarction, a new catheterisation, a balloon angioplasty, a new heart operation), major non-cardiac health events ('e.g., cancer'), major non-health events ('e.g., death in the family') and the number of occurrences of cardiac re-hospitalisation exceeding

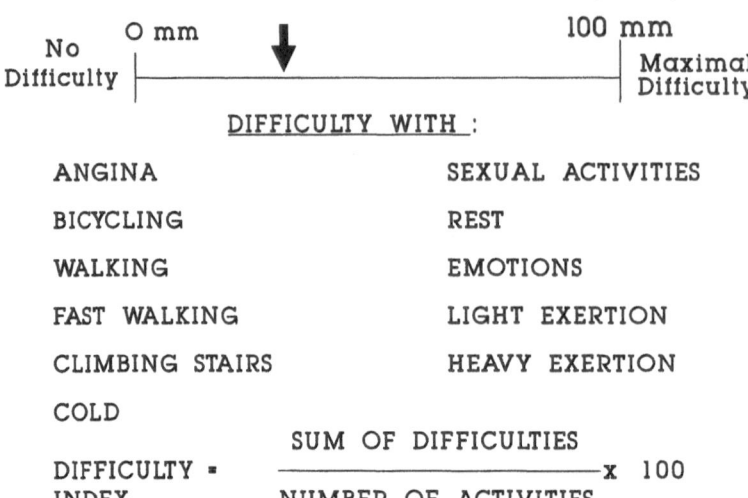

Figure 17.1. The difficulty index.

2 days. Changes in angina, health, family intimacy, sexual satisfaction, family income and work-capacity were also only asked at 5 years. Relevant to the physiological outcome are the variables angina and health.

Intellectual function
Data regarding immediate post-operative confusion were recorded by a single item as: definite confusion, doubtful confusion and no confusion [8].

Emotional state: This consisted of *personality tests* and *psychological tests.*
   Personality versus psychological state in differently aged CABG patients. Previous research has shown how patient personality can affect the results of CABG. For instance, Mahler [9] recently showed how patients with a higher desire for information regarding their health (sensitive to slight problems) but a lower desire for behavioural involvement with their recovery (requesting medications, self-treatment, etc.) had a poorer psychosocial outcome 4 months after surgery.
   In our study, the patient was only tested for personality type before the operation. Although the CABG event itself could have accelerated the changes in personality mentioned above, personality was not assessed at follow-up times because it was kept in this study only as a preoperative risk factor. For outcome, we instead relied on the change in the psychological state by other appropriate questionnaires.

Personality tests done in this study. The *Jenkins Activity Survey (JAS)* assessed the type A personality score with characteristics such as sense of time urgency, impatience, hard-driving, competitiveness, hostility and aggression [10]. The *Marlowe-Crowe Scale* is a scale of social adjustment, subconscious defensiveness and social approval [11]. And, finally, the *Trait Anxiety on the Trait scale of the State Trait Anxiety Inventory* was employed, using the Nederlands version [12]. As pointed out earlier, persons anxious by disposition may be anxious even for not very distressing symptoms and may have a suboptimal outcome.

Psychological questionnaires. The clinical importance of studying the psychological aspect in CABG patients has found additional support in recent times in the re-evaluation of the benefits of cardiac rehabilitation, in which it was found that the area with the greatest potential for improvement is psychological.

We used four psychological measures at the preoperative time and at 1, 4 and 12 post-operative months. The (a) *State sub-scale of the State-Trait Anxiety Inventory (STAI)* [12] has 20 items. (b) *Hopkins' symptom check list-90 (HCL-90)* [13] has been more popular for psychological assessment in Belgium and the Netherlands, perhaps because of available translations. It is very long; in 90 items patients are questioned about 8 psychological features: anxiety, depression, agoraphobia, somaticism, insufficiency, suspicion, hostility, sleep and psychoneuroticism. The scale's somatic content is probably more suitable for psychiatric patients. (c) *Erdman's HPPQ (Heart Patients' Psychologic Questionnaire)* [14, 15] assesses 4 variables which are asked in 52 questions: (i) well-being, (ii) invalidity, (iii) bad mood, and (iv) social constriction. This questionnaire was used at all follow-up times and provided very useful information. (d) *Maastrichte Vragenlijste voor Hartpatienten* [16] has 13 questions to register tiredness (and contrarily, vitality).

At 5 years, it was felt that the administration of all these scales as done until the 1-year follow-up was an excessive respondent burden (total items = 195 items) and may partly explain why the response rate in previous follow-ups (especially at 1 year) became somewhat poor. Therefore, it was decided that for the 5-year follow-up, questionnaires which (a) had less relevant questions, (b) were not sensitive to slight emotional upset (non-psychiatric level), (c) were too lengthy, (d) were less well known, or (e) provided limited information, should be omitted. All four scales, therefore, underwent a combined 4-Factor analysis of the results. As mentioned in Results, this revealed that all dimensions of the SCL-90 loaded on the first factor; on this scale, additionally, the responses of patients even before operation were within 'normal' limits on all dimensions and slight improvement post-operatively would be impossible to detect. This 90-item scale was therefore not repeated at 5 years. The Maastrichte Vragenlijste was also not used, as it took 13 items to arrive at a single conclusion on tiredness; as we required a separate score on depression, we instead used the *Hospital Anxiety & Depression scale* [17] in its place. Thus, psychological questionnaires given at the 5-year follow-up were (1) Erdman's HPPQ (52 items), (2) STAI-state anxiety (20 items) and (3) Hospital Anxiety and

Depression Scale (14 items). The total number of psychological questions (excluding personality questions) asked at 5 years had thus decreased from 195 to 86.

Performance of social roles

A key subcomponent in patients with a mean age around 60 years is work and a work-related social sphere. Apart from questions on education level, system of employment (e.g. self-employed?), marital status, system of medical insurance, religion, etc., before the operation and until 1 year post-operatively, patients were asked if they were working, unemployed, on sick-leave, on pension, etc., if invalidity was because of heart reasons, their time away from work, etc. A similar question was asked at 5 years.

Social interaction was determined by 3 ordinal questions before operation and until the 1-year follow-up: (1) contact with family; (2) contact with friends, and (3) an evening out for relaxation; with the possible responses: (at least) every day, once a week, once a month, less often and never. Obviously, no scores are possible either for longitudinal comparison or across age groups. Therefore, at 5 years all patients were given a 7-item social resources scale of the Older Americans Resources Schedule [18] to acquire subscores on interaction, dependability of social support and the affective component, i.e. loneliness.

General satisfaction

Conceptual understanding of the structure of this domain and its important role in quality of life assessments is discussed in more detail in the next chapter. As inclusion of scales of general satisfaction in a quality of life study is only a recent development, this component was not separately assessed preoperatively or at follow-up times until 1 year. At 5 years this was done by a Delighted-Terrible Faces scale [19], details about which are available in the next chapter. From this scale we derived a Health-Related Quality of Life (HRQOL) score.

Generic scale

We used the instrument EuroQOL [20] which contains five questions on whether patients had problems with mobility, self-care, daily activities, pain (or symptoms) and mood. Details are also available in the next chapter.

All calculations of this study were made by the computer program SAS.

Results

Operative mortality in both younger and older patients of this study was 0%.

At the 5-year follow-up of the 135 young patients (<60 years of age), 10 could not be traced and were lost to follow-up (follow-up was 92.6% complete). Among the remaining 125 patients, 7 had died (94.4% surviving at 5 years). Of the 118 known to be alive, 114 returned completed questionnaires. Of the 122

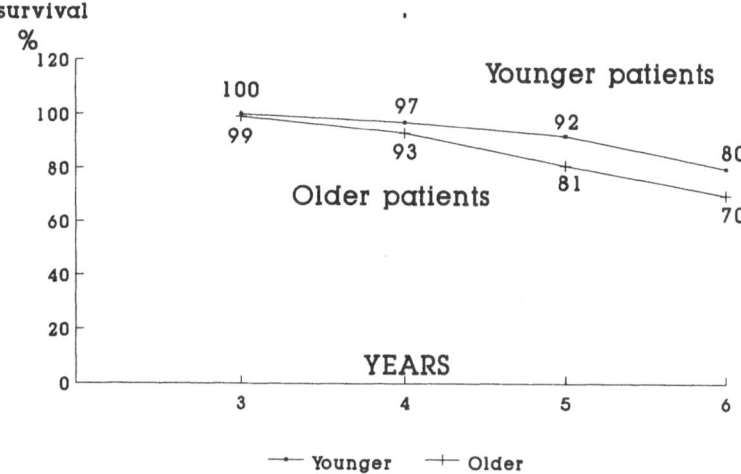

Figure 17.2. Actuarial survival of younger and older patients.

older patients (+60 years old), 7 could not be traced and 14 had died. Ninety-four patients returned the filled out questionnaires. Actuarial survival of younger patients (aged 53 years before operation) was 100% at 3 years, 97% at 4 years, 92% at 5 years and 80% at 6 years. Actuarial survival of older patients (aged 59 years before operation) was 99% at 3 years, 93% at 4 years, 81% at 5 years and 70% at 6 years (Figure 17.2).

Projected survival of the general Belgian population at age 53 in 1989 was 97% at 3 years, 96% at 4 years, 95% at 5 years and 94% at 6 years. The ratio of survival of younger patients versus an equally young population, respectively, was: 103%, 101%, 97% and 85%. Survival of a 59-year-old Belgian population, respectively, was 92%, 89%, 86% and 83%, the ratio being 108%, 104%, 94% and 84%. Thus, for both younger and older patients survival is better than for an age-adjusted population up until 4 years, after which time survival decreased for patients.

Preoperative and operative data

The proportion of women was 15.5% versus 8.1%, in older versus younger patients ($p = .06$). Marital status and education were similar in the two groups. Preoperatively, both age groups had similar medical details: about 85% of patients in both groups had NYHA Class III or IV angina ($p = $ NS), 25% had > Class I dyspnea ($p = $ NS), about 63% had had previous myocardial infarction ($p = $ NS), anginal complaints existed for about 30 months ($p = $ NS), among 12 medications older patients were more often taking digitalis or diuretics ($p < .05$), about 62% of both groups had 3-vessel disease, 14% had left main coronary artery disease ($p = $ NS), and about 65% had abnormal ventricular function ($p = $ NS). The number of grafts received (mean = 3.77) or use of internal mammary artery (in 95% patients) was similar. Regarding complications, older patients required inotropes more frequently but other complications were similar.

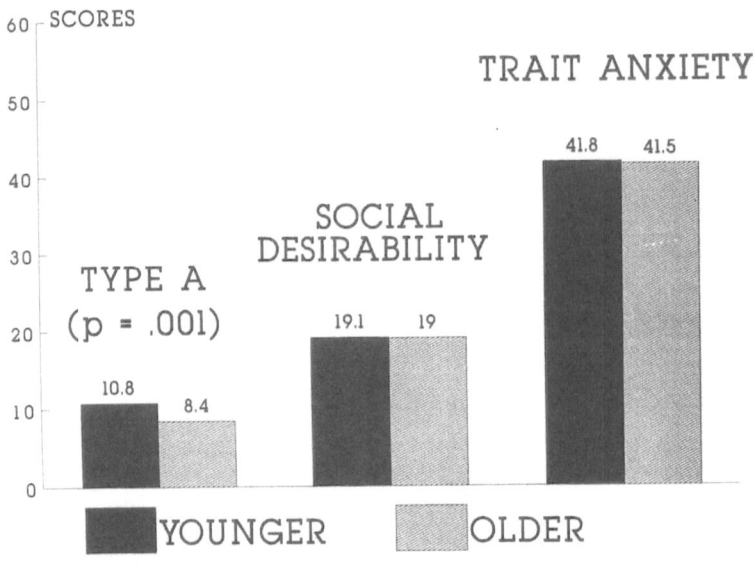

Figure 17.3. Preoperative personality.

In personality tests, more younger than older patients had a **type A** personality ($p = 0.001$); the Marlowe-Crone scale scores and trait anxiety **scores** were similar (Figure 17.3).

Functional disability. Preoperatively *experienced* difficulties **among 11** exertions (including angina, physical status and emotions) on the **visual** analogue sçale were most often sexual activities and the difficulty **index was** similar. However, older patients *expected* post-operatively more (**$p < .05$**) difficulties in 7 out of 11 exertions (walking, fast walking, cold, stairs, **sex, rest** and light exertion) and had a higher difficulty index of expectation **(Figure** 17.4).

Number of risk factors. Ten medical and three social risk factors were **identified** which could affect quality of life. The mean number of both kinds of risk **factors** was similar in younger and older patients.

Follow-up data

Functional outcome.
At 4 months, 1 and 5 years, severity of angina on the visual analogue **scale and** the difficulty index had reduced remarkably from preoperative levels **and** similarly ($p = NS$) for younger and older patients (Figure 17.5).

Older patients had more difficulties in walking at 4 months; in **walking, fast** walking and sex at 1 year; and in fast walking only at 5 years.

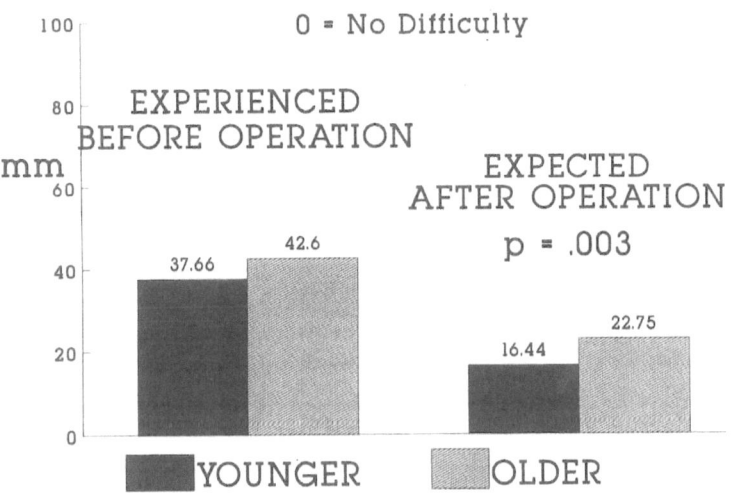

Figure 17.4. Preoperatively experienced and expected difficulty index.

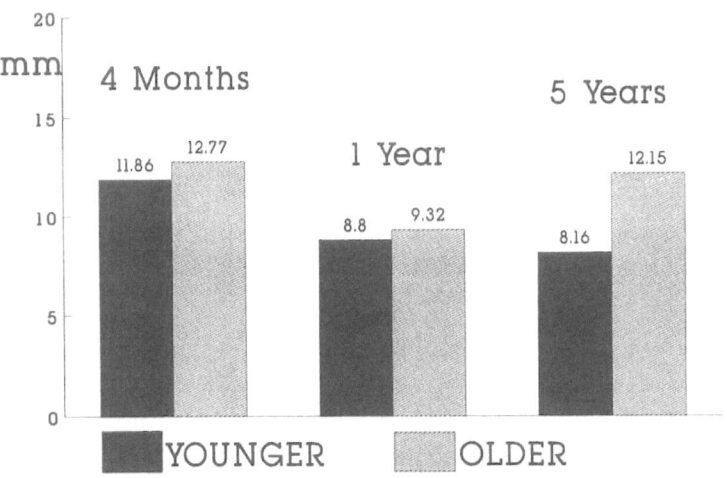

Figure 17.5. Reduction in difficulty index.

Psychologically. On the *symptom check list* (*HSCL-90*) younger and older patients had no differences in 8 dimensions before operation and at 4 months, but younger patients had more suspicion and hostility than older patients at 1 year. On the *Maastrichte Questionnaire* older patients had more tiredness before operation but there were no differences at 4 months or at 1 year. These two questionnaires were not repeated at 5 years.

On the *Erdman's-Heart Patients Psychological scale*, before the operation older patients had similar well-being and mood, but perceived more invalidity than younger patients as well as perceived social constriction. A steady improvement and normalization was noted in all four dimensions of this scale for both younger and older patients at all follow-up times compared to the preoperative levels. Between the two groups no differences were seen at 4 months, although improvement in well-being was greater in the older patients. At 1 year, older patients reported significantly better well-being and marginally significant better mood than younger patients. Improvement was greater for elderly patients until 1 year. Between 1 and 5 years, elderly improvement remained stable, but it was better for younger patients. At 5 years, the older patients perceived significantly more invalidity than younger patients (Figure 17.6–9).

State Anxiety (*Spielberger*) was similar in older and younger patients before operation and at 4 months, but at 1 year younger patients felt significantly more anxious than older patients. At 5 years there was no difference (Figure 17.10).

On the *Hospital Anxiety & Depression scale* at 5 years, no differences were noted on anxiety or depression in younger and older patients, with clinical

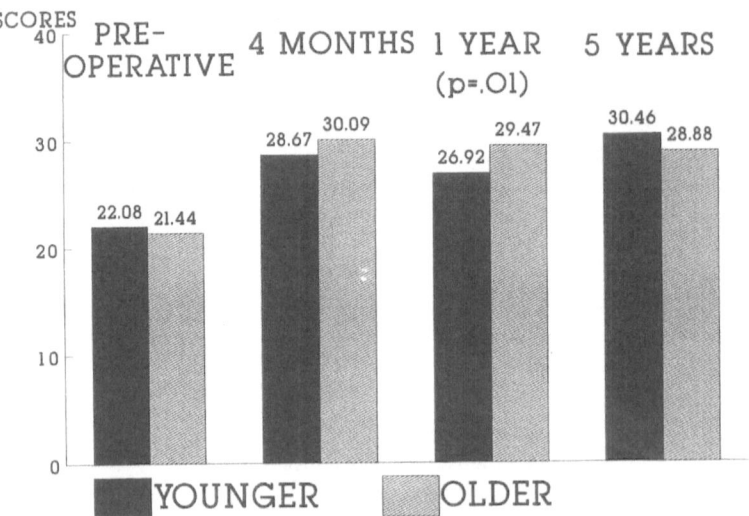

Figure 17.6. Well-being on Heart Patients' Psychological Scale.

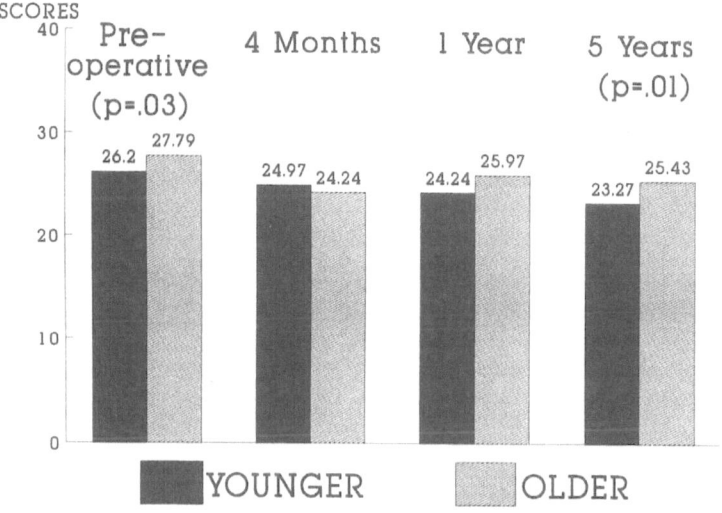

Figure 17.7. Invalidity on Heart Patients' Psychological Scale.

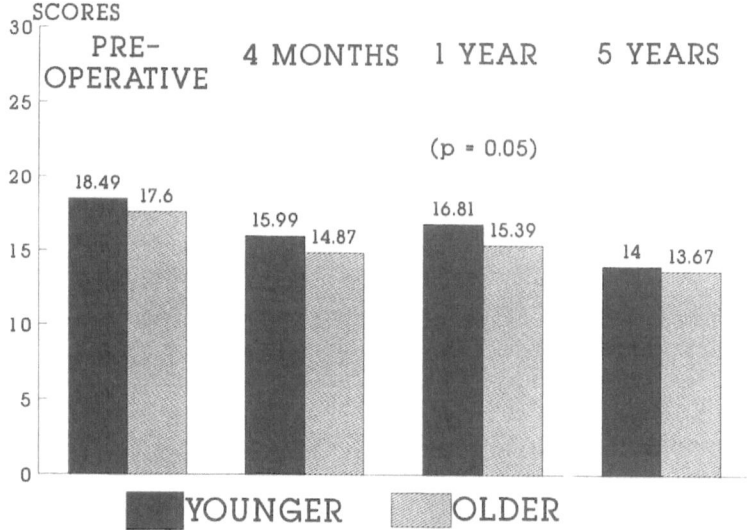

Figure 17.8. Bad mood on Heart Patients Psychological Scale.

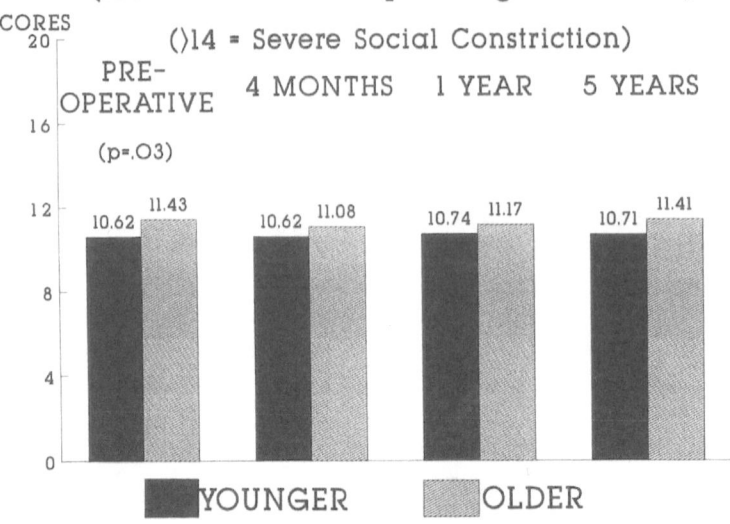

Figure 17.9. Social constriction on Heart Patients Psychological Scale.

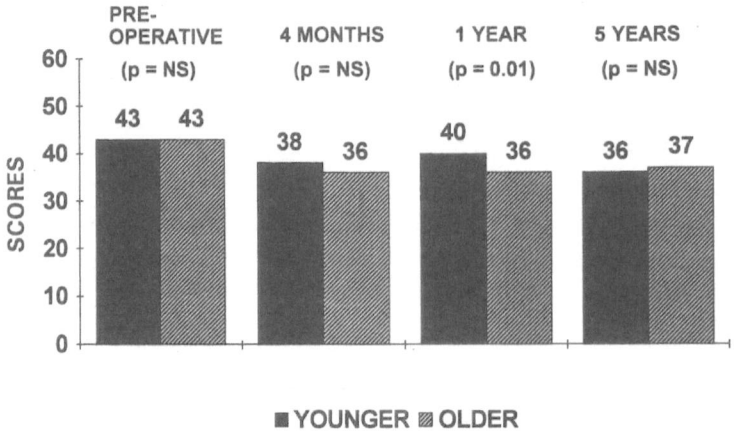

Figure 17.10. State Anxiety on Spielberger Scale.

anxiety seen in about 6% of patients and clinical depression in about 3% of patients in each group.

Social outcome. Of the younger patients, 73% were working prior to the operation, and about 16% of the older patients (*p* <.0001). At 5 years, 48% of the younger patients and about 7% of the older patients were still working. No patient who was not working before operation was working at 5 years.

Obviously, because of retirement the number of patients not working for non-health reasons was far higher for older than younger patients ($p < .0001$). Regarding social contact, there were no differences between age groups in the frequency of contact with friends or family, or the amount of outdoor relaxation before operation or at 1 year, but at 4 months highly significantly ($p = 0.009$) fewer older patients were going out for relaxation. At 5 years all social subscores and total scores were similar on the *OARS*.

Patient perceived change. There was no significant association between age group and whether patients perceived themselves at 5 years to have improved, stayed the same or deteriorated, over their preoperative status in angina, health, family intimacy, sexual satisfaction, work capacity or family income.

Among the questions asked only at 5 years, younger patients *perceived* themselves to be in better health, with less confusion, and had had similar occurrences of cardiac, health and non-health events and cardiac re-hospitalisation. At 5 years, their satisfaction with 8 areas of life, i.e. life, operation, health, achievement, problem solving, family life, pleasure and standard of living, was similar on the Delighted-Terrible Faces Scale, and the HRQOL scores derived from these satisfactions were also similar as were total EuroQOL scores.

On a multivariate regression analysis of the preoperative 10 medical and 3 social factors for predicting (R-square) the total EuroQOL scores at 5 years, the most predictive items resulting in a poor EuroQOL score were a high expected difficulty index, followed by high experienced (preoperative) difficulty index, high trait anxiety, number of social risks and, finally, number of medical risks.

Discussion

Age itself is just a number; its association with changes in body functioning is what gives it meaning. In comparing the outcome of younger and older patients, therefore, it is important to know the number and type of risks with which the two age groups face an operation and, of these, which are influential on the outcome. In this study, in almost all respects older and younger patients had similar risks. This cannot be explained by patient selection: although only electively operated patients were included, there was no further selection, as is evidenced by the 85% incidence of NYHA Class III + IV angina in both younger and older patients and > 60% incidence of myocardial infarction, 3-vessel disease and 'abnormal' ventricular function. Probably the reason for higher risks among older patients in all other clinical studies which we recently reviewed [21] is because the patients in those studies were older than the patients in the present study. However, this non-difference of risk is useful for our longitudinal investigation because any difference in post-operative outcome must be the effect of chronologic age alone – there was a difference of 13 years between the mean age of the two populations. The only preoperative difference was that more elderly patients were on digitalis and diuretics, although their NYHA dyspnea classes were similar.

One of the most striking findings of this study was that, despite the fact that older and younger patients had a similar difficulty index both before the operation and at 5 years, at both times the older patients perceived themselves to be more invalid than younger patients. They also expected more difficulties than younger patients, although this pessimism was unwarranted, as their performance matched that of younger patients on the same scale at all follow-up times. In sum, it could be said that older and younger patients began with the same risks, physical capacity, mood and social contact, but perceived themselves to be more invalid and tired before operation with less expectations of recovery. Equally important is the finding that not only were expectations low among the elderly, but that these expectations are the most important in predicting long-term health-related quality of life. This parallels what many previous studies noted in research on return to work after CABG – the positive effect of the expectation and will of the patient in returning to work [22, 23]. A recent study showed how dispositional optimism before CABG was a predictor of better coping, less denial, better physical recovery, faster return to normal life activities and, finally, a better quality of life [24]. Therefore, preoperative encouragement leads to improved long-term functioning and less frustration, and is especially required in the elderly as they are more pessimistic about their current and future health.

Upon analyzing separately the components of quality of life, the most convincing observation regarding the non-effect of advancing patient age was the functional component, i.e. longitudinal change in difficulty index. The mean age at operation of all patients (younger + older) who either improved versus deteriorated was the same (p = NS), i.e. 58 to 59 years, and this was the mean age of all patients. Psychologically the elderly patients had a better state at 1 year; between 1 and 5 years the improvement continued for younger but remained steady for older patients. Among social scores, it was interesting to find that patients (younger + older) who were seeing fewer friends before the operation (versus those who met friends more frequently) continued to have significantly poorer social interaction scores on the OARS at 5 years; additionally, the 5-year mean social scores predicted both the 5-year HRQOL and EuroQOL scores significantly. The social domain is also related to return to work. None of the patients not working before operation returned to work in our study. In a Milwaukee study of 9,905 patients, patient age was found to have minimal effect, unless near retirement age, when the chance of retiring was greater than for the general (non-operated) population [25]. Another large U.S. study (n = 2,229) found that after age 65, 'the desire to relax and enjoy life' became the dominant reason for 'disability' [26]. Thus, either working or not working could both mean a better or worse quality of life.

Finally, as the HRQOL and EuroQOL scores of our younger and older patients were similar at 5 years, we can conclude that this is unaffected by advancing patient age.

References

1. Kornfeld D, Heller S, Frank K, Wilson S, Malm J. Psychological and behavioural response after coronary artery bypass surgery. Circulation 1982; 66(suppl III): 24.
2. Zyzanski S, Jenkins D, Klein M. Medical and psychosocial outcomes in survivors of major heart surgery. J Psychosom Res 1981; 3: 213.
3. Gundle M, Reeves B, Tate S, Raft D, McLauren L. Psychosocial outcome after coronary artery surgery. Am J Psychiatry 1980; 137: 1591.
4. Bass C. Psychosocial outcome after coronary artery bypass surgery. Br J Psychiatry 1984; 145: 526–32.
5. Walter PJ. Return to work after coronary artery bypass surgery. Berlin: Springer Verlag, 1984.
6. Sergeant P. Changing pattern in age distribution of coronary bypass patients and their possible early influence in early and late events. Proceedings of the 3rd World Congress of the International Society of Cardiothoracic Surgeons; 1993 Jan 25–27; Salzburg.
7. Rose GA, Blackburn H. Cardiovascular survey methods. Geneva: World Health Organization, 1968.
8. Guadagnoli E, Cleary PD. Age related item non-response in surveys of recently discharged patients. J Gerontol 1992; 47: 206–12.
9. Mahler HIM, Kulik JA. Health care involvement preferences and social-emotional recovery of male coronary bypass patients. Health Psychology 1991; 10: 399–408.
10. Jenkins CD, Zyzanski SJ, Rosenmann RH, Cleveland GL. Association of coronary prone behaviour with recurrences of coronary heart diseases. J Chron Dis 1971; 24: 601.
11. Crowne DP, Marlowe D. A new scale of social desirability independent of psychopathology J Consult Psychol 1960; 24: 349–54.
12. Van der Ploeg HM, Defarres PB, Spielberger CD. Zelf Beoordeling Vragenlijste. Een Nederlandstalige Bewerking van de Spielberger State-Trait Anxiety Inventory. Lisse, The Netherlands: Swets and Zeitlinger, 1982.
13. Derogatis LR, Lipman RS, Rickles K, Uhlenhuth EH, Covi D. The Hopkins symptom check list: a self-report symptom inventory. Behav Sci 1974; 19: 1–15.
14. Erdman RAM. Medisch Psychologische vragenlijste voor hartpatienten. Lisse, The Netherlands: Swets and Zeitlinger, 1982.
15. Erdman RAM. A medical psychological questionnaire to assess well-being in cardiac patients. Hart Bulletin 1982; 13: 143–7.
16. Appels A, Hoppener P, Mulder P. A questionnaire to assess premonitory symptoms of myocardial infarction. Int J Cardiology 1985; 17: 15–24.
17. Zigmond AS, Snaith RP. The Hospital Anxiety & Depression Scale. Acta Psychiatrica Scand 1983; 67: 361–70.
18. Blazer D. Social support and mortality in an elderly community population. Am J Epidemiol 1982; 115: 684–94.
19. Andrews FM, Withey SB. Social indicators of well being: Americans' perceptions of life quality. New York: Plenum Press, 1976.
20. EuroQOL: a new facility for the measurement of health related quality of life. Health Policy 1990; 16: 199–208.
21. Mohan R, Amsel BJ, Walter PJ. Coronary artery bypass grafting in the elderly – a review of studies on patients older than 64, 69 or 74 years. Cardiology 1992; 80: 215–25.
22. La Mendola W, Pellegrini R. Quality of life and coronary artery bypass surgical patients. Soc Sci Med 1979; 13A: 457.
23. Walter PJ. Is employment after coronary artery bypass surgery a measure of the patient's quality of life? In: Walter PJ, editor. Quality of life after open heart surgery. Dordrecht, The Netherlands: Kluwer Academic Publishers, 1992: 203–15.
24. Scheier MF, Magovern GJ, Abott RA. Dispositional optimism and recovery from coronary artery surgery: the beneficial effects on physical and psychological well-being. J Pers Soc Psych 1989; 57: 1024–40.

25. Anderson AJ, Barboriak JJ, Hoffman BG, et al. Age & sex specific incidence and main factors. In: Walter PJ, editor. Return to work after coronary artery bypass surgery. Berlin: Springer Verlag, 1985.
26. Johnson WD, Kayser KL, Pedraza PM, et al. Employment patterns in males before and after myocardial revascularization surgery – a study of 2229 consecutive male patients followed for as long as 10 years. Circulation 1982; 65: 1086.

18. Health-related quality of life five years after coronary bypass surgery at age 75 or above

A research approach to item selection

PAUL J. WALTER, RAVINDER MOHAN and CHRIS CORNELISSEN

Introduction

As the population has aged, ethical dilemmas have arisen over society's responsibility towards the health care of its old and very old citizens. Because of disproportionate disability and disease in old age, the +65-year-olds consumed 30% of U.S. health care costs although they constituted only 13% of the population [1]. Further, reluctance is high for spending on +80-year-olds, as they are not only non-productive and more dependent, but they have already lived longer and have fewer years of life to gain from intervention [2]. Marked by a focus on identifying inappropriate interventions [3] and public concern over a rise in coronary bypass operations [4], 1993 has been a year of health care reform.

Operative mortality, morbidity [5] and costs are significantly higher in older patients [5]. With increasing technical experience, reports of operations in old [6] and very old [7, 8] patients are increasing. Early institutionalisation of many elderly is often due to disability experienced in everyday life because of angina [9], and those living at home find that their family has to share the burden [10]. Several studies have shown that coronary disease is more extensive and angina more likely to be unstable in older patients [11] and, in one study among consecutive octogenarians who underwent coronary angiography, 39% had post-infarction angina and another 27% had unstable angina [12]. If not operated on, not only is their risk of hospital mortality substantially high, but costs of their emergent reanimation after myocardial infarction become prohibitive. Greater demands for investing in these operations would make sense, however, if an improvement could be shown in the longer-term, health-related quality of life, i.e. more independence in mobility and self-care, less hospitalisation, more integration in society, greater self-satisfaction, etc. [13]. On reviewing recent developments in quality of life measurement methodology, this investigation intends to take full, practical and timely advantage of the new understanding in quality of life research.

The aim of this research was to study the 5-year quality of life outcome of all patients who were 74 years or older when they underwent an isolated coronary

195

P.J. Walter (ed.), Coronary Bypass Surgery in the Elderly, pp. 195–210.
© 1995 *Kluwer Academic Publishers, Dordrecht.*

artery bypass operation at our hospital. A comparison was made with (a) CABG patients representing the usual age at which CABG was done 5 years ago (i.e. a mean age of 59 years at operation) and (b) age-adjusted 'normal' populations, whether or not they had coronary disease.

Patients and methods

Pre- and post-operative clinical details of all patients (n = 137) who were 74 years or older when they underwent isolated CABG (mean age at CABG = 77 years) between January 1986 and August 1990 at the University Hospital of Antwerp have been published previously [14]. Briefly, 127 patients survived the 30-day hospital stay, i.e. an operative mortality of 7.2%. A follow-up done for the current study was at a mean of 66 months (about 5 years) after the operation, i.e. patients who answered the questionnaires of this very old population to date were all older than 80 years old (with a mean age of 82 years), and will be referred to as Population A. At the same time, almost identical questionnaires were answered by a younger, control population of 257 selected (neutral risk) patients who underwent isolated CABG at a mean age of 59 years, between January 1987 and January 1989 at our hospital. All of them survived the 30-day hospital stay. At present, their mean follow-up is 58 months (about 5 years), and their mean follow-up age, 64 years (Population B).

This study was a cross-sectional comparison of the health-related quality of life of these two populations by a mail questionnaire at 5-year follow-up. Older patients were also compared with three general populations of similar age.

A standard questionnaire to assess the quality of life after open heart surgery whether in the young or old patient does not exist. We therefore decided to select items suggested by research to be relevant for CABG patients. Selection was done on the basis that we would have a minimum of self-designed questions (use of well-known questionnaires with satisfactory validity and reliability is preferred), and applicability that would cover a very elderly as well as a younger population, for both cardiac patients and a healthy population. Questionnaires would be both disease- (and domain-) specific, as well as generic, as advised earlier [15]. Quality of life would be assessed under the domains: physiological state, intellectual state, emotional state, performance of social roles and general satisfaction [16], and each domain would be separately assessed by a questionnaire meant only for that domain. An emphasis would be given to CABG-related events, e.g., cardiopulmonary symptoms, cardiac events and re-hospitalisation, etc., and questions evaluating change (after operation) would also be included.

Questionnaires used at the 5-year follow-up

Functional status
The physical domain is the most essential determinant of quality of life, especially in the elderly, in whom failing health might interfere with their capacity for independent living. Although closely related to symptomatic status, functional performance is a distinct concept of physical health, especially in elderly patients who might be asymptomatic because of refraining from activities common to younger patients or who might not recall specific symptoms in detail. Disability in old age is also more heterogeneous than in younger persons. It is usually measured by two personal self-maintenance scales called the Activities of Daily Living (ADL), which asks about the unaided performance of six basic personal-care activities [17], i.e. eating, toileting, etc., and the Instrumental Activities of Daily Living (IADL), which include home management and independent living. We chose a Dutch scale [18] which comprises 5 basic ADL and 5 household ADL. Using this scale we were then able to compare the disability of our octogenarian patients with that of 293 elderly 'healthy' persons older than 80 years, living at home in The Netherlands, who answered the scale in a longitudinal study to assess the requirement of socio-medical support. Medical details such as severity of angina or dyspnea, cardiac events after the operation and frequency of confusion were also asked, and these items have been reported elsewhere [19].

Emotional state
A core domain of quality of life is the psychological. The transition from being middle-aged to becoming an old person is associated with a period of status and role losses among the elderly. Loss of physical health is also a reason for chronic emotional upset. Several instruments exist to measure mental health, as its definition is controversial. In the seventies, it was realised that the benefit of coronary artery bypass surgery was closely associated with the psychological outcome, when several patients failed to feel more energetic about their everyday activities and work after operation, even though they did not have angina and their objective exercise capacity had been restored. The psychological state would be interesting to study in the older patient since work considerations do not apply. Although several scales have been developed for detection of anxiety and depression, Snaith [20] and others [21] have criticised the fact that these scales often include items pertaining to somatic attributes such as appetite, which could be more dominantly affected by physical disease than mental health.

We chose the Hospital Anxiety and Depression scale for this study. It was developed by Zigmond and Snaith [22] and assesses anxiety and depression in 14 items (7 each), with purposeful exclusion of all questions which could relate both to somatic and emotional reasons, e.g., headache, and all questions assessing pure neurosis and anhedonic depression; n.b. the authors advise prescription of anti-depressant medication to patients with high depression scores. The scale has been validated for both cardiac patients [23] and an elderly population [24]. Its validated translations were available from its developer, R.P. Snaith (personal communication).

Performance of social roles

A constant interaction between an organism and its environment is essential for maintaining life. Regarding the relationship with family, friends and the community, the literature was searched for possible social scales. Several of these scales have been developed by social gerontologists because of increasing dependence on social support with advancing age. Bowling makes a theoretic distinction between the concepts of social interaction and social support [25], although the two are closely related. The affective component is also crucial as an improper social interaction may be stressful rather than relieving stress. Orth-Gomer [26] reviewed the dimensions, requirements and shortcomings of several popular social scales. We selected the instrument 'Social support scale' of the Older Americans Resources Schedule (OARS) [27], which consists of three components (in 7 items only): social interaction, dependability of social support and affective component of support, indicating loneliness. We did not use the Social Health Battery of the Rand Health Insurance experiment [28] (although it too had only 11 items and similar dimensions and face content) because it was in principle developed only for adults aged 14 to 61 years of age. The Medical Outcomes Study and its currently popular short form (SF-36) were also developed from the Rand experience and were not used in this study because of advanced patient age.

General satisfaction

Satisfaction as a distinct and key element in quality of life considerations has been particularly advanced by social gerontological research. Three very well-known early studies on quality of life in society established a precedence in the essential use of measures of life satisfaction in any such evaluation [29–31]. We used the Delighted-Terrible (D-T) Faces Scale, as it has high correlations with the Cantril scale, the Bradburn affect-balance scale, a visual analogue scale of satisfaction, and the Neugarten's scale. The scale's correlation with the Neugarten's LSIZ was also high in 662 persons aged 85 years and older in the community [25]. The D-T scale has an affective component as well as an cognitive component in the self-appraisal of quality of life. After experimenting with 123 concerns (selected out of 800) on about 5,000 Americans with 68 global measures of happiness and satisfaction (including Neugarten's LSIZ, Cantril's ladder scale, a circles scale, a D-T scale without faces, a Faces scale, etc.) Andrews and Withey [29] recommended the D-T scale as the best. The faces have clear expressions and transcend language and cultures.

The questions we asked with this scale were most of those found to be of core relevance by Andrews and Withey and suggested by Bowling [25] as well. As also suggested by them, we included items of relevance to our investigation, e.g., satisfaction with the CABG operation. Satisfaction was therefore asked in eight areas: with life as a whole, experience of the operation, health, self-accomplishment, handling of problems, family life, pleasure and fun, and living standard. It is also possible to get a sum score on *general satisfaction* with this scale after adding the responses to all the items chosen [25, 29]. Whether this is really possible would depend on knowing whether all of these items were measuring a single dimension. We could confirm that this was the case by doing a Principal component analysis on responses by our patients. A mean of these satisfactions on the D-T scale was considered a *'quality of life'* score. A health-related quality of life *(HRQOL)* score was then derived as a sum of four equally contributive factors: (a) the 'quality of life' score, (b) life satisfaction, which is at the core of all global QOL investigations, (c) satisfaction with health, and (d) satisfaction with operation.

Generic measure
For this we chose the EuroQOL [32], an instrument consisting of five questions on mobility, self-care, daily activities, symptoms or pain and mood (anxiety or depression). Each part consists of three possibilities roughly described as (a) 'No problem', (b) 'Require some help', and (c) 'Severe problem or impossible'. One of the largest EuroQOL evaluations was the Rotterdam survey (n of respondents = 869), which arrived at a parametric relation between difficulties in each dimension and its relative contribution to a total health (EuroQOL) score [33]. Based on these relationships we could calculate a total health score for each of our patients.

Questions on change
Finally, in questions on change we asked about improvement, no change or worsening, occurring after the operation in six life areas: health, angina, family intimacy, sexual satisfaction, family income and work capacity.

All these questions together comprised only 54 items for both populations (excluding the 10 ADL items asked from only population A patients). Only 13 of these items (related to occurrence or not of health events in the last 5 years after the operation) were self-designed. When required, translations and back translations were done by different language experts.

Formatting the questionnaire
Following the advice of Lu Ann Aday [34], we numbered the questions, indented every subpart of a question, gave sufficient space between answers, tried to maintain a consistent pattern in asking questions, aligned the response codes to be circled along the right margin of the paper, used a dotted line between the question and the answer, used a vertical format only, used closed-ended questions only, tried not to split questions between pages and used a large and clear type in printing the questions. The questionnaire was comprised of an eight A4-size page booklet with a yellow cover and 'interest-getting' title as well as a 'neutral but eye-catching illustration' (the emblem of our department). The questionnaire was accompanied by a cover letter to the patients, expressing the hope that they were in good health and ending with a thank you for their time and effort. An aggressive attempt was made to complete the follow-up,

including calling each non-responder by telephone and searching their whereabouts.

All calculations of this study were made by the computer program SAS.

Results

Survival

Follow-up of Population A was 89% complete, i.e. of the 127 operative survivors, the survival status of 113 patients was known. Of them, 77 patients answered the questionnaires, 26 patients had died after the operation, 10 were known to be alive but did not answer our postal questionnaire (refused to answer or promised on the telephone to send a reply but did not). Fourteen patients were considered completely lost to follow-up, i.e. because (a) questionnaires were returned marked either 'address unknown' or 'address changed' (addresses collected from the patient dossiers), current whereabouts could not be found despite consultations with the local municipal authority (*gemeentehuis*), and (b) a correct telephone number also could not be found by the telephone company when searched according to the address mentioned in the dossier. The replies of 77 patients of population A are the subject of the quality of life investigation.

The follow-up was done in September 1993 – thus the first calculation is at 3 years. Actuarial survival of Population A patients was 97% at 3 years, 88% at 4 years, 82% at 5 years, 55% at 6 years and 47% at 7 years.

Of the population B patients (n = 257), none died when in hospital (operative mortality of 0%). At the 5-year follow-up, 240 patients were successfully contacted again (follow-up was 93.3% complete). Eighteen of the followed-up patients had died (92.5% were surviving). Actuarial survival of these patients was 99.6% at 3 years, 95% at 4 years, 90% at 5 years and 81% at 6 years (Figure 18.1).

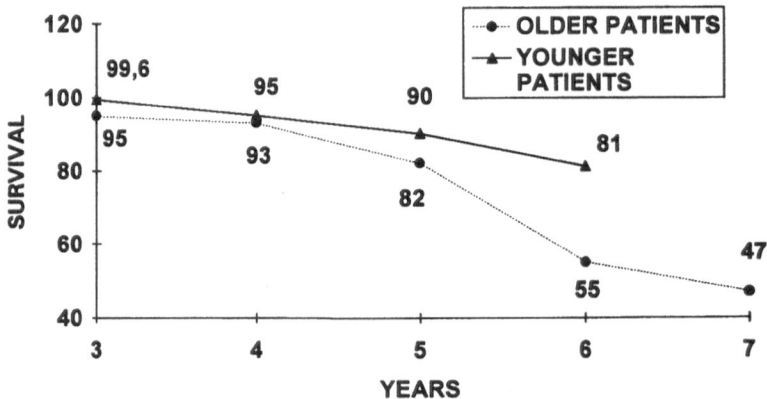

Figure 18.1. Actuarial survival of younger and older patients.

Comparison of 'quality of life' of populations A and B at 5 years

Of Population A, 87.7% (n = 77) and, of younger patients (Population B), 95.4% (n = 208) answered the questions themselves. Three of the five older patients who had not replied themselves could not read and 2 could not understand what was asked of them. But of the 4 younger patients for whom someone else had replied to questions by proxy, only 1 could not read the questions and 3 could not understand them.

Nationality. Population A: 37 (48.1%) were Belgians (Dutch-speaking) and 40 (51.9%) were Germans. Population B: 66 (31.7%) were Belgians (Dutch-speaking) and 142 (68.3%) were Germans.

Gender. Population A: 29 (37.6%) were women and 48 (62.3%) were men. Population B: 30 (11.7%) were women and 227 (88.3%) were women.

Self-perception of current health. (Question asked: In general, how is your health at this moment?) Approximately 73–75% of both younger and older patients perceived their health to be excellent or good. Also, there was no significant difference in health perception between age groups.

Social status. The entire population of A and B patients were living at home. Significantly more younger than older patients were married. On the OARS, older patients had similar interaction scores as younger patients, although 34%

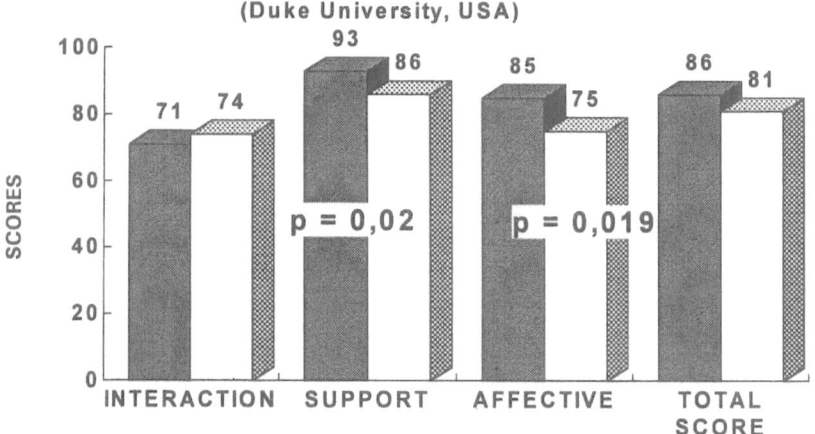

Figure 18.2. Social scores on the OARS scale.

of them were living alone. However, significantly more older patients perceived a lower dependability of social support and felt more lonely. A total score derived from these 3 sub-scores showed that overall social resources were similar in younger and older patients (Figure 18.2).

Satisfaction and the HRQOL score. On the Delighted-Terrible Faces scale, older and younger patients had similar satisfaction in all eight areas, except that older patients were highly significantly more satisfied with their CABG operation experience and were marginally more satisfied with their living standard (Figure 18.3). The calculated HRQOL score was similar in both younger and older patients (Figure 18.4).

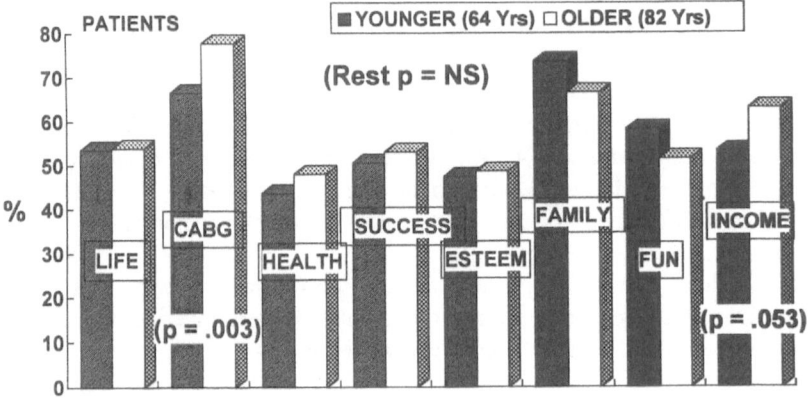

Figure 18.3. Satisfactions on the Delighted-Terrible Faces Scale.

(Delighted-Terrible Faces Scale)

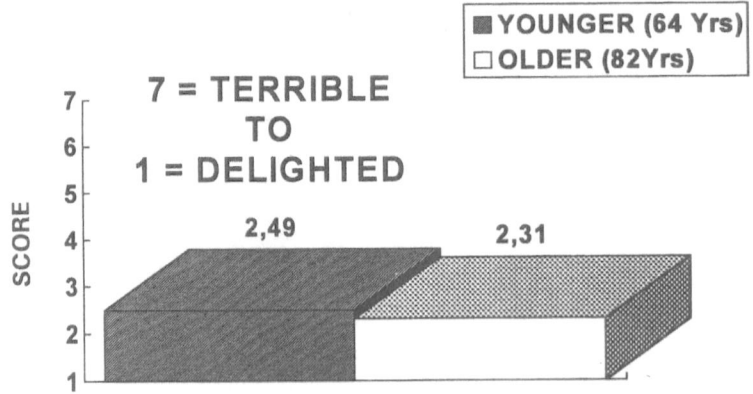

Figure 18.4. Health-related Quality of Life Score.

Hospital Anxiety & Depression Scale

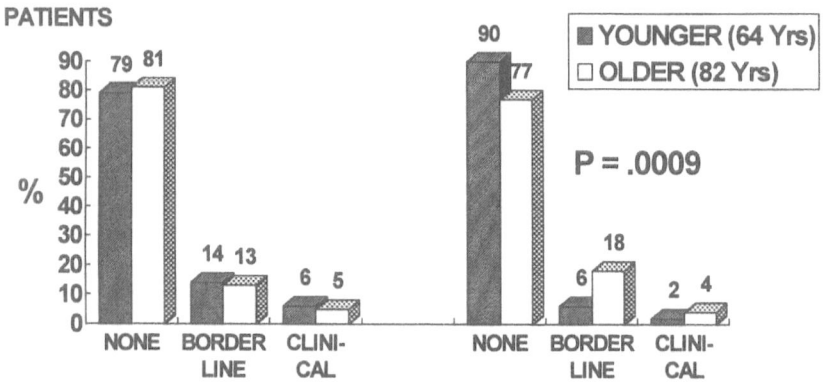

Emotional state. On the Hospital Anxiety and Depression Scale, approximately 80% of both younger and older patients were not anxious, but approximately 22% of older patients had at least borderline depression (4% clinically depressed); thus, depression was significantly more frequent in older patients (Figure 18.5).

EuroQOL. Population A had significantly more problems with mood than population B, but difficulties regarding other variables (mobility, self-care, activities of daily living and symptoms or pain) were similar (Figures 18.6, 18.7). The total EuroQOL health scores were also similar in both age groups.

Self-assessed change after operation. No differences between older and younger patients were found in change after the operation (improvement, unchanged, worsening) in any of the six areas tested.

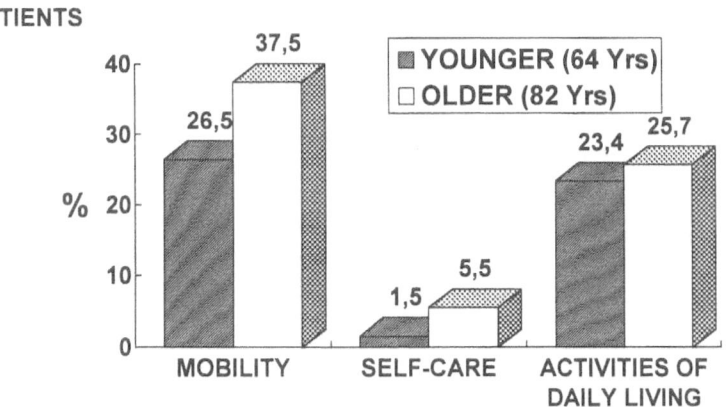

Figure 18.6. Difficulties on EuroQOL (a).

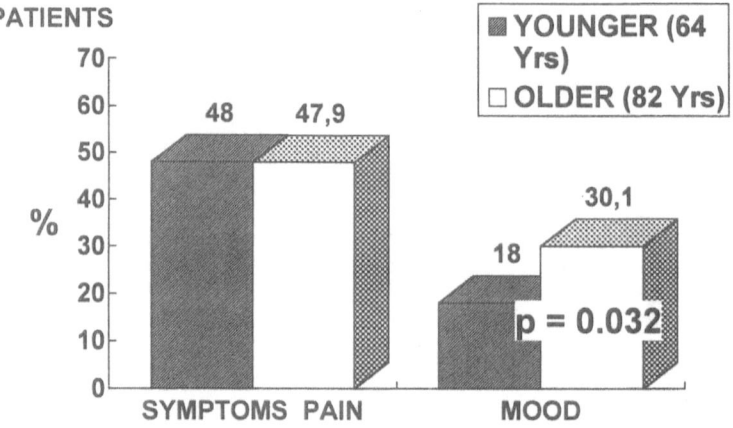

Figure 18.7. Difficulties on EuroQOL (b).

Further comparisons

Older patients were also compared with 3 general populations:
1. An American 'geriatric' population (n = 2193) which, however, was not so old (> 60 years old) [35]: Even in comparison to this group, our octogenarian patients had better *self-health perception*, reported better *improvement in health in the last 5 years* (for patients this was after the operation) and had better *social resources scores on the OARS*.
2. The Rotterdam EuroQOL survey, from which we chose only the 10 octogenarians in the survey: In comparison our octogenarian patients had marginally better *EuroQOL scores* (personal communicated survey data, Figure 18.8).

MEAN EUROQOL RATINGS
>80 yr Patients vs >80 yr Population

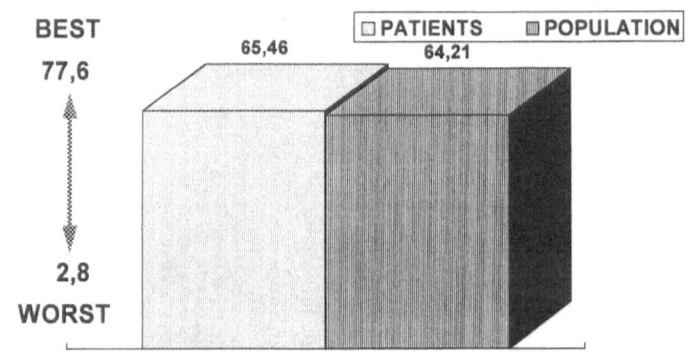

Figure 18.8. EuroQOL score comparison with 'healthy' octogenarians.

3. A Dutch +80 year population (n = 293) [18] was compared on *Basic and Household Activities of Daily Living Scores*: In both, our octogenarian patients did significantly better ($p < .01$) than the octogenarian general population. Mean basic activity limitation scores were 0.17 ± 0.55 for population A and 0.47 ± 1.02 for the Dutch general population (maximal limitation = 5, minimal limitation = 1).

Discussion

The surgical ability to operate on older and older patients has been reported as an achievement as the mean patient age at CABG has mounted steadily, ever since the procedure began in the late 60's. That the operation will lengthen life is a vague promised currently offered to almost every CABG patient. Older patients of this study usually did not seek operation; it was forced on them because of compelling indications which predicted early impending death. Their 5-year actuarial survival, better than that of an age-adjusted general population, is proof that the operation both saves and extends life.

But is old age worth extending? Because of the survival benefit of CABG, reports of operations in even older patients, i.e. over the age of 75 and 80 years have been met with some consternation [36]. In recent years, there has been controversial reappraisal of all prevailing medical practice which prolongs the misery of old age by modern technology. A group of philosophers and politicians, who have attracted wide press attention in the United States, strongly take the view that the health care of the elderly should be rationed: their case is based on the arguments that human life span is limited, that death is preceded by old age, and that when one becomes old, it is neither wise nor without expense for science to heroically fight the inevitability of death [37–39]. Katz *et al.* [40], for instance, predict 'active life expectancy', i.e. that of the average 16.5 years remaining after age 65, 6 will be spent in disability and dependency and, after age 85, of the remaining 7.5 years, 4.5 years shall be in such a state. As heterogeneity in function is far more marked in advanced than younger age [41], one must be circumspect with generalising. Care refused for cost alone is clearly unethical. However, in a climate of cost-containment, even elective surgery with known benefits must undergo the test of appropriateness to disqualify as a 'heroic treatment'. As both the elderly and CABG are high cost areas, their combination invites the potential for rationing.

This investigation was intended to develop a methodology for assessing the health and quality of life as a result of these operations in elderly patients, so that a case could be made for or against these pressures of rationing.

A mail questionnaire was used because a majority of our patients were German nationals who had come from Germany only for the operation and had returned after it was performed, and would therefore be difficult to trace for an interview. Also, in a face to face or telephone interview it becomes difficult to ask specific or embarrassing questions. On the other hand, in a self-administered questionnaire, the vision of the elderly may be too poor to read, their motivation, literacy or intelligence insufficient for understanding, they may not be able to write the answers, etc., and we would not know if they had self-answered or not. We encouraged the patients to seek help from others in answering, report to us if help had been enlisted and explain why, i.e. if questions could not be read, understood or answers written. Every non-respondent who had a telephone was called personally and, as it has been found that return rates are higher [42], we used reply paid envelopes. A recent study found that with proper format and planning, regarding not only the length but also the appearance of the questionnaire, the use of postal questionnaires in an elderly population was as reliable as an interview [43]. In contrast to social studies, we expected and received satisfactory response rates because we knew our patients well.

Regarding duration of follow-up after CABG, it has been advised that as graft attrition takes a few years to manifest, at a minimum, follow-up must be of 4 to 7 years [44]. However, even in younger CABG patients, the duration of a quality of life follow-up has rarely been more than a year. According to a review by King [45], 'Timing of assessment of postoperative quality of life has varied across studies, ranging from 6 weeks to 3.5 years after surgery'. Previous investigations in elderly patients were all limited to 1 year, often had no comparisons with younger patients, and sometimes only included electively operated patients or those not so old (e.g., > 65 or > 70 years) were studied.

In evaluating the quality of survival of our patients at 5 years, demographically the older patients were remarkably different from younger patients: they were all older than 80 years at the 5-year follow-up with a mean age of 82 years (older than younger patients by 18 years), their female sex proportion was thrice, 41% of them were widowed and 34% were living alone, although none were institutionalised.

On comparing the *functional capacity* of these octogenarian patients (n = 77) with a Dutch, general octogenarian population (n = 293), again older patients seemed to be doing better. Considering that more than two-thirds of deaths in such an old population are due to cardiac reasons and that their disability is often due to angina [10], the better functioning of CABG patients could reflect a continuing benefit of the operation. As reported elsewhere [20] for these populations, there was no difference in anginal or dyspnea symptoms, or in the incidence of cardiac events (in frequency of cardiac re-hospitalization > 2 days, occurrence of myocardial infarction or a new coronary angiography, angioplasty or operation). On a single item asking about frequency of confusion, mentally the older patients had reported significantly more confusion. However, 90% of them had completed our questionnaires themselves (of those who had not, 60% could not because of bad sight). To function well intellectually is one of the most important factors in the ability to enjoy a full and rewarding life. Especially in the elderly, it became important to study the soundness of the faculty of their reasoning and memory, as it is known to deteriorate with age. The strongest argument against CABG in the elderly is that elderly patients have many times more neuropsychologic complications than younger patients; however, in absence of clinical neurological deficit, improvement is usually complete within 6 months, depending on the emotional state, which is often used as an excuse to avoid work. Therefore, at 5 years, the issue of cognitive state was not as an aftermath of extracorporeal circulation, but the possible intellectual decline occurring due to age per se. Despite its importance, the cognitive state could not be measured satisfactorily, as it is impossible to do this without an interview. Self-administered questions exist, but these must be completed in the presence of an investigator.

Regarding *social status*, younger patients had higher social interaction but not significantly more. However, the dependability of social support for octogenarian patients (often widowed and living alone) was significantly lower than for younger patients; affectively, too, they were significantly less content with their social resources. However, their total social scores, which are derived from all of these three components, were not different from younger patients. Older patients reported a better improvement in family intimacy and work capacity after the operation than did younger patients, but not significantly more. Also, a fifth of the elderly and approximately a fourth of the younger patients reported a worsening in work capacity, inclusive of household work and hobbies. Surprisingly, more elderly than younger patients reported an improvement in sexual satisfaction. Family income was mostly unchanged for both groups.

Thus, both physically and overall socially, the older patients' state appeared to be no different from younger patients. However, although their anxiety on the Hospital Anxiety and Depression Scale was similar to younger patients, depression was significantly higher (the mean was about twice that of younger patients), with 4% of older patients exhibiting clinical depression of a score that is recommended to warrant anti-depressive treatment. On the generic scale, EuroQOL, the elderly patients also had significantly more difficulties with mood than younger patients, corroborating the depression observed on the HAD, but in the other four physical dimensions no differences were seen with younger patients. Total EuroQOL scores of the younger and older patients were also similar, but the scores of octogenarian patients were marginally better than an octogenarian general population.

The mean health-related quality of life (HRQOL) scores were not significantly different for older and younger patients. The health-related quality of life score correlated strongly with both anxiety and depression, and more with depression than anxiety in both younger and older patients. The reason of depression could not be attributed to any one dimension. Depressed (borderline + clinical) versus non-depressed older patients had worse physical scores (scoring done by a criteria combining severity of cardiac symptom, events, re-hospitalisation and disability), worse social scores on the OARS, worse EuroQOL and worse HRQOL scores. There was no difference in depression in those living alone or with others. Despite more frequent in some elderly patients, their numbers were small (clinical depression in 4% patients) because this did not affect the comparative health-related quality of life score of older versus younger patients which ultimately remained similar, as did the EuroQOL score. Possibly depression is not the only determinant of patient-perceived and patient-judged, health-related quality of life. In old age, people are known to be more tolerant of stress, whether physical, social or emotional, and although this might be severe enough to depress them, they may accept such moodiness as an inevitable accompaniment of aging and continue to judge that they are happy about life and their health in general.

Regarding the higher incidence of cognitive dysfunction in older patients, first, the validity of this finding is disputable (only 1 item was asked) and, second, whether this difference is because of extracorporeal circulation 5 years ago or because of advanced age cannot be said. One could doubt the validity of self-report by a population found probably to have more confusion, but we found very few mistakes in their answering questions set in a format which changed with every dimension. In those who returned the questionnaire incomplete, non-response was maximal (5 to 10%) for questions on change (it could be difficult to remember the status 5 years ago) for both younger and older patients; it was less than 5% on all other questions. Additionally, patients had been encouraged to accept the help of others in answering whenever difficulty arose.

Finally, taking patient-perceived satisfactions as an indication of quality of life, 5 years after CABG, 27.9% of octogenarian patients perceived their HRQOL between 1 to 1.99 (where 1 = 'Delighted' and 2 = 'Pleased'), 57.1% between 2 and 2.99 (where 3 = Mostly satisfied) and the remaining 14.8% between 3 and 3.99 (where 4 = Neutral). No elderly patient had a poor HRQOL score (5 = Mostly dissatisfied, 6 = Dissatisfied, 7 = Terrible). For younger patients, scores were between 1 and 1.99 for 14.1% patients, 67.3% between 2 and 2.99, 17.1% between 3 and 3.99, 1.5% between 4 and 4.99 and 0.5% between 5 and 5.99.

Thus, even though coronary bypass surgery in very old patients is often done only as a semi-urgent procedure to save life, the benefit both in survival and quality of life matches or even exceeds that in younger patients. Perhaps because of refusal or postponement of surgery, either due to physician-perceived excessive multi-organ senescence or because of lowered occupational worth, these patients may have long suffered symptoms, dependence and hopelessness and feel justifiably satisfied about the kind of life which the operation permits.

In conclusion, the operation can save, extend and transform the life of these very old patients. Instead of increasing the threat by delaying surgery, assessment of their operative risk must be realistic and balanced against the risk of mortality and of a worsening quality of life without operation. It must also be contrasted against the chance of longevity of the operative survivor and the quality of life possible because of the operation. This study makes distinct the medical appropriateness of the operation from cost-considerations which also merge in decision-making and resource allocation. Its findings are therefore an important ethical argument for prioritizing elderly patients equally in waiting lists for coronary bypass surgery.

References

1. Wenger NK, Marcus FI, O'Rourke RA. Cardiovascular disease in the elderly. J Am Coll Cardiol 1987; 80A–7.
2. Lockwood M. Quality of life and resource allocation. In: Bell JM, Mendus S, et al, editors. Philosophy & medical welfare. Cambridge: Cambridge University Press, 1988: 50.
3. Pheleps CE. The methodologic foundations of studies of the appropriateness of medical care. New Engl J Med 1993; 329: 1241–53.
4. Cowley G. What high tech can't accomplish. Newsweek 1993; Oct 4: 34.
5. Dudley RA, Harrell FE, Smith LR, et al. Comparison of analytic models for estimating the effect of clinical factors on the cost of coronary artery bypass surgery. J Clin Epidemiol 1993; 46: 261–71 .
6. Loop FD, et al. Coronary artery bypass graft surgery in the elderly. Cleve Clin J Med 1988; 55: 23–34.
7. Edmunds LH Jr, Stephenson LW, Ratcliffe MB. Open heart surgery in octogenarians. N Engl J Med 1988; 313(3): 131–6.
8. Bashour TT. Coronary artery bypass grafting in the over 80 population. Prog Cardiol 1993; 5(1): 117–29.
9. Vetter NJ, Ford D. Angina among elderly people and its relationship with disability. Age Ageing 1990; 19: 159–63.
10. Chappell NL. Aging and social care. In: Binstock RH, George LK, editors. Handbook of aging and social sciences. 1990: 438–54.
11. Mohan R, Amsel BJ, Walter PJ. Coronary artery bypass grafting in the elderly – a review of studies on patients older than 64, 69 or 74 years. Cardiology 1992; 80: 215–25.
12. Kowalchuk GJ, Siu SC, Lewis SM. Coronary artery disease in the octogenarian: angiographic spectrum and suitability for revascularisation. Am J Cardiol 1990; 66: 1319–23.
13. Cassell CK. Certification – another step for geriatric medicine. JAMA 1987; 258: 1518–9.
14. Mohan R, Walter PJ, Vandermast M, et al. Isolated coronary artery bypass grafting in patients 75 years of age or older. Thorac Cardiovasc Surg 1992; 40: 365–70.
15. Patrick DL, Deyo RA. Generic and disease-specific measures in assessing health status and quality of life. Medical Care 1980; 27: S217–32.
16. Walter PJ. Quality of life after open heart surgery. Dordrecht, The Netherlands: Kluwer Academic Publishers, 1992.
17. Katz S. Studies of illness in the aged: The index of ADL – a standardised measure of biological and psychosocial function. JAMA 1963; 185: 914–9.
18. Fredriks CM, te Wierik MJ, Visser AP, Sturmans F. Functional status of the elderly living at home. J Adv Nurs 1990; 16: 287–92.
19. Mohan R. Too old for coronary bypass surgery? Health-related quality of life in older patients 5 years after operation. PhD thesis, University of Antwerp, Belgium, 1994.
20. Snaith RP. The Hospital Anxiety and Depression Scale. Quality of Life Newsletter 1993; 6: 5.
21. Kutner NG, Fiar PL, Kutner MH, et al. Assessing anxiety & depression in chronic dialysis patients. J Psychosom Res 1985; 29: 23–31.
22. Zigmond AS, Snaith RP. The Hospital Anxiety and Depression Scale. Acta Psychiatr Scand 1983; 67: 361–70.
23. Channer KS, Papochado M, James MA. Anxiety and depression in patients with chest pain referred for exercise testing. The Lancet 1985; 820–3.
24. Kenn C, Wood H, Kuckyji M, et al. Validation of the Hospital Anxiety & Depression scale in an elderly psychiatric population. Int J Geriatr Psychiatry 1987; 2: 183–93.
25. Bowling A. Measuring health: a review of quality of life measurement scales. Milton Keynes, UK: Open University Press, 1991.
26. Orth-Gomer K, Unden AL. The measurement of social support in population surveys. Soc Sci Med 1987; 24: 83–94.

27. Blazer DG. Social support and mortality in an elderly community population. Am J Epidemiol 1982; 115: 684–94.
28. Ware JE, Brook RH, Davies-Avery A, et al. Conceptualisation and measurement of health for adults in the Health Insurance Study, Santa Monica, CA, USA: Rand Corporation, 1980.
29. Andrews FM, Withey SB. Social indicators of well being. New York: Plenum Press, 1976.
30. Campbell A. The quality of American life. New York: Russell Sage, 1976.
31. Cantril H. The pattern of human concerns. New Brunswick, New Jersey: Rutgers University Press, 1965.
32. EuroQOL – a new facility for the measurement of health related quality of life. Health Policy 1990; 16: 199–208.
33. Sintonen H, editor. Proceedings of EuroQOL conference; 1992 Oct; Helsinki.
34. Aday LA. Designing and conducting health surveys. San Francisco: Jossey-Bass Publishers, 1989.
35. Fillenbaum GG. Validity and reliability of the Multidimensional Functional Assessment Questionnaire: the OARS methodology. Durham, NC, USA: Duke University, Centre for the Study of Aging & Human Development, 1978.
36. Edmunds LH Jr. Uncomfortable issues [editorial]. Ann Thorac Surg 1990; 50: 173–4.
37. Callahan D. Setting limits: medical goals in an aging society. New York: Simon & Schuster, 1987.
38. Daniels N. Am I my brother's keeper – an essay of justice between the young and the old. New York: Oxford University Press, 1988.
39. Lamm RD. Saving a few, sacrificing many – at great cost. NY Times 1989; August 8: 39.
40. Katz S, Branch LG, Branson MH, et al. Active life expectancy. New Engl J Med 1983; 309: 1218–24.
41. Rowe JW, Kahn RL. Human aging: usual and successful. Science 1987; 237: 143–9.
42. Newland CA, Waters WE, Stanford AP. A study of the mail survey method. Int J Epidemiol 1977; 6: 65.
43. Victor CR. Some methodological aspects of using postal questionnaires with the elderly. Arch Gerontol Geriatr 1988; 7: 163–72.
44. Wenger NK, et al. Overview: assesment of quality of life in clinical trials of cardiovascular therapies. In: Wenger NK, et al., editors. Assesment of quality of life in clinical trials of cardiovascular therapies. New York: Le Jacq Publishing Inc., 1984: 1–22.
45. King KB, Porter LA, Norsen LH. Patient perceptions of quality of life after coronary artery surgery: was it worth it? Res Nurs Health 1992; 15: 327–49.

PART SIX

Rehabilitation

19. Rehabilitation following coronary artery bypass graft surgery at elderly age

NANETTE K. WENGER

Introduction

The emerging pattern in coronary artery bypass graft surgery is operation at older age and in patients with more severe coronary atherosclerosis, greater ventricular dysfunction, and more frequent co-morbid medical illnesses. Often these older patients have had prior coronary artery bypass graft surgery, as well as antecedent percutaneous transluminal coronary angioplasty. Operation at elderly age encompasses a higher percentage of female patients in the operated cohort as well, owing to the older age at onset of clinical manifestations of coronary disease among women.

Exercise training and coronary risk reduction are the major modalities of rehabilitative intervention designed to enhance the functional status of patients following coronary artery bypass graft surgery at all ages. The goals of coronary rehabilitation are to extend the post-operative period of disability-free and dependency-free survival, both by limiting recurrent coronary events and by enhancing and maintaining the level of physical functioning. The potential of rehabilitative care to confer benefit may be even greater in older than in younger coronary surgical populations, owing to the higher risk for disability at elderly age.

No data regarding disablement are available for the specific subset of patients following coronary bypass graft surgery at elderly age. However, among coronary patients in general older than 65 years of age, limitation of physical activity is present in 51–70% of men, and in 40–74% of women. Elderly women with angina are at significantly higher risk for diminished functional capacity than are elderly men [1]. After age 70 years, owing to angina, heart failure, or combinations of these problems, activity limitation is described in greater than 60% of men and 80% of women. Heart failure predicted disability only in women in the Framingham cohort [2]. At ages older than 75 years, up to 76% of men with coronary heart disease are considered disabled.

P.J. Walter (ed.), Coronary Bypass Surgery in the Elderly, pp. 213–221.
© 1995 *Kluwer Academic Publishers, Dordrecht.*

Exercise rehabilitation

Until recent years, exercise rehabilitation of coronary patients was often arbitrarily restricted to those younger than 65 years of age. Few or no elderly coronary patients were enrolled in clinical trials of exercise rehabilitation. However, with the changing demography of the coronary population, such that the majority of coronary events are encountered beyond age 65 years and that half of all myocardial revascularization procedures in the U.S. are performed in this age group, an increasing proportion of elderly coronary patients are currently enrolled in structured exercise rehabilitation programs [3]. There is relatively uniform documentation, albeit derived predominantly from observational studies [4–8] that the improvement in functional capacity as a result of exercise training at elderly age is comparable to that among younger coronary patients. Furthermore, such exercise rehabilitation is both feasible and can be accomplished with safety. It is important to remember the admonition of Dr. Paul Dudley White [9] that '. . . exercise of almost any kind, suitable in degree and duration . . . can and should play a useful role in the maintenance of both physical and mental health of the aging individual . . . ' Despite this wisdom, physicians commonly underestimate the habitual activity level of their elderly patients and often prescribe excessive bed rest and activity limitation for many medical and surgical problems, including coronary atherosclerotic heart disease, and following myocardial revascularization procedures.

A number of additional factors, unrelated to coronary disease or coronary bypass graft surgery per se, contribute to the decrement in habitual levels of physical activity at elderly age [10]. Apart from cardiovascular symptoms, a number of non-cardiac limitations can decrease both the habitual physical activity level and the resultant exercise capacity of elderly coronary patients. These include psychologic factors such as anxiety, depression, fear, and lack of motivation; musculoskeletal instability; arthritis and other orthopedic problems; decrease in peripheral muscular strength owing to the lesser skeletal muscle mass with aging; co-morbid problems such as peripheral vascular disease, decreased pulmonary function, and neurologic disorders; and often inappropriate admonitions by family, by friends, and by medical personnel. This decrement in habitual physical activity is substantially greater among elderly women than among elderly men [11].

A number of physiologic features of normal aging also influence the lessened habitual activity level at elderly age. Aerobic capacity decreases with aging, such that any specific activity entails a greater percentage of the lowered functional capacity [12]. As a result, patients overestimate the work intensity of a particular task; the same activity is progressively perceived as requiring increased work. Further, the aged ventricle is characterized by decreased compliance, which may be accentuated in the presence of diabetes and hypertension. The poorly compliant ventricle has as its clinical counterpart exercise-induced dyspnea, with dyspnea appearing even at low intensities of exercise. This dyspnea may be misinterpreted by medical personnel as due to ventricular systolic, rather than diastolic, dysfunction, and prompt recommendations for further limitation of activity. Finally, the aging changes in the lungs increase the work of breathing, adding to the perception of excessive work intensity [13].

As with younger individuals, exercise training-induced adaptations at elderly age are primarily mediated by peripheral mechanisms. They include an increase in oxygen extraction by trained skeletal muscle, a lessened myocardial oxygen demand (due to a lesser heart rate and systolic blood pressure response to any submaximal exercise intensity), and a resultant increase in the anginal threshold and decrease in exercise-induced angina. A comparable increase in maximal oxygen uptake occurred in elderly male and female coronary patients following exercise training [7]. The improved exercise tolerance can reverse prior limitations of activity due to angina pectoris.

Post-operative exercise training is of particular importance in elderly patients, owing to their typically complicated clinical course following coronary artery bypass graft surgery. The perioperative course at elderly age is characterized by frequent and multiple complications, including an increased requirement for ventilatory support, for temporary or permanent pacemaker implantation, for use of aortic balloon counterpulsation, for treatments for bleeding and infections, and the like. All these entail an increased period of immobilization at bed rest, as well as a more protracted hospital stay, both of which exacerbate the problem of physical deconditioning due to inactivity. A marked decrease in post-hospital exercise tolerance is often encountered, even in previously active elderly coronary bypass graft surgery patients. If not advised that this activity limitation is a reflection of the deconditioning response, rather than their underlying coronary disease, patients are likely to inappropriately perceive their coronary disease as being excessively severe or their coronary artery bypass surgery procedures as having been unsuccessful.

Guidelines for the conduct of exercise rehabilitation at elderly age [14] include the provision of a longer duration of warm-up and cool-down activities. Warm-up activities involve flexibility and range-of-motion exercises to enable cardiorespiratory readiness for exercise. The prolonged cool-down period is requisite for dissipation of the heat load, given the decrease in skin blood flow and less efficient sweating mechanism at elderly age, as well as to enable subsidence of the exercise-induced peripheral vasodilatation. Additionally, because of the slower return of the exercise heart rate to resting values than at younger age, more rest time is required between components of exercise training. A gradual increase in the intensity and duration of exercise is prudent both to limit injuries and to avoid discomfort. High-impact activities such as running and jumping should be avoided, even for previously physically active elderly individuals, to limit musculoskeletal complications; elderly women are more prone to jogging injuries than are elderly men [15].

Contemporary guidelines suggest benefit from a lower intensity of physical activity than previously recommended, typically 60–70% of the maximal heart rate achieved at exercise testing; these lower intensity recommendations are likely to promote adherence, in that exercise-related discomfort is less likely to occur [3]. Furthermore, exercising farther from a potential ischemic threshold limits the risk of adverse outcomes, particularly when exercise is unsupervised. In this regard, brisk walking is an ideal aerobic stimulus for elderly patients in that it requires no special equipment, skills, facilities, or training. Whereas brisk walking often provides an inadequate stimulus at younger age, the exercise intensity is adequate at elderly age to enable a training response [16, 17]. Enclosed shopping malls offer a temperature- and humidity-controlled environment, as well as a level surface for walking, and encourage the companionship of co-exercisers as well. Although at younger age monitoring of the pulse rate or the rating of perceived exertion is recommended to control the intensity of exercise, the 'talk test' is a more feasible and effective control mechanism for elderly patients. Patients are instructed to exercise only to an intensity that permits them to continue to converse with an exercising companion [11].

In recent years, improvements in exercise tolerance as a result of exercise training have been documented in patients with left ventricular dysfunction, without apparent deterioration of left ventricular performance [8, 18]. Additionally, strength training, previously considered contraindicated for coronary patients, can be safely instituted once a reasonable level of aerobic performance has been attained. The increase in muscle mass and muscular strength and function can further improve aerobic capacity and enhance physical work capacity and endurance.

Exercise rehabilitation can increase the physical performance of elderly coronary patients, thereby prolonging their duration of an active lifestyle and maintenance of functional independence. Elderly coronary patients have comparable exercise trainability, e.g., improvements in functional capacity, exercise hemodynamics, exercise tolerability and exercise safety, to younger patients in similar exercise rehabilitation programs. Exercising elderly coronary patients describe an improved sense of well-being and lessened anxiety and depression, comparable to favorable psychologic response described in exercising healthy older men and women [19, 20]. Thus, rehabilitative exercise training following coronary bypass graft surgery is associated with favorable life quality outcomes that are both personally beneficial and cost-effective.

Multifactorial coronary risk reduction

Rehabilitative care also involves education and guidance for multifactorial coronary risk reduction, as well as for the maintenance of recommended therapies. Modifiable coronary risk factors are highly prevalent at elderly age and continue to influence the recurrence of coronary events. Despite the paucity of data regarding the efficacy of post-operative coronary risk reduction at elderly age, extrapolation from results in populations of non-operated elderly coronary patients appears reasonable [21], particularly since persons known to

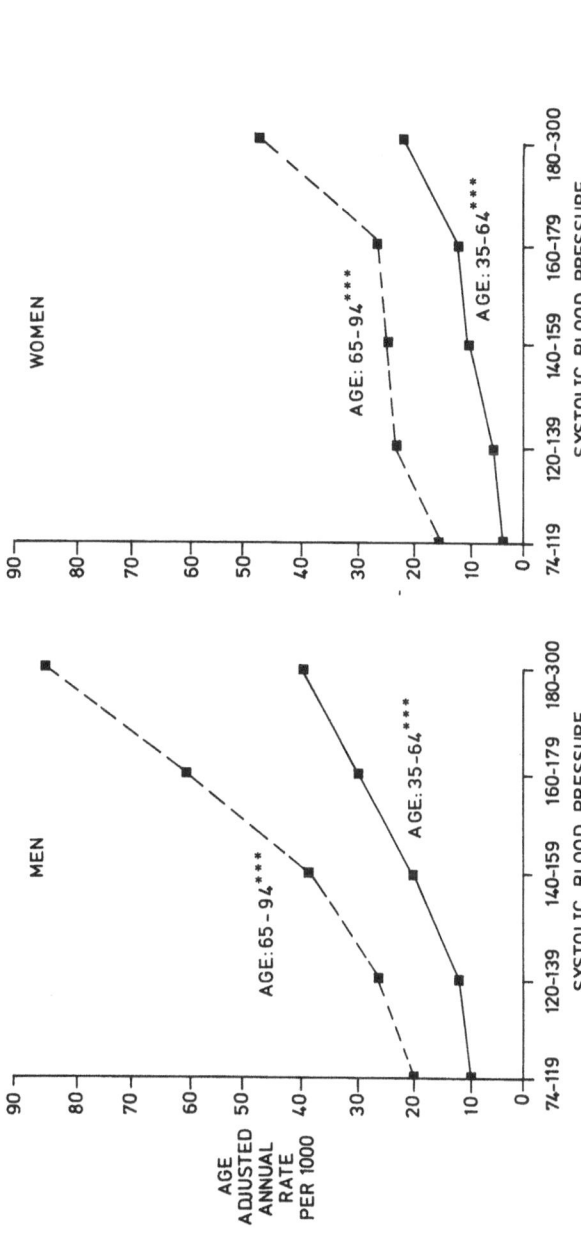

Figure 19.1. Risk of cardiovascular disease by age, sex, and level of systolic blood pressure, from a 30-year follow-up in the Framingham Study. ***p <0.001 (Wald statistic for logistic regression analysis). (From Vokonas PS, et al. J Hypertens 1988; 6(suppl 1): S5. Reproduced with permission.)

have coronary heart disease are at the highest risk for recurrent coronary events and thus have a greater likelihood of benefit from effective preventive interventions. Stated otherwise, secondary preventive care is likely to impart greater benefit at elderly age due to the excess of coronary morbidity and mortality in this population [22]. Lifestyle changes to accomplish coronary risk reduction should be undertaken when feasible, with medications added as needed.

Post-infarction hypertension, based on Framingham data [23], confers a five-fold increased risk of recurrent coronary events, and the adverse impact of hypertension increases with increasing age. Isolated systolic hypertension, prevalent at elderly age, carries a comparable adverse prognosis to combined systolic and diastolic hypertension. Sodium restriction is an important component of care. Based on data from the Systolic Hypertension in the Elderly Program (SHEP) trial [24], the ease of control of isolated systolic hypertension with low-dose chlorthalidone and added beta blocker as needed can be recommended (Figure 19.1). Hypercholesterolemia predicts an increased likelihood of reinfarction, coronary death, and all-cause mortality, with a 4- to 18-fold greater absolute benefit of cholesterol-lowering described in older patients with defined coronary disease than in younger healthy and coronary populations. Hypercholesterolemia appears to accentuate the loss of vasodilator reserve in atherosclerotic coronary arteries. Cholesterol-lowering at younger age has been documented to decrease the progression of athero-sclerosis, both in native coronary arteries and in coronary artery bypass graft conduits (Figure 19.2) [25–27]. Based on data from the CASS Registry, smoking cessation has a beneficial effect in elderly coronary patients. Smokers have a 70% excess risk of 6-year mortality, and a 50% excess risk of myocardial infarction and death. Among younger patients in the randomized Coronary Artery Surgery Study [28], continued smoking following coronary artery bypass graft surgery appeared to nullify the surgical benefit. Elevated blood sugar levels and obesity, as additional coronary risk attributes, confer greater absolute risk at older than at younger age.

Rehabilitative programs can provide guidance to elderly patients after coronary artery bypass graft surgery to encourage adherence to medical regimens; can offer social support which, per se, may improve coronary risk; and can aid in the reintegration of elderly coronary surgical patients into their pre-illness community and societal roles, including return to work when appropriate.

Coronary rehabilitation at elderly age in the 1990s

Considerable data identify a lesser frequency of referral to and of participation in structured rehabilitation programs at elderly than at younger age [4, 21], with the differential being most prominent for elderly women with coronary disease [7]. The reasons for differences in physician referral patterns remain uncertain,

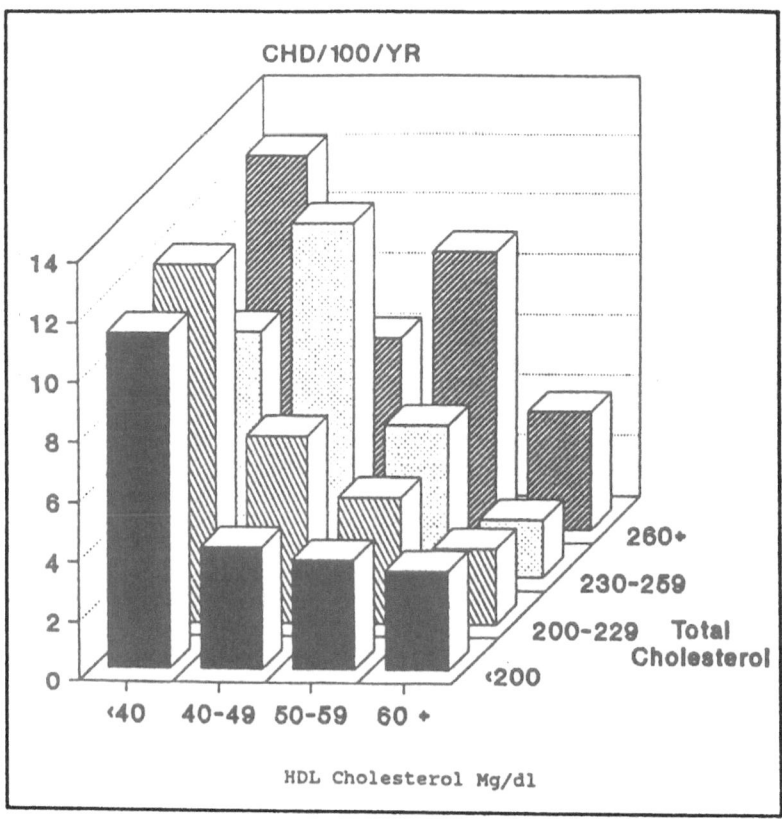

Figure 19.2. Relation of coronary heart disease (CHD) rate and total high-density lipoprotein (HDL) cholesterol concentrations (ages 50 to 79 years). (From Castelli WP, et al. Am J Cardiol 1991; 63: 12H. Reproduced with permission.)

as do the components attributable to problems with transportation, to financial or insurance limitations, or to societal factors that may limit the desirability or acceptability of exercise at elderly age. However, physicians report recommending independent exercise to elderly patients following a coronary event to aid in their recovery.

Recent documentation among younger patients of the feasibility, safety, and efficacy of home-based rehabilitation [26, 29], using telephone follow-up for coronary risk reduction and other counseling, as well as to encourage adherence to an exercise regimen, may offer promise for a more cost-effective and acceptable intervention at elderly age. However, testing of this hypothesis is requisite among older age coronary patients, including those after coronary bypass graft surgery.

Many years ago, the poet Longfellow wrote:

For age has opportunity no less
Than youth itself, though in another dress,

And as the evening twilight fades away,
The sky is filled with stars, invisible by day.

Were Longfellow to return today to view elderly patients following coronary bypass graft surgery, he would find them to be a population not only eminently visible by day, but the focus of increasing attention to the components of their care most likely to cost-effectively improve both their survival and the quality of their lives. Rehabilitative care of elderly patients following coronary bypass operation has the potential to limit deterioration of functional capacity and to prolong the duration of an independent, active, and energetic lifestyle.

References

1. Nickel JT, Chirikos TN. Functional disability of elderly patients with long-term coronary heart disease: a sex-stratified analysis. J Gerontol 1990; 45: S60–8.
2. Pinsky JL, Jette AM, Branch LG, Kannel WB, Feinleib M. The Framingham Disability Study: relationship of various coronary heart disease manifestations to disability in older persons living in the community. Am J Public Health 1990; 80: 1363–8.
3. WHO Expert Committee. Rehabilitation after cardiovascular diseases, with special emphasis on developing countries. World Health Organization Technical Report Series 831. Geneva: WHO, 1993.
4. Ades PA, Hanson JS, Gunther PGS, Tonino RP. Exercise conditioning in the elderly coronary patient. J Am Geriatr Soc 1987; 35: 121–4.
5. Ades PA, Grunvald MH. Cardiopulmonary exercise testing before and after conditioning in older coronary patients. Am Heart J 1990; 120: 585–9.
6. Ades PA, Waldmann ML, Poehlman ET, et al. Exercise conditioning in older coronary patients. Submaximal lactate response and endurance capacity. Circulation 1993; 88: 572–7.
7. Ades PA, Waldmann ML, McCann WJ, Weaver SO. Predictors of cardiac rehabilitation participation in older coronary patients. Arch Intern Med 1992; 152: 1033–5.
8. Williams MA, Maresh CM, Esterbrooks DJ, Harbrecht JJ, Sketch MH. Early exercise training in patients older than age 65 years compared with that in younger patients after acute myocardial infarction or coronary artery bypass grafting. Am J Cardiol 1985; 55: 263–6.
9. White PD. The role of exercise in the aging. JAMA 1957; 165: 70–1.
10. Shephard RJ. Habitual physical activity levels and perception of exertion in the elderly. J Cardiopulm Rehabil 1989; 9: 17–23.
11. Wenger NK. Coronary heart disease in the elderly. In: Wenger NK, Hellerstein HK, editors. Rehabilitation of the coronary patient, 3d ed. New York: Churchill Livingstone, 1992.
12. Fleg JL, Lakatta EG. Role of muscle loss in the age-associated reduction in VO_2 max. J Appl Physiol 1988; 65: 1147–51.
13. Redden WG. Respiratory system and aging. In: Smith EL, Serfass RC, editors. Exercise and aging: the scientific basis. Hillside, NJ: Enslow Publishers, 1981.
14. Shephard R. The scientific bases of exercise prescribing for the very old. J Am Geriatr Soc 1990; 38: 62–70.
15. Pollock ML, Carrol JF, Graves JE, et al. Injuries and adherence to walk/jog and resistance training programs in the elderly. Med Sci Sports Exerc 1991; 23: 1194–200.
16. Bruce RA, Larson EB, Stratton J. Physical fitness, functional aerobic capacity, aging, and responses to physical training or bypass surgery in coronary patients. J Cardiopulmonary Rehabil 1989; 9: 24–34.
17. Larson EB, Bruce RA. Exercise and aging. Ann Intern Med 1986; 105: 783–5.

18. Coats AJS, Adamopoulos S, Radaelli A, et al. Controlled trial of physical training in chronic heart failure: exercise performance, hemodynamics, ventilation, and autonomic function. Circulation 1992; 85: 2119–31.
19. Taylor CB, Sallis JF, Needle R. The relation of physical activity and exercise to mental health. Public Health Rep 1985; 100: 195–202.
20. Blumenthal JA, Emery CF, Madden DJ, et al. Cardiovascular and behavioral effects of aerobic exercise training in healthy older men and women. J Gerontol 1989; 44: M147–57.
21. Lavie CJ, Milani RV, Littman AB. Benefits of cardiac rehabilitation and exercise training in secondary coronary prevention in the elderly. J Am Coll Cardiol 1993; 22: 678–83.
22. Castelli WP, Wilson PWF, Levy D, Anderson K. Cardiovascular risk factors in the elderly. Am J Cardiol 1989; 63: 12H–9.
23. Kannel WB, Sorlie P, Castelli WP, McGee D. Blood pressure and survival after myocardial infarction: The Framingham Study. Am J Cardiol 1980; 45: 326–30.
24. SHEP Cooperative Research Group. Prevention of stroke by antihypertensive drug treatment in older persons with isolated systolic hypertension. Final results of the Systolic Hypertension in the Elderly Program (SHEP). JAMA 1991; 265: 3255–64.
25. Blankenhorn DH, Nessim SA, Johnson RL, Sanmarco ME, Azen SP, Cashin-Hemphill L. Beneficial effects of combined colestipol-niacin therapy on coronary atherosclerosis and coronary venous bypass grafts. JAMA 1987; 257: 3233–40.
26. Haskell WL, Alderman EL, Fair JM, et al. Effects of intensive multiple risk factor reduction on coronary atherosclerosis and clinical cardiac events in men and women with coronary artery disease: The Stanford Coronary Risk Intervention Project (SCRIP). Circulation 1994; 89: 975–90.
27. Watts GF, Lewis B, Brunt JNH, et al. Effects on coronary artery disease of lipid-lowering diet, or diet plus cholestyramine, in the St. Thomas' Atherosclerosis Regression Study (STARS). Lancet 1992; 339: 563–9.
28. Hermanson B, Omenn GS, Kronmal RA, Gersh BJ, and participants in the Coronary Artery Surgery Study. Beneficial six-year outcome of smoking cessation in older men and women with coronary artery disease. Results from the CASS Registry. N Engl J Med 1988; 319: 1365–9.
29. DeBusk RF, Miller NH, Superko R, et al. A case-management system for coronary risk factor modification after acute myocardial infarction. Ann Intern Med 1994; 120: 721–9.

Discussions

Discussion: M. Schneider

Schulte: In one of your slides you were showing the development of the patients over the age of 80 years, and you showed that in 1990 it was at a certain level and it was then decreasing at the year 2000. What is the reason for this development?

Schneider: The reason of the relative decrease of the share of the very elderly aged 80 years and older between 1990 and 2000 is the drop of the birthrate during World War I. This has considerably shaped the population pyramid. The reduction can also be found in national forecasts.

Wenger: Let me make a comment, if I may, on the issue of relative costs. It is very easy to identify coronary bypass graft surgery as a cost because it is one large single item, but that item is not the alternative to no cost. I hope that in our discussions over the next days we examine alternative costs, because what we will have to examine is the cost of care for the patients not operated and that will include hospitalizations, drugs, office visits, long-term custodial care and the like. Unfortunately, in any health economic analysis, the ultimate economy is death and that really is not the goal of what we are about. So we have to examine the relative costs in operated and non-operated elderly patients, because it is not simply coronary bypass graft surgery cost versus no cost.

Hoffmeister: Dr. Schneider, you said that there will be an increase in the prevalence of coronary heart disease and of cardiovascular disease at all in the next time. I agree with you but I think it is different if you look on standardized total populations or on different age groups. There is an increase in the old and very old population which is not the case in the younger (younger means under 70) population. Do you agree?

Schneider: I have mentioned Sweden, because the regular questionnaires on the health status of the Swedish population have shown a strong increase in the well-being of the elderly. The elderly have more improvements in health-status

P.J. Walter (ed.), Coronary Bypass Surgery in the Elderly, pp. 223–257.
© 1995 *Kluwer Academic Publishers, Dordrecht.*

than the general population. This means morbidity is compressed during the lifespan, but it is not so much to reduce prevalence because life-expectancy is increasing faster than morbidity declines. This is, I think, the central point. Therefore, we should compare the epidemiological data of more countries concerning this subject. The investigation for Germany should be compared with other countries and maybe we will come to better conclusions.

Let me answer the question of relative costs. I do not know of cost studies which are also looking at the cost rehabilitation and long-term care after coronary bypass grafting for the elderly. One way of looking at costs is to look at the costs of alternative procedures for bypass grafting, another approach is different follow-up procedures after coronary bypass surgery. Principally, both approaches should be combined. There are huge variations of costs depending on the kind of rehabilitation. In the European countries we can observe great variations in the kind of rehabilitation after myocardial infarction. For example, in Germany most is done in special rehabilitation hospitals. In other countries, like Sweden or the U.K., more rehabilitation is provided in the acute hospitals and in ambulatory care. All of these types of rehabilitation result in different costs. From the total costs of the treatment of cardiovascular diseases the direct costs of coronary bypass surgery are only a minor part.

Mohan: In the discussions we are going to have in the coming days, I believe there are two points which are relevant and important when we are looking at the future. Firstly, let us not run away with our imaginations that life expectancy is going to go on increasing. From what I read, even in the coming 30 years, life expectancy is to increase only up to about 82–83 years. At the moment, that is probably in Japan, and even in the next 30 years, it shall increase by only another 3 or 4 years. So the need for coronary surgery in the elderly will not be in a much older population. We should not be thinking that we have to decide on whether to operate or not on patients 100 or 110 years old because that will not be the case. What I mean to say is that the patients will not come any older; what we have to decide is whether or not to operate on patients who are, let us say, 80 years or older. Secondly, you mentioned that the prevalence of cardiovascular diseases in the elderly has been decreasing. I only wish to reaffirm that two-thirds of deaths in the elderly are due to cardiovascular causes. So even though the prevalence will decrease the requirements for coronary surgery in an elderly population will continue to be high.

Schneider: One remark to life expectancy. Presently, in Japan, Sweden and in Switzerland, all countries with high life expectancy, a further increase in life expectancy can be observed. But in other countries, like in the Netherlands or in Denmark, we do not have this increase in life expectancy. Thus, there are possibilities to influence it. In Denmark, one hypothesis is that the limited increase in life expectancy compared to other countries. The continuing strong increase in life expectancy in a lot of countries should make us cautious with statements which see no need for bypass surgery in higher age groups in the future.

Discussion: H. Hoffmeister

Laczkovics: I would like to make a comment concerning life expectancy and reflecting what the participants said in the first session. I've looked at a statistical analysis of the Federal Republic of Germany for the last 100 years, and what you said about life expectancy is true for the newborn age. A hundred years ago you had a life expectancy for about 35 years and that's going up to 74 years now. But if you look at ages 60, 70, 80 or 90, the relative increase is not very impressive. I'll just give one example concerning people aged 90 and older. There were some small figures of 90 100 years ago. The relative life expectancy was +1, so if you compare this with the population of 90 today, their relative expectancy is therefor +3 or +4. The relative increase in this age is not tremendous in my eyes. So I sympathize with what the colleague over there said that we probably have not to deal with an extremely old population in the future but more with an incredibly increasing number of just normally old people.

Hoffmeister: I agree with your figures. But what is a big increase or not in a high age is another question. It is clear that the mean bulk of the increase until 1960 comes from the younger age groups, but in the last decades we have to realize that the relative increase results more from the older age groups. What we see in Germany and other European countries is that just in these age groups relative to the other ones, there is a larger growing of life expectancy and it seems to continue. On the other hand, we will not come to a situation where people in the next 20 or 30 years will have life expectancies of 100 or 110 years. This will not be the case. We are doing well already now, and we cannot enhance lifespan very much.

Fontan: I am not sure that you replied entirely to the question of your title. Could you clarify the answer to your title?

Hoffmeister: I feel that we have to focus on the elderly. When I was confronted with the title my answer was: when you have good health care and a very healthy population you will find severe diseases mainly in the old and very old group of the population. There is no other possibility, aside from accidents which occur in younger people, too. But I feel, the first thing we have to realize is that we've lived a very long time in good health in all Western populations, and at the end of this life (and hopefully it is very late in life) we will suffer from some chronic or other disease. But the distance between getting the disease and dying from this disease has not grown. That is the point which I wanted to focus on.

Fontan: Does your title mean that we have to focus just on what is the future of the elderly person or do we have to focus on health care in this category of patients?

Hoffmeister: No, we do not have, in my mind, to focus on containing health care costs in the elderly. This is very clear. But we have to focus on the elderly, and this is needed more in the future.

Mohan: To your question: 'containing health care costs: why focus on the elderly?' It has two aspects to it. A positive and a negative aspect. The positive aspect is that in the elderly there are more costs and you have to look at them. The negative aspect is: why should you look only at the elderly? The elderly have as much a right as younger people in getting health care even if it comes for them at a higher cost.

Discussion: Keon

Stalpaert: I have a question concerning the increase in the incidence of sternal dehiscence. Was it related to the use of the LIMA?

Keon: It may well be and perhaps bilateral mammaries are not a great idea on a frail elderly patient. As you know, this didn't withstand statistical analysis, but it is higher.

Stalpaert: You are using both arteries?

Keon: Where possible, yes.

Fontan: I noticed in one of your slides that there was no single-vessel disease in the coronary artery bypass graft patients but there were certainly patients with single-vessel disease. Does that mean that all of them were left under medically treated group?

Keon: It just happened that in the cohort pulled out here, there were no patients over 70 who were operated for single-vessel disease. There were a few patients below age 70 that were operated on for single-vessel disease. If you're looking at our overall experience, there are a small number of patients with single vessel disease still being operated upon, but a very small number.

Erickson: I wonder if, by chance, you will enter some quality of life assessments into your studies as you continue to follow these persons at the heart institute? If so, you could tell us what you plan to implement?

Keon: There is a group at the heart institute in the primary and secondary prevention centers and the rehabilitation center that are doing this. I didn't ask them for their data because I wouldn't dare to speak on it, anyway, I don't know enough about it. But there are people in our institution that are doing this – Dr. Dafoe's group. And I'm very interested in what is going to unfold here with subsequent speakers, because, obviously, that is truly an important subject. My subjective impression of this is that for some reason, elderly patients do very well with AC bypass. They don't seem to occlude their grafts. They don't come back for reoperation. Perhaps it's because we are more rigid with the selection criteria, but they seem to get a tremendous benefit from the operation as opposed to some of the younger patients. I think perhaps in this younger age group, particularly the young people in their 30's who are heavy smokers, hyperlipidemic and so. We should perhaps not even be operating on them, because they do come back very early with problems.

Stalpaert: I would like to ask you were these patients operated with the same technique and what was your technique?

Keon: Well, there are seven surgeons in our institution. They were all trained by myself.

Stalpaert: Thus they just do what you do?

Keon: They do exactly what they are told; isn't that utopia? But, on a serious note, we have tended to try to standardize our procedures and, as a matter of fact, they keep me educated now, so I tend to do what they do. The cardioplegic technique that we are interested here in the '93 group, the 300 cohort group is crystalloid cardioplegia (St. Thomas solution). It's a 19 mmol potassium solution. Earlier on we used a number of cardioplegic solutions. We have not used warm blood cardioplegia, even though it is highly toted in Canada. I'm not a great believer in it at this point in time.

Stalpaert: I have seen that there was a high reoperation rate. What was the reason for this operation, because you also do a lot of endarterectomies. Was it mainly the closing of these endarterectomies or was it rather disease of the venous bypass?

Keon: I'm very glad that you asked that question, because many of the audience don't know that we have been arguing about endarterectomies for 20 years. There is a paper in the literature in the Journal of Thoracic and Cardiovascular Surgery at our institution that shows autopsy follow-up on our endarterecomies. It clearly demonstrates that endarterectomized vessels stayed patent much longer than the vein graft that is put in proximal to the endarterectomy, and indeed, you can go back in on these patients 10 years later and graft the original endarterectomized vessel even though the vein graft is occluded. So, although there is some perioperative morbidity and mortality associated with endarterectomy, once the patient gets by that initial early period, the vessels do not appear to be affected by atherosclerosis nearly as quickly as the saphenous vein that is inserted proximally.

Stalpaert: So it was mainly the venous bypass disease.

Keon: Yes, it is the vein graft that occludes.

Schubel/berlin: I think it's not a problem to operate on a patient of 80 years who is in good condition and who has good coronary arteries. We all, I think, have good results, but in my opinion, the problems are the patients who are overweight, they have problems with renal failure or pulmonary obstructive disease, and these patients frequently are in the intensive care unit for many days or weeks. The problem is: can you better the life quality for these patients? I think it is not to say all patients over 70 years are in one group. I think we must differentiate between patients with and without additional diseases, and the main problem in my opinion is renal failure and pulmonary obstructive disease.

Keon: Well, we agree, we saw a higher incidence of renal failure in the patients over 70. It was not statistically significant but it was there. The incidence of chronic obstructive pulmonary disease, however, was considerably lower in the patients over 70 than under 70 and the incidence of hyperlipidemia and hypercholesterolemia was dramatically lower, although not statistically significant. But I think it is going to show statistical significance very soon.

Wenger: Have you had the opportunity to differentiate your 70 to 75 year old from 75 to 80 year, from older than 80 within that older cohort, to say if there really is a difference among them?

Keon: We had a quick run at it, and I couldn't see anything there so I didn't take it any further. I think we need more numbers.

Discussion Fontan

Schulte: In your abstract, you said in your conclusions: 'Selected octogenarians can undergo cardiac surgery etc. . . . .' and you described the problem to have a fight about the contraindications for those patients. You already answered the question. But can you give any selection criteria you would announce precisely in those age groups?

Fontan: As far as the heart itself is concerned we make the decision as in younger patients. In addition, we carefully take into account the pulmonary, renal, cerebral, psychological and general situation of the patients in order to neutralize, as much as possible, the hospital mortality of non-cardiac cause. So, selected octogenarians does not mean selection from the heart but selection from the general condition of the patient.

Walter: I have noticed in your slides that one of your patients died because of suicide, which raises the question of psychological evaluation and post-operative counseling. We have found in our own study that the best predictor for long-term survival was the expectation of the patient before operation. How important do you think it is to investigate the patient's expectation, intellectual functioning and psychological state? Could you please say some words about this?

Fontan: I think that you are right. The more you expect preoperatively or the more you expect from any event in life, the more you are rewarded if the post-operative or the post-event situation fulfills your expectations. I am not sure that in our institution we do as well as you do here in the preoperative evaluation of the patients in this field and certainly we have to learn from your clinic in this domain.

Stalpaert: What is the percentage of these octogenarians where they have done a PTCA and other kinds of operations?

Fontan: Among the 102 patients who had isolated coronary artery bypass graft and none of them had a PTCA.

Stalpaert: Certainly I think in some of these octogenarians they will do a PTCA instead of an operation.

Fontan: So you are asking me . . .

Stalpaert: The ratio between PTCA and coronary surgery. Is this 50–50 or 70 for PTCA and 30 for surgery or vice versa?

Fontan: I cannot reply to your question because I know the figures for the surgery. I don't know the incidence of patients over 80 years of age in whom our cardiological colleagues perform PTCA but I know that they are reluctant after that age.

Stalpaert: They are reluctant?

Fontan: Yes. Because most of them have multiple-vessel disease, surgery is a better solution to achieve complete myocardial revascularization.

Stalpaert: I should think, maybe it is better to do PTCA in these octogenarians than to do an operation. If possible.

Fontan: As surgeons we know that with ageing, the arteries, including the coronary arteries, become more calcified. That is a good reason to be cautious to dilate the coronary arteries and, as you may know, the results are not that good.

Mohan: The question of patients' selection recurs in this discussion again and again. It would seem at least, many people would think, that in such old patients, only selected patients might be operated. I find in the literature, that there are far more urgent than elective operations in the elderly, which would mean that these in fact would be less selected than the younger patients. As far as PTCA's are the literature shows, that especially in the elderly firstly the risk PTCA equals or is even more in terms of mortality than CABG-operations and secondly because their disease is generally more diffuse, it is difficult to cross the obstructions.

Evans: We all recognize that you are only examining a subset of the patients who might benefit from surgery. You are selective and, therefore, the external validity of your results cannot be ascertained. Today, with a population-based approach to health care, the issue of external validity is of paramount importance.

Most of us are also aware of the extreme pressure being placed on research. It is difficult to predict in advance which patients will maximally benefit. Therefore, in an effort to identify the most appropriate patient population, we may be less selective. The tendency is to focus on age, but this is probably a small matter. General health status is a more significant issue.

Both Professor Fontan and Professor Keon have presented data that are intended to go beyond age per se. In this regard, they each want to more clearly define the appropriate candidate. If we do not run some risk, there is unlikely to be any change in the services we provide or the way in which they are delivered. While we must minimize the level of economic inefficiency associated with technological innovation, we cannot be excessively conservative. There is little to be gained by inaction, and a great opportunity may be lost.

Schneider: My question goes a little bit beyond the subject of presentation. The *budget global* has caused great cost containment pressure in general on hospitals in France. How has it affected the access of patients to operations in French hospitals? Is there any selection effect or would you say there is no link between cost containment and patient access through the *budget global*?

Fontan: There is no effect. I have reported an experience of a private institution which is not, so far, affected by *the budget global*, in which, actually, the costs are much lower than in a hospital affected by the *the budget global*.

Schneider: But this means that you may have a selection of patients in the elderly according to social status in French Hospitals.

Fontan: It is not the case at all. In this regard in France there is no difference between a private institution and a university hospital, because in a private institution the Social Security covers the patients costs.

Wenger: Do you have any idea of selection process until you are asked to see the patient? Because so much relates to how much the specialist communicates both to the general practitioner and to the patients. There may be very different referral if the general practitioners are comfortable with good outcomes and the patients who return to them, or if elderly patients and society in general, non-medical society, have a favorable perception of what happens at elderly age. Do you think this differs in communities, in countries, and how that accounts for the patients you see?

Fontan: I think it is a question of continuing post-graduate education between the cardiac surgeon and the cardiologists and then the general practitioner. Postgraduate education in cardiology and cardiac surgery is well developed in our area in southwest France and we ourselves organize several sessions yearly. I don't know exactly how much it has affected the referral of our patients but it certainly did. We have provided the cardiologists with much information, not the general practitioners directly. But, as I said in my presentation, when we made the follow-up enquiry recently, we found that most of the general practitioners were enthusiastic about the good results achieved, surprisingly to them, in these old patients. I think that the first steps had to be done, afterwards the results will speak for themselves.

Keon: Can I be allowed a question and a comment? There is one indication for surgery that I think none of us are addressing and perhaps we should be. Certainly it is very important in our own institution, and that is the inability of the medical staff to discharge the patient. Frequently these elderly patients are on the medical wards and the cardiologists keep insisting that if they are not operated on they are going to be there for a very long time. I would like you to comment on that, Dr. Fontan, if you would.

Fontan: Do you mean that the patient is going to die without an operation or has a slight chance to survive with a very risky operation but with the high chance of dying after the operation?

Keon: No, I think the problem arises that you get a patient, aged 87 for example, with tight aortic stenosis, calcified aortic valve or left main coronary stenosis in a medical bed. They cannot get the patient out of that medical bed. So they are saddled with the dilemma of keeping this patient in the hospital for weeks or months or having a surgeon.

Fontan: I think that if there is no absolute contraindication, as I will discuss in my presentation, the patient should be operated upon.

Discussion Flameng

Fontan: You used any blood cardioplegia.

Flameng: No, never.

Fontan: Don't you think that could make a difference? Intermittent cross-clamping has some potentially deleterious effects because each period of ischemia is followed by a period of non-pressure-controlled reperfusion. Even after a short period of occlusion there is a risk of reperfusion injury either of the myocytes or of the endothelium. From our studies blood cardioplegia makes a difference, particularly when it is combined with refined modalities of reperfusion.

Flameng: Yes, I agree completely, but I must honestly say we don't have any experience with blood cardioplegia at all. For regular coronary bypass surgery – and you know that we perform a lot of these operations – we never use any cardioplegia, so we always do intermittent cross-clamping. The total ischemic time is rather short, so it's only for the distal anastomosis that the aorta is cross-clamped and you end up with very decent total ischemic periods. Also, there is always systemic cooling to 28°.

Fontan: You say that but you don't know what the myocyte feels.

Flameng: That is correct. I hope that they don't complain.

Keon: We have published out of our muscle mechanics lab that in isolated atrial trabeculae if they are arrested at 5° Centigrade with St. Thomas' solution and 20 Meq of potassium, they can be stored for 12 hours at 12° C without any chance in either compliance or contractility. So you don't damage the myocytes at all with up to 12 hours of storage at 12° C after an arrest. I'm convinced that all of the damage that we see as cardiac surgeons is due to reperfusion, and it concerns me that we're getting into complex reperfusion techniques in these older patients when we prolong the time of surgery. I believe that, as evidence unfolds, it will be demonstrated that probably the safest type of cardioplegia for these elderly patients is one shot of crystalloid cardioplegia at about 5° C achieving arrest and then store the myocardial temperature at 12 °. All of the other modalities including warm blood, I believe get into reperfusion injury, approaching a no-reflow phenomena that was described so many years ago.

Flameng: Thanks for the comments, because this is exactly what we do.

Stalpaert: We have used this intermittent cross-clamping only for surgeons who are very fast. If you can do a distal anastomosis in 6–7 minutes then it's no problem and in selected patients you have a hospital mortality of 1%. But if you are not so fast, then I suggest to these surgeons to use cardioplegia if they need 12–15 minutes to do a distal anastomosis, which is the big difference. Either you have a surgeon who is fast or another one who is slower.

Discussion Vidne

Fontan: I think your results are the best in the world as far as I know, and I think immediately that it comes to mind that a selection of patients on a cardiac basis had been made, according to the results. But, they are still excellent results.

Vidne: Yes, we have done a selection of patients on a cardiac basis, besides other general criteria. As an example, patients with porceline aorta or diffuse calcification of the coronary arteries were not accepted for surgery. I think that in this very selective group of patients surgery should be offered to patients with good probability from the cardiac aspect, since they are generally impaired in other organ systems.

Fontan: This is correct.

Discussion Chruscz

Pintor: The problem is, you speak about charge. We know there is some difference between charge and costs. Would you please explain if you have considered this difference?

Chruscz: The charge is made as a contract between the clinics and the health insurance. This has nothing to do with the real expenses for a patient.

Maynard: In that case what we have here are numbers which are related to resource costs and therefore we are not clear what the relationship is between these administered prices and the resource consequences to the procedure. How is this information being used and what use is it in making decisions about resource allocation?

Chruscz: What I pointed out at first is that there must be a stronger look at the data sources and the data availability to get much more information on these real costs.

Mohan: I found in your figures that although the number of ischemic heart disease patients per million population was not very different in the younger and older age groups, the number of operations done in especially +80 year olds decreased very very steeply. This would give the impression, that although the number of ischemic heart disease patients are more, they are not being operated.

On the contrary I find, at least in the literature, that in consecutive octogenarians undergoing coronary angiography, the incidence of unstable angina was extremely high. More than 70% of patients had such severe angina that something had to be done about it, that means they would undergo either a PTCA or an operation. Because these patients would die otherwise. My question is: what was the percentage of these patients of ischemic heart disease who had angiography but not heart surgery? That would show whether there is bias in selecting patients for surgery.

Chruscz: To answer your last question, we know that the number of heart surgeries is about 10% of all hospital cases of ischemic heart disease in 60–69 year old people. This proportion drops to 5% in the group of people 80 years and older.

Corallo: In a social system like what we have in the majority of the countries in Europe, I think that we should consider that the elderly have paid taxes for many years, so they have prepaid the costs of their operation and medical assistance. We should consider that, don't you think so?

Chruscz: I agree with you and it is not the decision of a health insurance company to decide whether elderly patients will undergo a bypass operation or not. It's a decision for the physician.

Harris: I just wanted to follow-up on this last point. I think it is very dangerous to justify treating the elderly on the grounds of their contribution because this leaves no basis for treating newborns.

Laczkovics: I have just calculated that those patients up to the age of 60 made about half a billion DM and I wonder how many of them could have returned to work. I do not charge the other social insurances because one has to balance both charges, both expenses. I know that the German health insurance does not pay for unemployment or invalidity but nevertheless we have to learn in Germany much more about looking at the entire cost and not just the cost for the treatment. Can you give us some information about this?

Chruscz: No, I'm afraid I can't. There is no real information on that special group of people.

Maynard: This is quite a complicated issue: reducing expenditure on social security is not a saving but a transfer of income. Social security transfer payments are not a real resource cost. The measure of welfare relevant for health care decisions is the change in the length and quality of life, not the financial contribution of individuals. If finance is the only consideration, the elderly, for instance, are of little value. It is essential to be clear about the objectives of policy so that evaluation of the 'success' of health care interventions is appropriately identified, measured and valued.

Discussion Stason

Maynard: Could I ask you a question in relation to this subject? You seem to be getting quite significant changes, savings and costs. Are these 'once and for all' savings (like with DRGs) or are they continuous and cumulative?

Stason: There is a forever upward pressure on the costs of health care in the United States. To achieve continued savings, incentives will need to continue and intensify. You are really asking two questions: What will happen when this demonstration comes to an end? What will happen to costs if global pricing continues? If global pricing comes to an end, prices will move to whatever the market permits at that time on a fee-for-service basis. I sense enthusiasm, however, (or at least acceptance) to continue and extend global pricing. We'll have to see how this plays out and what the effects are.

Cleary: Were there provisions built to protect against or adjust for case selection in the demonstration?

Stason: All patients who fell into DRG 106 and 107 in each hospital were entered into the demonstration. So, in this sense, the demonstration includes a 100% sample of eligible patients. There is some possibility that hospitals upcoded patients to fit criteria for the more expensive DRG 108 in order to avoid the demonstration. DRG 108 includes patients who received CABG and also a second cardiovascular procedure. We haven't evaluated whether this happened, but I do know that, for the period we have examined so far, case severity has increased, not decreased. Thus, it doesn't seem likely that case selection has been a major factor.

Cleary: But what about institutional selection, with which we are very concerned about, come health care funds?

Stason: Case-mix severity varies significantly from one hospital to another. We have no good knowledge, however, whether these differences represent favorable case selection by some hospitals, differences in referral patterns, or differences in selection criteria among communities or market areas. Unfortunately, we have no way to obtain these data given the limitations of the study.

Wenger: You mentioned that there was a lesser use of consultants. Do you have any breakdown as to that change? What types of consultations were less frequently obtained? Next, is there any evidence of substitution of non-physician personnel for prior position roles?

Stason: I can provide only anecdotal answers. We do not have systematic information at the present time. Anecdotal evidence suggests less use of respiratory specialists during intensive care and less use of cardiologists and nephrologists during the post-operative period. Regarding the substitution of non-physician personnel, we have seen more delegation to nurses for implementation of 'same-day' CABG surgery and perhaps more delegation of responsibility during surgical ICU care.

Corallo: We employed the system of Victor Parsonnet for stratification of mortality. I wish to know if there is some comparison from your system of prediction and a spectrum of mortality.

Stason: We collect detailed information on co-morbidity status as well as on the severity of underlying cardiac disease. We haven't formally converted co-morbidity data to Parsonnet scores, but we do consider many of the same variables, such as the presence of congestive failure, renal failure and age in our own regression analyses for hospital mortality. We also are examining co-morbidity scores in our evaluation of the appropriateness of CABG surgery using an explicit system similar to that used by RAND.

Discussion Kellet

Stalpaert: It is very nice, of course, this mathematical decision-making, but I think you overestimate the chance of getting a stroke because in the thousands of patients we have operated upon, the percentage of stroke was 0.4 %; so that's really not good decision-making in my opinion.

Kellet: Well I appreciate what you are saying but the only thing is that when you go to look at the literature you find that as people get older, the incidence of stroke during bypass surgery does go up. It doesn't really matter if you don't believe the figure I quoted. You could always redo the decision analysis. You could even, for example, totally eliminate the chances of stroke and see if it makes any significant difference to the expected outcome.

Stalpaert: But in your figures I see . . . dying is 0% , success is 100%, but stroke is 50%. But that's not true.

Kellet: Those figures you quoted are the quality of life adjustments and not the chance of stroke. Not only does a stroke, at say, 80 have an excess mortality rate caused by the stroke itself, but on top of that the quality of life with a stroke is much less than the quality of life without one, so you adjust the calculated life expectancy downwards. I can appreciate that you may feel that the quality of life with a stroke may be even less than 50% or you might feel it's worth more. The point is you can put in different quality adjustment values and redo the analysis and see if it makes any big difference to the outcome and then adjust your decisions accordingly. Even though people may get hung-up on quality adjustments, in most situations if you put in reasonable adjustments, it doesn't make an enormous difference to the expected outcomes.

Stalpaert: Well, but from a practical point of view, if you have such a patient, in that case it was your father, but it can be another patient, and he has angina. If he is going very well with drugs at his age, we should wait and see. On the other hand, if he is unstable, also with drugs, then I think you should say: 'Well, you make up your mind. In this situation the chance there is to get an infarction is very high'. So the patient himself will have to make the decision, 'I will be operated upon', not the doctor.

Kellet: I couldn't agree with you more. In fact my father actually picked a mathematically incorrect option. I think all the decision analysis should do is outline as fairly as possible the range of possibilities for the patient. So it is just the same as if you are buying a car. People buying a car are entitled to know the miles per gallon, the speed of the car, what the price is, etc. But you end up selling them a Mercedes, a Ford or whatever it is. The final decision is obviously up to the customer, is it not?

Stalpaert: Yes, I agree.

Keon: It would seem to me that the reliability of your system would be highly dependent on the specificity of the information that went into it at the front end. I could see potential for the methodology being very valuable. I think the risk of diminishing value as when there is no objective data being fit in the front end.

Kellet: Well, the advantage the system has is that it helps you by redoing the analysis several times (i.e. by sensitivity analysis). Thereby you can actually work out what bits of information are absolutely critical to any decision. Furthermore, if the chance of a stroke, for example, was very very critical, you may find yourself having to tell your patient 'Look, we don't know what to do in your case because we really don't know precisely enough what the chance of your having a stroke is. There is just not enough evidence in the literature or our own clinical experience'. I expect, however, that in real life you will usually not find that the stroke rate over a plausible range is not likely to make very much difference to the final outcome.

Dr. Keon, you said something earlier on this morning which I felt I should have challenged because I didn't want to make too many enemies before I gave my talk. You mentioned that age was a small item when considering the management of a patient. In my view it isn't a small item. The age-specific excess mortality rate of elderly people is high, even if they are in perfect health. If you are 40 years of age and you've got nothing wrong with you, your chance of dying in the next year is almost negligible. On the other hand if you are 80 and even if you are in perfect health, your situation is still a serious one. You are looking at about an 8% chance of dying in the next year. So as I mentioned earlier in my talk, even in an 80 year old if you are totally cured of ischaemic heart disease and hence removed all possibility of dying from that condition, there are still lots of things left over to die from.

Keon: But you're looking at a regression analysis or life curve. I was speaking of 30-day mortality.

Kellet: Yes, OK, that might be. But in terms of putting the whole picture, I think patients are not interested in upfront risk of dying. I think people are also interested in 'how much longer have I got left to live?'

Keon: How do you explain the fact that our statisticians looking at 10,000 operations, concluded that age is not an indicator for 30-day mortality?

Kellet: I just think it shows you the limitation of statistics over common sense.

Evans: Clinicians typically think that every case is uniquely different from every other case. We refer to this as the 'clinical mentality' which, in very clear terms, is at odds with the 'statistical mentality'. Statisticians believe in measures of central tendency, whereas clinicians frequently refer to the exceptions rather than the averages. Therefore, when I see data modeled according to the procedures you describe, I am unsure of their clinical utility, given a lack of clinical relevance. In short, John, while I like your approach, I am not sure it is 'user friendly' in the minds of practicing physicians. People do not necessarily change their behavior based on data.

Kellet: Could I just answer that by asking you a question? Do you think it is right when patients in their 70's and 80's are going for an operation that they should be made familiar with the risks and that those risks and perils should be spelled out to them as explicitly as possible?

Evans: Yes, I think what you describe is a very important clinical decision-making activity. I think your approach better enables patients to understand their treatment options, provided you qualify your results accordingly. However, once you have offered all the possible caveats, I am not sure how much you have left that is worthwhile to offer. Perhaps you have overly confused the patient, or you have been too certain with your data. Clearly, we want patients to make informed decisions, but we can influence them based on our own assumptions about the data we provide.

Kellet: Yes I think there is. I think a lot of elderly people are actually more petrified of strokes than even of sudden death. I think they are also interested in how much longer they are going to live.

Wenger: That is a very important item that probably should be factored into the decision-tree. It is not simply mortality rate. It is symptomatic and functional status as it relates to mortality rate. The time will come for your father or any other prototype patient with severe symptoms and the effect of the symptoms in limiting usual daily activities where will becomes greater than the fear of stroke risk. Because as long as he can function within the limits of personal value, stroke risk becomes the issue. When he cannot walk across the room because of angina or shortness of breath, stroke risk fear relatively lessens. Somewhere in the model we need not only survival data but the value system of functional status. That is what we all use in advising patients about surgery, patients who have a high risk at surgery. But it substantially depends on the limitation of function with which they approach their surgical procedure.

Kellet: I agree with you but I think the other thing, that bit of information missing, is what is the natural history of coronary artery disease not treated by surgery and how much it has been improved by the new drugs that have become available. Because even the studies where they have looked at the natural history, like the CASS study, don't give this answer, as a lot of the initially medically managed patients subsequently underwent revascularization. Therefore even though we have managed coronary artery disease for hundreds of years, I think currently we don't know the natural history of the disease if managed purely medically. My dad has actually done very well, and is as well now as he was 6 years ago. I don't know, however, how typical he is.

Harris: Two points: I liked your car analogy but it is an important dysanalogy in one way. With the car, the customer is doing the purchasing. It is the doctor that is doing the referral for this procedure, not the individual with the heart problems. If you adapted your scenario so that the decision analysis was done by the patient and it was the patient's decision, whether they got referred or not, I would find it much more acceptable and I think the car analogy would then be a good one. On the issue of fear of stroke, there is another way of dealing with this, which we ought to consider, and that is excepting a combination of advance directives plus voluntary euthanasia to cope with the outcome, if that's the most feared outcome. Then the best option is to go for the procedure that offers the best outcome and enables him or her to give an advanced directive that, in the eventuality of stroke, they can have voluntary euthanasia, and that copes with both problems.

Discussion Walter/Mohan

Corallo: I have two questions. The first one is: in your experience, after a 5-year follow-up, what do you think about the presence of a preoperative cardiovascular factor X of risk for development of psychiatric or psychological disease in the post-operative period? And, secondly: Did you use the state or the trait scale of the Spielberger Anxiety Inventory in the previous study?

Mohan: In answer to the first question: we have published the comparison of preoperative risks between younger and older patients[1] and have also published a review of other studies in this regard.[2] We found that older patients in almost all studies, including ours, have more risks, both cardiac and non-cardiac. After the operation, neuropsychologic complications are significant more for the older patients. For the second question: yes, as we have just presented, we compared both trait and state anxiety on the Spielberger scale in longitudinally evaluating the outcome of our older and younger patients.

Amsel: I have a question for Dr. Mohan. You showed in one of your slides that there was, of course, some mortality at 5 years, especially in the older patients. Did you find any difference in the quality of life scores between patients who proved to be five-year survivors and patients who proved not to be? If this were so, it might have influenced your results, e.g., if more unhappy patients died in the meantime than happy patients, then your results at 5' years would have turned out to be better for the latter group.

Mohan: We did not investigate the quality of life between 1 and 5 years. That is when we might have longitudinally be able to know if there were happier or unhappier patients at one year and who, during the interval between 1 and 5 years may have subsequently died.

Fontan: What is your explanation for confusion and depression in these elderly patients?

Mohan: Older patients, as a group, would be likely to be more confused, and we do know that with advancing age, there is a general decrease in all kinds of cognitive functioning and this includes memory, intelligence and reasoning. We think that this may be one reason why our older patients also had these problems. If you want to know whether coronary bypass surgery and the extra corporal circulation had contributed to this confusion at five years, we do not know. But I doubt that very much, because neurological complications post-operatively did not match with psychological or cognitive deficit at the 5-year follow-up.

Shumaker: I cannot resist commenting on the assumption that confusion and decline in cognitive function are a necessary component in aging. Although it is true that some people suffer from dementia as they age, this is not true of the majority of older people. Further, recent data from studies conducted by Dr. Deborah Best, a professor in psychology at the Wake Forest University (North Carolina, USA), underscore the role that assumptions play in actual performance. In a series of laboratory-based studies, Dr. Best has demonstrated that older people assume that as they age they will decline in their cognitive functioning and, based on this self-attribution, they perform less well on tests of cognitive function than younger people. However, this attribution can be manipulated with verbal feedback such that the cognitive performance of the older person is improved upon by merely altering their self-attribution (e.g., telling the older person that his or her ability is at a particular level). These data support the fact that by making assumptions about the cognitive skills of our older patients we can influence the level at which they perform. And, if we hold 'ageist' attitudes about the cognitive abilities of the elderly, our influence will be negative. The concept you are discussing is referred to as self-efficacy in the field of psychology. An example of the application of self-efficacy to the expectations of bypass surgery patients comes from a study conducted by Dr. Susan Gortner of the University of California, San Francisco. Dr. Gortner hypothesized that one could experimentally alter the self-efficacy of post-bypass surgery patients and that by increasing positive self-efficacy immediately following surgery, the patients' short- and long-term outcomes (i.e., morbidity and HRQL) would improve. In her randomized, clinical trial, no differences were found between the enhanced and non-enhanced self-efficacy groups. However, studies in other patient populations (e.g., osteoarthritis, post-MI) have shown significant positive effects of efficacy manipulations and this is an area that merits further attention in the post-bypass patient population.

Mohan: I would just like to make two comments on that. We used only a single item, as you know. We simply asked, 'Do you feel confused or disoriented?' This is because we had earlier planned to use all those scales like the Mini-mental scale but we had been told by experienced investigators, like Ann Bowling, that it would be a mistake to ask older patients these kinds of scales because they could give offense. For example, it might not be appropriate to ask 'which year is it now' by mail. Intellectual function is almost impossible to determine by mail and we therefore took a question from Dr. Cleary's questionnaire which was: 'Do you feel confused or disoriented?' As far as the effect of aging on intellectual function is concerned, I have gone through the studies which have been done and it seems indeed, that there is a decrease in response speed, but of course there is contradictory information in other ways. As you know, older patients are said to be wiser and so in the real life experience, they say that it could even improve. But when it comes down to things like mathematics and learning new tasks involving speed, older patients show a decline.

Corallo: Prof. Walter, how can life and social expectancy modify the life satisfaction in the elderly patients?

Walter: Well I think if a patient or a person has a vision of his life in the future he will be much more directed and aimful, and has a better inspiration of how his life would become in the future. This would be my explanation, that older patients often have a vision of the kind of their life in the future, in what they expect from it, and with definite expectation they can better manage things which might happen to them in the future, and enjoy the added lifespan after surgery, thus improving their life satisfaction.

Kellet: I would return to the confusion in the elderly. I think we should distinguish between delirium and dementia. An awful lot of elderly people become confused when they get sick and their mini-mental scores are really quite low, and then we just do the sort of sample of that patient coming into our hospital. It is actually quite frightening when you are asking people basic bits of information like who they are, where they live and things like that. I haven't noticed any of these people becoming offended. We have to know were they live, etc. But with any acute illness like pneumonia infection or whatever it is, a lot of elderly people are really quite out of it for quite a long time. Have you no measure of that in your post-cardiac patients or is it a temporary situation?

Mohan: I told you about the intellectual function, that was the only item we had. But I would like to say something else. Dr. Shumaker also made another point. She said: 'We have problems in the elderly about their income, we have problems in their mobility'. From our study, I got the impression that they do have these problems, but they seem satisfied with it. There is generally a higher satisfaction despite several of their limitations in all these spheres.

Kellet: Let me just sharpen this up a little bit. If a patient doesn't know that it is 1994, is he really in a position to be able to tell whether he should have bypass surgery or not? There is a substantial number of people in this older age group that won't know what year it is. Or maybe not that many? I think you need to know answers to that kind of question.

Mohan: I did mention earlier in the discussion that we did allow patients to consult their spouse or whoever is at home to be able to help them with the questions. Indeed patients may be confused but they could know the answer to Mini-mental type questions through such help – thus such questions cannot be given by mail. And I come back to the point of satisfaction: I'm not saying that it is alright if a person is confused and doesn't know what he is really doing, but we found that they are satisfied and then it is alright.

Fontan: You conclude your presentation by a suggestion that preoperative counseling can enhance the expectation of post-operative well-being, the strongest predictor of better quality of life after 5 years. Could you clarify what you mean by counseling and do you have that already organized in your department? How do you do it and who should be in charge of doing this counseling and on which basis?

Mohan: We took 10 medical factors and 3 social factors from the preoperative variables we had. These, we thought, could be the most predictive of their health-related quality of life at 5 years. And from these and other factors we found that the most predictive was a higher level of expectation of difficulties after the operation. That is in close association with the fact that the older patients were having about the same difficulty index as the younger patients and, in fact, that continues to be so after the operation. Also, their difficulties were the same. What is really happening is that their difficulties are the same before the operation and after the operation, but they perceived themselves more invalid before the operation and this affects what is happening at 5 years. Their quality of life is lower. It cannot be pure chance; therefore I'm saying it is possible, that in case they are explained that their abilities or their disabilities and their chances of recovery are similar to younger patients, maybe they feel more reassured and then might show better QOL scores at 5 years. This probably should be continued during the follow-up, also. They need to be reassured constantly that they are not doing as badly as they think. The preoperative counseling could be done by a psychologist but we do not have a clear program of psychological counseling at the moment.

Shumaker: In psychological literature, there is something called self-efficacy, which is basically what you are talking about, and that is basically increasing those expectations about their ability, their efficacy in particular fields. There was a study conducted by Dr. Susan Gortner, where she did exactly what you are proposing. She actually tried to enhance self-efficacy in post-bypass-surgery patients. Although the groups were not separated by age, her notion was that if we could increase peoples' self-efficacy immediately following surgery, that their short- and long-term outcomes would improve. There is another literature in post MI-patients showing that to be the case. Unfortunately, in the post-CABG patients she got no difference with it. She had an intervention group and an non-intervention group and they bring no differences in short- and long-term outcomes. But there were a lot of problems with that and the study was done on South African territory in a small population, and it is a difficult thing to manipulate, it is difficult to lean upon. I just want to mention that there has been some study done on it.

Walter: When we were examining the results of our study in detail, it became evident that the expectation of difficulties after the operation was the strongest predictor of the outcome after the operation.

We had the experience that preoperative counseling had a very positive effect on the patient's mood stability to enter the perioperative period. The informative talk of the surgeon with the patient about his functional and social abilities gives him a chance to look with great hope into the future and to make plans for a 'new life' after the operation. Patients become depressed during the long period of disease and are very happy to know exactly what kind of expectations they may have. This certainly will improve their short- and long-term outcomes.

Erickson: When you are analyzing data from a follow-up study, it is important to consider whether or not you are using only the survivors at any point in time or if you are using the initial cohort, keeping track of not only the survivors but also persons who have died during the follow-up period. In general, the health status or health-related quality of life of the survivor group will be higher than that of survivors plus non-survivors. With the survivor-only group, any statement about health is conditional on the fact that persons have survived. This enables us to say, given that theses persons survived, they have the following average health status level. The fact that some people will die over the course of a longitudinal study is one of the reasons for using a utility-based measure such as the EuroQol, the Quality of Well-being Scale, or the Health Utility Index, the type of approach that I used in my presentation. Since a utility-based measure incorporates death in its scoring algorithm, this type of measure allows you to estimate not only the quality of life of the survivors but also that of the total cohort. We used a modified version of the HUI for persons with hypertension, a condition that is usually considered to be quite benign. When we accounted for the fact that persons die over a 10-year period, the quality of life of the cohort of persons with hypertension dropped remarkably.

Evans: The more I study quality of life, the more I am convinced we have gotten it all wrong. For over 20 years I have been involved in quality of life studies of transplant recipients. We have used both subjective and objective indicators. When I look at the tools we have used, I find them very suspect. I am unsure how they truly relate to patient's lives. While I don't like to use anecdotes, I will offer one in hopes of making a critical point.

Many of the quality of life measures we use are not generic or universal to all conditions to the extent that they should be. Moreover, when we interpret the results, the implications may be entirely counter-intuitive. If, for example, we evaluated quadriplegics, our conclusion would probably be that life is no longer worth living. In other words, if a person has only minimal ability to physically function, much of what is important in life is no longer possible. What else is there? In short, our perception may have no basis in reality for the person we are attempting to evaluate. People apparently aspire to something more than we are willing to credit them.

As an example, I will use a very well-recognized figure from Formula I racing to illustrate my point. I am sure many of our European colleagues are aware of Formula I racing in general and Frank Williams in particular. Frank Williams is the owner of the Williams Grand Prix Team. He is also quadriplegic, the result of an automobile accident several years ago. To many people unfamiliar with Frank's achievements, his existence would probably constitute very little. Some might even argue that Frank Williams is nothing more than a head stuck on a body. Yet, Frank Williams owns and manages one of the most successful Grand Prix teams in the world, despite his physical condition.

Frank Williams' wife recently wrote a book on her life with Frank before and after the accident. The title of the book is 'A Different kind of Life'. She conveys the message as to how difficult it was for both Frank and her to adapt to the remarkable changes that occurred following the accident. Frank has done well, despite his physical limitations.

Based on experiences such as this, I think we have to take a careful look at the quality of life concepts we try to operationalize for empirical analyses. I think there are two existential concepts these measures fail to grasp – *meaningful life* and *purposeful existence*. In the final analyses, perhaps these two concepts capture all that is necessary to assure us that the value of life is independent of our functional status and our interpretation of our ability to function. Moreover, it suggests that even some of our subjective concepts, such as well-being and life satisfaction, are also too removed from our life experience.

I can assure you that there is little in the quality of life literature that is consistent with my existential impressions. I realize a meaningful life and a purposeful existence are not easy concepts to operationalize. However, even though difficult to measure, they still serve as the basis for the motivation to live. This, I believe, grants them the status of unsurpassed importance. Thus, before we waste further time on dealing with methodological issues, perhaps we should better understand those concepts that are critical to living and dying at a time when life appears to have a price we are unwilling to pay to sustain.

Notes

1. Mohan R, Amsel BJ, Walter P. Coronary artery bypass grafting in the elderly – a review of studies on patients older than 64, 69 or 74 years. Cardiology 1992; 80: 215–25.
2. Mohan R, Walter PJ, Vandermast M, Amsel BJ, Vanaken D. Isolated coronary artery bypass grafting in patients 75 years of age and older: is age per se a contraindication? Thorac Cardiovasc Surgeon 1992; 40: 365–70.

Discussion Wenger

Corallo: As far as I experienced in my center, cardiac arrhythmias after CABG are very frequent. But they didn't cause a reduction or a slowing of patients' active training.

Wenger: Early perioperative arrhythmias have no relationship to the late arrhythmias. We find that early perioperative arrhythmias are primarily supraventricular in character. In our center, the surgeons have convinced me that when they initiate atrial pacing for these patients, at least for the first days or until they leave the intensive care unit, at an atrial rate between 90 and 100 bpm, there is a lesser occurrence of supraventricular arrhythmias. If you look at well populations in regard to ventricular arrhythmias, very excellent studies of 24-hour Holter monitoring in elderly individuals without apparent underlying cardiovascular disease show ubiquitous single ventricular ectopic beats, very frequent pairs, triplets and bigeminy and frequent runs of non-sustained ventricular tachycardia. There are elderly individuals without disease. Therefore it becomes very difficult to find the signal of disease against this huge amount of background noise. I expect that with collective experience in the very limited efficacy of anti-arrhythmic drugs, most of us want sustained or symptomatic ventricular tachycardia before we stop exercise or before we start intensive drug therapy. So we watch these patients carefully, watch their baseline, but have a far higher threshold of intervention than at younger age.

Discussion Maynard

Kellet: There are just two comments or questions I would like to raise. One was that you mentioned the fact that older people age at different rates. I guess one of the things I'd like to bring you back to is the fact that as people get older they do actually start to approach a common endpoint. Whilst you can die young or old if you are 6 years of age, by the time you are 80 you're going to die as an old person and the amount of range of time you have to play with is considerably less. I can remember when I was a medical student there was all this controversy about what age you should try and resuscitate people and it was shrouded with confusion, ethical considerations and all sorts of things. Eventually clinical studies were done. It turned out that the results on attempted resuscitations on people over 80 were remarkably poor. From a pragmatic point of view, therefore, trying to resuscitate octogenarians is usually a waste of time. This opinion is purely based on the clinical facts and has nothing to do with ethical, economic or other considerations.

The other point I'd like to raise is the whole question of 'quality of life'. How much is this a feature of fashion and how much do we gain by talking about certain things to change people's perception of what they need to have a good quality of life?

Maynard: The question of quality of life measurement is very complex. The major issues in this area are: 1) from where are the descriptors derived which describe physical, social and psychological well-being, energy, pain and other pertinent values in quality of life? And, 2) how are different combinations of these descriptors valued?

There are two types of quality of life measure. There are a half-dozen generic measures and there are hundreds of disease-specific measures. The descriptors for these measures are generally derived from studies of what communities and societies regard as relevant aspects of quality of life (QoL). Thus the researchers who created measures such as that used by Rand from which Kaplan's Sickness Impact Profile (SIP) and Ware's Short Form 36 (SF36) were derived, used descriptors derived from the literature and from surveys or community values. The tendency to 'pluck descriptors from the air' has to be avoided, but testing of the relevance of the descriptors inevitably leads to some ad hoc revision of scales.

The valuation of combination of descriptors is done using a variety of techniques: e.g., time trade-off and standard gamble. There is debate about both the QoL descriptors and the valuation techniques, with no agreement as to what is best in terms of validity and responsiveness. This absence of a 'gold standard' quality of life measure means that the best recommended practice for studies is to use both a generic and a disease-specific instrument.

The application of these measures in clinical trials is increasing rapidly, especially in trials of pharmaceuticals. This interest in Qol measures in the pharmaceutical industry is enhanced by the requirement in Australia for all new drugs to be registered with the reimbursement commission with data on cost effectiveness. The commission uses these data to determine whether new drugs will be reimbursed by Medicare in Australia. Similar requirements have emerged in Canada, England and Italy and there is an international interest in the creation and application of guidelines for good practice in economic evaluation, including the development and application of QoL measures. Such developments are highlighting the strengths and weaknesses of these measures. They inform the process of identifying good medical practice but are, as yet, experimental and unlikely to remove the need to use judgment to supplement the results of this difficult and contentious work.

Discussion Harris

Keon: You came very close to addressing the issue of human rights. Certainly Canadian doctors, in my opinion, contravene human rights frequently as they are enshrined in our constitution, and I believe in the American constitution, also, and I'm not sure what the British one says but . . .

Harris: We don't have a constitution, fortunately and unfortunately. Some of us wish we did.

Keon: It clearly states in ours that you cannot discriminate against a citizen on the basis of age, so I believe a doctor who tells a patient that he will not treat him on the basis of age is contravening his human rights.

Harris: I would be interested to know whether they would also hold that an allocation of resources away from a procedure on the grounds that the benefit was less because the sufferers were old would also be unconstitutional in Canada and in the U.S.A., as I believe it should be, although I doubt yet whether it is. That is why I am in favor of a constitution. I think that equal protection is one of the first requirements of any constitution and should be required to counterbalance the progress of quality. That is why I have to appeal to the 17th century philosopher Thomas Hobbes for my argument because I have no constitution to appeal to.

Kellet: First of all: in Ireland we have got a constitution, too, and my advice would be you shouldn't write anything down. It creates all kinds of problems. I'm not sure exactly what you have in mind, but I appreciate it might be of value to people who are making policy decisions but not for practicing doctors, especially those dealing with something like coronary artery disease. They are trying to help patients make a choice between a treatment that 'possibly doesn't work, might work, might work a little, and might work a lot' and that the patient 'doesn't want, might want it a little, and might want a lot'. The final decision will depend a lot on how you frame the benefits and risks to the patient. You understand what I'm saying? I bet I could talk your granny into a bypass if you wanted me to and I bet I could talk her out of it, also. It would just depend on the way I would express the risks and benefits to her.

Harris: That's why doctors should be kept away from patients!

Kellet: Well, I appreciate that, I just wonder how you get around that problem. I can understand that politicians could do the same thing but I'm not sure that they would be any better. I think that most doctors who are actually dealing one-to-one with an individual patient actually do have that individual's concerns and best interests as their primary goal. What is the best way to tell people the facts about their illness and treatment options without framing it in such a way that you bring out your own prejudice?

Harris: That is a practical question. Of course there is a lot of literature on non-directive counseling and a lot of literature on how to set up the conditions for informed consent, so that that sort of thing doesn't arise. I'm not an expert. But I'd like to look at another dimension of what you said and that is: the issue of whether or not there is sufficient benefit to make a procedure worthwhile. Some of you may know, recently there has been a cause célèbre in the U.K., which I alluded to in my paper, about whether or not people who smoked heavily were eligible for CABG. And some doctors in Wythenshaw hospital, very near to where I work in Manchester, refused to treat patients on the grounds that they were smoking. This caused a national furor and, among other things, the ethics committee of the British Medical Association, on which I sit, agonized on this over the space of three of our meetings. And they drafted a statement which wanted to have it both ways. On the one hand they wanted to hold that it is unethical to discriminate against people on the basis of lifestyle and, hence, it follows that it is unethical to discriminate against smokers. On the other hand, the statements said it is also unethical to give a treatment which stands only a poor chance of benefiting. And they were quite happy with this until I pointed out to them that this would preclude cardiac massage at the curbside in an accident where there is very little chance of the cardiac massage resuscitating the person, but it just might do it. And to declare it unethical – an attempt to do such a thing – on the grounds that the benefit was very remote in terms of statistics or possibilities was going a little far. And that seems to me to be *nub.* of the issue. If there is enough benefit for the patient rationally to want it for himself or herself, then I believe there should be an equal and open competition for that benefit even though other patients might get a greater benefit in terms of life years if those same resources were deployed elsewhere.

Kellet: Can I just come back to you. We can well imagine that there will be unlimited amounts of money that will go into this health care system that you are devising. What actually happens, however, if you are in a time and place situation: you've got a four bed coronary care unit and you have got four people having acute infarcts and a fifth one comes in. How do you square that one? What do you do? Because more money right at that moment is not going to help you.

Harris: Have you got any coins in your pocket? You toss one.

Kellet: That is the ethical way of doing it, is it? I am just interested to know.

Harris: This is a serious point, and a very good ethical reason. What you have to do is adopt a selection procedure which does not discriminate in anybody's favor, which does not prioritize any particular sort of individual. What you have to do is to show no preference. You have to value each at par, and if you can't treat all, then any random method is a method that values each at the same level which shows no preference to any. But if I am in favor – and Allan mentioned coin tossing that he adopted from his written presentation – then I'm in favor of tossing coins or drawing straws.

Kellet: Would you feel it was reasonable to ask the patient what he would prefer?

Harris: That is fine, if any of them wanted to say 'Oh, no, in that case I'd rather you counted me out'. That is fine, everybody is entitled to contract out.

Kellet: How would you frame that request to them?

Harris: Well, I'm about to toss a coin. If anybody wants to volunteer, that is fine. Why not? It is their life, not yours.

Keon: I can't believe what I am hearing here: an Irishman and an Englishman debating a subject which George Bernard Shaw clearly answered a hundred years ago.

Mohan: You did suggest one other method to decide on unfairness and that was that it would be unfair ethically to take away a treatment which someone wanted, and there is David Callahan's argument about elderly people, that because they have lived the life the younger people have not, they should feel guilty in wanting to live longer, and they should not want that. So it is okay if you refuse that treatment to them.

Harris: Well, that is a matter for them, not a matter for Calahan, in my view. It depends how you analyze the wrong what you do in taking a life. This is something I haven't had time to argue about today. But the way I analyze it, the wrong of killing is in taking away from that individual a life that they want to continue, and that is how you can make sense of the difference between suicide and voluntary euthanasia on the one hand and murder on the other. What differentiates the most is, in the one case, you are taking away from somebody something that they want and, in the other case, you are taking away from somebody something that they don't want. If you analyze the wrongness of killing in that way then that wrongness remains present so long as people want to live, however much life they have already consumed.

Mohan: So, as long as someone is able to show that older patients are happy with the operation they took five years ago, you think there is every ethical reason to be able to insist that they must get their operation.

Harris: I must have an equal chance to get it and not have the chances fixed, and an equal chance is to go into an equal competition. Where there are not enough resources for all, some fair procedure most be adopted.

Erickson: I would like to take issue with some of your comments on QALYs, because much of what you are saying is due to the life expectancy component of the calculation rather than the quality adjustment component. Quality-adjustment factors for a given health state are the same for all persons. Thus, when you see a difference in QALYs between people in the same health state, the difference is due to life expectancy. Thus, many of the arguments that people make against the use of QALYs, including your comments here, also apply to the use of life expectancy, which is a much used and respected indicator of health status and health-related quality of life.

Harris: That can't be right. Because in the case that I gave you of the two sisters . . . assume that they are the same age. Now, assume something I didn't put into the case, that they have the same life expectancy after the treatment, but one can only be restored to very poor quality of life by any objective standard and the other will be restored normal life. If quality adjustment is to mean anything it must give a lower quality score to the chairbound pain-ridden sister, even though her life expectancy in terms in numbers of years is the same. Otherwise I just fail to understand what the quality adjustment part could possible amount to. It must give her a lower quality score and, if it does, and the person with the most qualities is to be preferred, then she loses out.

Erickson: If you design the example so that life expectancy between two individuals is the same, then I agree, that logically the differences are attributable to the quality adjustment factors.

Harris: Then let us forget the quality part of it all together and just call it an 'aly'.

Discussion Evans

Cleary: I have a couple of comments. One: I think it is very important to distinguish between waste and efficiency. There is a class of treatments for which the risks outweigh the benefits and, in terms of allocating resources, I think most us would agree there are classic procedures that are unnecessary, in fact harmful, and we can eliminate them without dilemma. Secondly: I think it is extremely important to distinguish between the situation in which you are making decisions among treatments for a comparable condition versus between treatments for different conditions. The former would be something I think we are concerned with here. If a person has ischaemic heart disease, there is medical management versus PTCA versus CABG, and that is a case in which Qalys or quality of life or various metrics can be very useful in resolving the relative weighting of different outcomes. I think that is very different than when you are talking about an allocation decision where you decide not to provide, for example, renal dialysis over 65. Third: I think some of the presentations sounded somewhat nihilistic, as if it is an either/or situation. I don't think that is the case. I think we combine ethical criteria and some of these effectiveness rules. What I mean is you can bound certain situations, you can allow the rule of rescue, you can allow minimal quality of life, and within a bounded set of conditions you can make decisions about the relative effectiveness within those constraints. So, for example, you can say that this is an age-stratified determination and you can actually eliminate what you called age discrimination. I think there are a variety of conditions irrespective of which perspective you take, whether it is a social welfare perspective or a human capital perspective where you come to the same conclusions. Although there are some dilemmas which may be unresolvable, application of some of these techniques may result in better decisions from a variety of perspectives than we are doing now, which are a sort of non-decision. Finally, I stand to be corrected by the economist, but I think the reason we have tied insurance to employment has more to do with the historical conditions around WWII and wage and price controls but I may be wrong. I think it had to do with economic circumstance at the time rather than the broad significance you attribute to that.

Evans: On the latter point, I would suggest that we in America trump-up rhetorical explanations to support a capitalistic ideology. Since World War II we have had plenty of time to divorce health insurance from employment. We have chosen not to do so because we refuse to accept the fact that we are implicitly valuing human lives. We ourselves cannot confront the inhumanity we now tolerate. Rather than patting Americans on the back, we should hit them in the head. Perhaps we could then get their attention.

I also share your concern about analyses based on a short-term 'episode of care'. The economics of health care must be conceived in terms of longitudinal analyses. While discrete episodes of care may have favorable economic consequences, a complete analysis of costs and outcomes over time may yield a dramatically different picture from that depicted by an episode of care analysis. For example, the economic consequences of hospital readmissions are not always factored into the equation.

Finally, within the context of managed care, patients are no longer an economic transaction. We assume full responsibility across the continuum of patient care. More importantly, the traditional medical model of disease is no longer applicable. We must now take care of patients with public health goals in mind. Unfortunately, I remain unconvinced of our commitment to public health. In the early 1970s we espoused the same rhetoric, but did not have the courage or wherewithal to follow through in our commitments as stated.

Discussion Cleary

Kellet: Could you look at your data and find out which patients were actually sent for angiograms out of the various subgroups, you know, Q-waves, non-Q-waves and so forth? Once they have been 'angioed', was there any differences between the different categories as to who got an intervention, either angioplasty or CABG? Do you have that data?

Cleary: Yes, we do, absolutely. I can tell you one thing we are going to do, and I can tell you what I think we know already. Dr. Wenger said that angio is a gateway procedure and that is absolutely right, and, across things like regional variability and racial variability and gender variability, I think a general statement is that the differential selection stet cath is much less than the selection process in the cath. That is arguable, and I'll open it up to the other experts in the room, but basically a general finding, and what we have seen is that once you are cathed, the conditional probability is not that different. So if you have three-vessel with left main disease it is a non-issue. You are going to be revascularized. For other situations appropriateness is almost impossible to operationalize. I agree with decision analysis but you really cannot second-guess clinicians. So what I have said is let's look at the diagnostic yield of cath. If it is a gateway procedure in which you really want to know how many three-vessel left main patients you have, and you can pick different criteria – if you are doing 50% more in Texas than in New York are you finding any more three-vessel left main disease? And when you take large populations, that is actually a reasonable question. You can ask, What is the detection rate, given different practice patterns? We now are going back to every cath that was performed in the first 90 days but not during the index hospitalization and getting the cath-results to look at the diagnostic yield in a different states.

Keon: I thoroughly enjoyed your presentation, and these have been a very interesting couple of days because, over the last two years in our own institution, the more I look at what is unfolding out of our databank, I've come to realize that all of our perceptions of CABG have been the reverse of scientific reality. In fact, in our institution, the worst results that we have are in patients age 35–45, any way you look at it. The in-hospital mortality, the long-term survival, everything. I think it has got absolutely nothing to do with the surgery at all. It is because they are diabetic, they are 3-pack-a-day smokers, hypercholesterolemics, hypertensives, and they are just walking disasters. And, somehow, this information is just beginning to unfold and it is fascinating for me to watch what you have just come out with. I enjoyed it very much.

Cleary: By the way, in addition to the risk stratification, and what I am calling propensity, you know that you do revascularization for different reasons. In some cases it is to save a patient and in some patients it is for symptom relief, and unless you know the indications of the surgery, you are comparing two things that are incomparable. So we really have to dig into these studies to look at the indication and risk stratification. Age probably doesn't get us there.

Wenger: There is, however, another aspect regarding elderly patients. Typically symptomatic indications in elderly patients are the trigger for operating on a patient at higher risk. Once you do the catheterization and define very high risk anatomic lesions you realize that, within this population, there is a large subset, and we have known this since Framingham, where there is silent ischaemia. These patients do not have symptoms in part related to the elderly age, in part to the concordance of diabetes and hypertension and the like. So that these may be some reasons why you see some discrepancy between the high-risk clinical stratification based on an incomplete, a non-Q-wave, infarction and pain and the catheterization-based. As you put the cath data together, it is likely to give us fascinating information; what I would like to see are the patients considered high risk based on cath who are not considered clinically at high risk. We have had the experience at the Emory University School of Medicine of reviewing some 10,000 patients going to coronary bypass surgery between 1974 and 1991, of whom some 3,000 were women. Once catheterization was accomplished there was no difference in referral, either age-based or gender-based. All the differences that went into determining who came to catheterization are unknown in a tertiary referral center, but catheterization seems to be the great equalizer.

Cleary: That is an excellent point. By the way, if there were more cardiologists instead of predominantly surgeons here, one of you would have said you have not adequately characterized the medical management in those two areas. However, one of the things we have done is, we measured drug use on admission, on discharge, and then, 2 years later, we asked patients the kind of drugs they were taking. We have actually done random samples of the physicians in the two states, and so, for example, the use of betablockers is lower and less adherent to what we would accept as guidelines in Texas. So you are looking at very complex patterns of medical managements, surgical indications, surgical techniques. It is a fascinating but very complicated kind of contrast when we do these kind of investigations.

Wenger: As one of the few card-carrying cardiologists in the audience, it is important to realize that surgical management is not surgical management in isolation. It is surgical plus subsequent medical management, in contrast to isolated medical management, in patients unoperated.

Discussion Caine

Caine: No, not really. Only the resource use of the study group is being compared to that of a younger group of patients. We're not attempting to compare the quality of life between the younger and the older age in this study but I have conducted a previous study of a group of 100 males undergoing bypass grafting who were all under the age of 60. We used the Nottingham Health Profile and very similar symptom scales and so there will be an opportunity to compare quality of life results from the two studies. I think the other important thing about outcome which has not been mentioned is the need for rehabilitation and this is something we are trying to introduce into our hospital. I certainly agree that better information beforehand and rehabilitation afterwards goes toward maximizing the benefits of this kind of surgery.

Wenger: I expect some of the descriptive studies suggest that elderly patients have less expectation of improvement *and* perhaps this is 'ageism' among health professionals and among patients themselves. This again may influence some of the replies; it may be important to then differentiate what the expectations are as compared with the observed and described improvements.

Caine: Of course having this sort of data on outcomes will hopefully help to better inform doctors to better inform patients as to what their expectations should be.

Cleary: We haven't finished those analyses. But we don't ask what their expectations were before. Later we say, Were the improvements you experienced greater than you expected or less than you expected? Age had small effects on the evaluation of functional improvement.

Caine: It is true.

Corallo: In a valvular group, what emotional impact does the fact to be obliged to take anticoagulant therapy have? Mainly in the first year.

Caine: We're certainly recording what drugs these patients are taking, but we're not asking them specifically how a certain drug is being tolerated. But, of course, we would be able to look at the data and see if there is any relationship between drug therapy and various aspects of quality of life.

Discussion Erickson

Cleary: Just a point of clarification, Dr. Erickson. Some of us had a question in the bypass–no-bypass comparison – how is the comparison group defined?

Erickson: You mean who were the bypass group?

Cleary: No, who were in the no-bypass group?

Erickson: The bypass and no-bypass groups are defined in terms of their responses to a question in the 1986 and 1987 questionnaires.

Cleary: So that's the entire population?

Erickson: This question divides the entire sample of approximately 10,000 people into two groups, one of which contains persons who reported having had a bypass operation. The other group consists of persons who reported that they had not had a bypass operation by the time of the interview.

Shumaker: I was interested in the relationship you presented on marital status and the probability of undergoing surgery. Do you have data on social integration or social support, since studies indicate that social support is predictive of access to health care? Sometimes marital status is used as a proxy for social support, with similar results.

Erickson: We probably do have some information on social support in the 1982–1984 survey because a very comprehensive data collection instrument was used in that survey. I'm less optimistic about having items on social support in the 1986 and 1987 follow-up surveys. In using these data to study the relationship of social support and health-related quality of life, however, one must be careful since the quality of life measures include a component of social function. So one has to be careful when we look at some of these independent – what you might think were independent variables – that we would not have the same measure on both the right hand and left hand side of the equation type of thing. But we can look at that and that was one of the interesting things that popped up: the marital status.

Wenger: One of the fascinating features is that these data I have just seen for the first time correlate with some clinical trial data. If we examine the cohort in the save study, which was a study that required infarction severe enough to result in a ventricular ejection fraction lower than 40%, which is a sizable infarction, the authors examined the pre-infarct characteristics of the population by gender. Fifty percent of the women, as compared with about a third of the men, before the episode of infarction had enough symptoms of angina that it interfered with their usual daily activities. Yet, despite that, twice as many men as women previously had been sent for coronary arteriography, which we now realize is the determinant of access to care for revascularization. This fits with your observational data.

Discussion Shumaker

Mohan: . . . more younger patients had completed the data themselves, but there was a very small difference.

Shumaker: I would have guessed that this would be the case, since older people are more likely to be married and in a marital relationship longer than younger people. If you think about your own lives, you can imagine receiving a questionnaire in the mail and sitting down with your spouse to chat about the contents and possible answers. For example, you might ask your spouse 'What do you think about that?' or, 'How do you think I should answer this?' This is simply human nature and I think this type of 'bias' in mail-out surveys is more likely to occur as one gets older and has been in a relationship for a longer period of time. There is a strong notion of protectionism between spouses. This is not something that just occurs in surveys on health-related quality of life. For those of you in clinical practices, I am sure you see this at times when patients come in with their spouses. The spouses will want to answer for the patients and protect them, just be there to take care of them and make sure that the health provider is not doing anything unkind or inappropriate with the patient. We cannot assume, however, that the way the spouse responds to queries is identical to the way the patient would have responded for him or herself. There are several studies that demonstrate spouses do not respond the same. That is, there is a general bias for physicians, nurses and spouses to under-estimate the quality of life of the patient. What the patient reports is usually better than that reported by a proxy. Unfortunately, however, this difference between proxy and patient reporting is not a constant error that can be corrected for statistically. Thus, we as researchers are forced to guard against proxy data as much as possible.

Erickson: We have looked at some of the issues regarding the use of self versus proxy respondents using data from the U.S. National Health Interview Survey (NHIS). The NHIS annually samples over 100,000 persons who are representative of the civilian, non-institutionalized population of the United States. About 40% of the responses from the adult population are from proxy respondents. We compared perceived health status ratings from self and proxy respondents. We compared perceived health status ratings from self and proxy respondents and found a definite bias. For persons 75 years of age and older, self respondents are more likely to report themselves in higher health status than when a spouse serves as a proxy respondent for the sample person. For younger persons, for example, 35 to 44 years of age, self respondents are more likely to report themselves in a lower health status than do proxy respondents.

Shumaker: And, that is an important question. That is, this particular item, 'In general, how would you rate your health?' has been demonstrated in a number of studies to be predictive of morbidity and mortality independent of clinical status. Thus, you have to wonder what you are capturing when you get proxy responses to this question. What is the proxy's perception of what is happening to the patient or target person? And, to what degree are the proxy's perceptions influenced by his or her mood, the degree to which the patient's behavior impacts on the proxy on a day-to-day basis, etc. If you are talking, for example, about a husband and wife where the husband is the patient and the wife the person providing data for the patient, she is also the person who is the primary caregiver for that patient; thus, her feelings about the patient and the degree to which he is capable of doing some things, and the degree that his needs impact on her life on a day-to-day basis are all encompassed in the way she responds to those questions. You are no longer capturing the patient's quality of life or his perceptions of the quality of his life. Rather, it is his wife's perceptions, filtered through her own moods and needs, that you have captured. This is not necessarily bad data, just a different type of data.

Index

Activities of Daily Living 169, 197
acute myocardial infarction 174
ageism 117, 146, 246
age-related
    costs 71
    problems 174
allocation of resources 111
anti-ageism 117
anti-oxidants 22
aortic valve replacement 41
anxiety 159, 188, 197, 207, 240
Australia 247

Belgium 179, 196
biological prosthesis 51
blood cardioplegia 232
body functioning 191
bypass surgery 79
    benefits 82, 179, 205
    choices 101
    cost-effectiveness 82
    economic consequences 121
    isolated 27
    need of 9
    patient selection 91
    social consequences 121
    trends 80

CABGTREE 95
Canada 247
cardiac arrhythmias 245
cardiac operations
    increase in 4
    need for 4
    variations of capacities 4
cardiovascular death
    proportions of 16
    rise in 72
care
    different types of 168
    patient-centred 86
    post-operative 38
    preventive 9, 21, 218

quality of 86, 251
cerebrovascular disease 17
charges 125, 233
choices 101
clinical
    evaluation 107
    results 25
    trials 102
cognitive dysfunctions 208, 240
combined bypass surgery 41
    risks 49
confusion 242
congestive heart failure
    definition 29
coronary atherosclerosis
    risk factors 6, 9
coronary revascularization 167
coronary risk reduction 213
    multifactorial 216
costs 74, 79, 223, 233, 235
    age-dependent 195
    effectiveness 79, 102, 251
        and mortality 84
    reduction 8, 71
    critical map 84

death causes 123
decision analysis 91, 236
decision strategies 91
demographic developments 3, 76, 214
Denmark 224
depression 159, 188, 197, 207, 240
difficulty index 187
disability 213
    scale 164
discrimination 118, 130, 247

economic changes 3
economic growth 7
elderly
    definition 130
emotional state 182, 197
equality principle 111

ethics 248
exercise rehabilitation 213
extracorporal circulation 55

France 55, 230
functional capacities 206, 214
Functional Status Questionnare 168

gender 33, 142, 255
Germany 16, 71, 195, 224, 225

habitual activity level 214
health benefits 82
health care
  access to 104, 255
  costs 20, 69, 122
  prioritising 111
  rationing 104
  utilization 20
health insurance companies 72, 234
health-related quality of life 137, 145, 155,
    167, 179, 197, 244
  changes after surgery 157
  definition 145
  improvement 172
  longitudinal effects 179, 195
  measurement problems 146
  quality of data 147
  scales 167
Health Utility Index 139, 244
Hospital Anxiety and Depression Scale 188,
    197, 207
hospital
  morbidity 56
  mortality 45, 56, 80, 84
hospitalization 19
  duration 58, 80
human rights 247
hypertension 22, 218

ICPM code 72
IMA 63
intellectual functions 182, 241
Ireland 247
Italy 247

Japan 5, 224

life expectancy 3, 5, 13, 72, 93, 205, 224, 225,
    237
  in developed countries 13
life satisfaction 149, 198, 208, 241

LIMA 61, 226
limitations
  in activities 170
  in performance of social roles 180, 198
longevity 6, 13, 157
longitudinal investigations 179, 195
long-term prognosis 41

measures 147
  ambiguity in 150
  condition-specific 168
  limitations in 167
  patient-based 167
  position effects of 151
  problems with 147
  proxy respondents 152
  sensitivity 150
  surrogate respondents 152
medical
  intervention 22
  progress 8
  technology 124, 205
Medicare 80, 125
Medicare Heart Bypass Center Demonstra-
    tion 81
  cost savings 83
mitral valve replacement 41
MONICA project 20
morbidity 6, 63, 195, 257
  perioperative 27
  post-operative 58
  trends in 19
mortality 6, 13, 45, 63, 93, 184, 236, 257
  age-specific 18, 195, 237
  cost-effectiveness of 86, 129
  decrease in 38
  early 165
  by younger patients 34
  perioperative 27
multiple valve replacement 41
myocardial infarction 18, 21

National Health and Nutrition Examination
    Survey 137
national priorities 114
Netherlands 224
New York Heart Association guidelines 29,
    62
non-cardiac complications 35
Nothingham health profile 159

octogenarians 55, 61, 206, 224, 229, 246

operative
  indications 55
  risks 58, 131
  variables 43
outcome measurement 102

patient-centred care 886
patient selection 38, 66, 191, 228, 233, 235,
  249
  with decision analysis 91
percutaneus transluminal coronary angioplasty (PTCA) 73
perioperative complications 35, 215
personality tests 182
physiological
  changes 49
  differences 218
  functions 181, 197, 214
post-operative
  care 38
  complications 50
  variables 43
preoperative
  counseling 242
  variables 43, 242
preventive care 9, 21, 218
primary operations 10
prioritising 111
procedural
  risks 58
  variables 35
psychiatric diseases 239
psychological questionnaires 183

QALY 101, 111, 114
quality of life 58, 79, 98, 118, 121, 137, 167,
  240, 246, 250, 254
  health-related 137, 145, 155
  measurement problems 147
questionnaires 157, 168, 183, 197, 199, 205,
  256

rationing
  by ability to benefit 105
  by age 101, 104
rehabilitation 213
  home-based 219
re-operation rate 10, 227
revascularization 61
risk factors 27, 35, 66, 186, 253

selection of patients 38, 66, 191, 228, 233,
  235, 249
social
  performance 180, 198, 207
  support 255
surgery
  age distribution 73
  benefits from 165, 179, 205, 230, 248
  denying 165
  improvements after 171, 186, 208
  increase in 71
  methods 29
  risks 41
  trends in 33, 202
  urgent 29
survival rates 155, 200
Sweden 6, 223
Switzerland 224
symptoms 161
Systolic Hypertension in the Elderly Program
  218

therapies 216
technology 124, 205
treatment choice 101

United Kingdom 164, 247

valve
  bypass surgery 41
  prothesis 50

waiting lists 165

Developments in Cardiovascular Medicine

1. Ch.T. Lancée (ed.): *Echocardiology*. 1979   ISBN 90-247-2209-8
2. J. Baan, A.C. Arntzenius and E.L. Yellin (eds.): *Cardiac Dynamics*. 1980
   ISBN 90-247-2212-8
3. H.J.Th. Thalen and C.C. Meere (eds.): *Fundamentals of Cardiac Pacing*. 1979
   ISBN 90-247-2245-4
4. H.E. Kulbertus and H.J.J. Wellens (eds.): *Sudden Death*. 1980   ISBN 90-247-2290-X
5. L.S. Dreifus and A.N. Brest (eds.): *Clinical Applications of Cardiovascular Drugs*.
   1980   ISBN 90-247-2295-0
6. M.P. Spencer and J.M. Reid: *Cerebrovascular Evaluation with Doppler Ultrasound*.
   With contributions by E.C. Brockenbrough, R.S. Reneman, G.I. Thomas and D.L.
   Davis. 1981   ISBN 90-247-2384-1
7. D.P. Zipes, J.C. Bailey and V. Elharrar (eds.): *The Slow Inward Current and Cardiac
   Arrhythmias*. 1980   ISBN 90-247-2380-9
8. H. Kesteloot and J.V. Joossens (eds.): *Epidemiology of Arterial Blood Pressure*. 1980
   ISBN 90-247-2386-8
9. F.J.Th. Wackers (ed.): *Thallium-201 and Technetium-99m-Pyrophosphate. Myocardial Imaging in the Coronary Care Unit*. 1980   ISBN 90-247-2396-5
10. A. Maseri, C. Marchesi, S. Chierchia and M.G. Trivella (eds.): *Coronary Care Units*.
    Proceedings of a European Seminar (1978). 1981   ISBN 90-247-2456-2
11. J. Morganroth, E.N. Moore, L.S. Dreifus and E.L. Michelson (eds.): *The Evaluation of
    New Antiarrhythmic Drugs*. Proceedings of the First Symposium on New Drugs and
    Devices, held in Philadelphia, Pa., U.S.A. (1980). 1981   ISBN 90-247-2474-0
12. P. Alboni: *Intraventricular Conduction Disturbances*. 1981   ISBN 90-247-2483-X
13. H. Rijsterborgh (ed.): *Echocardiology*. 1981   ISBN 90-247-2491-0
14. G.S. Wagner (ed.): *Myocardial Infarction*. Measurement and Intervention. 1982
    ISBN 90-247-2513-5
15. R.S. Meltzer and J. Roelandt (eds.): *Contrast Echocardiography*. 1982
    ISBN 90-247-2531-3
16. A. Amery, R. Fagard, P. Lijnen and J. Staessen (eds.): *Hypertensive Cardiovascular
    Disease*. Pathophysiology and Treatment. 1982   IBSN 90-247-2534-8
17. L.N. Bouman and H.J. Jongsma (eds.): *Cardiac Rate and Rhythm*. Physiological,
    Morphological and Developmental Aspects. 1982   ISBN 90-247-2626-3
18. J. Morganroth and E.N. Moore (eds.): *The Evaluation of Beta Blocker and Calcium
    Antagonist Drugs*. Proceedings of the 2nd Symposium on New Drugs and Devices,
    held in Philadelphia, Pa., U.S.A. (1981). 1982   ISBN 90-247-2642-5
19. M.B. Rosenbaum and M.V. Elizari (eds.): *Frontiers of Cardiac Electrophysiology*.
    1983   ISBN 90-247-2663-8
20. J. Roelandt and P.G. Hugenholtz (eds.): *Long-term Ambulatory Electrocardiography*.
    1982   ISBN 90-247-2664-6
21. A.A.J. Adgey (ed.): *Acute Phase of Ischemic Heart Disease and Myocardial Infarc-
    tion*. 1982   ISBN 90-247-2675-1
22. P. Hanrath, W. Bleifeld and J. Souquet (eds.): *Cardiovascular Diagnosis by Ultra-
    sound*. Transesophageal, Computerized, Contrast, Doppler Echocardiography. 1982
    ISBN 90-247-2692-1
23. J. Roelandt (ed.): *The Practice of M-Mode and Two-dimensional Echocardiography*.
    1983   ISBN 90-247-2745-6
24. J. Meyer, P. Schweizer and R. Erbel (eds.): *Advances in Noninvasive Cardiology*.
    Ultrasound, Computed Tomography, Radioisotopes, Digital Angiography. 1983
    ISBN 0-89838-576-8
25. J. Morganroth and E.N. Moore (eds.): *Sudden Cardiac Death and Congestive Heart
    Failure*. Diagnosis and Treatment. Proceedings of the 3rd Symposium on New Drugs
    and Devices, held in Philadelphia, Pa., U.S.A. (1982). 1983   ISBN 0-89838-580-6
26. H.M. Perry Jr. (ed.): *Lifelong Management of Hypertension*. 1983
    ISBN 0-89838-582-2
27. E.A. Jaffe (ed.): *Biology of Endothelial Cells*. 1984   ISBN 0-89838-587-3

28. B. Surawicz, C.P. Reddy and E.N. Prystowsky (eds.): *Tachycardias*. 1984
ISBN 0-89838-588-1
29. M.P. Spencer (ed.): *Cardiac Doppler Diagnosis*. Proceedings of a Symposium, held in Clearwater, Fla., U.S.A. (1983). 1983 ISBN 0-89838-591-1
30. H. Villarreal and M.P. Sambhi (eds.): *Topics in Pathophysiology of Hypertension*. 1984 ISBN 0-89838-595-4
31. F.H. Messerli (ed.): *Cardiovascular Disease in the Elderly*. 1984
Revised edition, 1988: see below under Volume 76
32. M.L. Simoons and J.H.C. Reiber (eds.): *Nuclear Imaging in Clinical Cardiology*. 1984 ISBN 0-89838-599-7
33. H.E.D.J. ter Keurs and J.J. Schipperheyn (eds.): *Cardiac Left Ventricular Hypertrophy*. 1983 ISBN 0-89838-612-8
34. N. Sperelakis (ed.): *Physiology and Pathology of the Heart*. 1984
Revised edition, 1988: see below under Volume 90
35. F.H. Messerli (ed.): *Kidney in Essential Hypertension*. Proceedings of a Course, held in New Orleans, La., U.S.A. (1983). 1984 ISBN 0-89838-616-0
36. M.P. Sambhi (ed.): *Fundamental Fault in Hypertension*. 1984 ISBN 0-89838-638-1
37. C. Marchesi (ed.): *Ambulatory Monitoring*. Cardiovascular System and Allied Applications. Proceedings of a Workshop, held in Pisa, Italy (1983). 1984
ISBN 0-89838-642-X
38. W. Kupper, R.N. MacAlpin and W. Bleifeld (eds.): *Coronary Tone in Ischemic Heart Disease*. 1984 ISBN 0-89838-646-2
39. N. Sperelakis and J.B. Caulfield (eds.): *Calcium Antagonists*. Mechanism of Action on Cardiac Muscle and Vascular Smooth Muscle. Proceedings of the 5th Annual Meeting of the American Section of the I.S.H.R., held in Hilton Head, S.C., U.S.A. (1983). 1984 ISBN 0-89838-655-1
40. Th. Godfraind, A.G. Herman and D. Wellens (eds.): *Calcium Entry Blockers in Cardiovascular and Cerebral Dysfunctions*. 1984 ISBN 0-89838-658-6
41. J. Morganroth and E.N. Moore (eds.): *Interventions in the Acute Phase of Myocardial Infarction*. Proceedings of the 4th Symposium on New Drugs and Devices, held in Philadelphia, Pa., U.S.A. (1983). 1984 ISBN 0-89838-659-4
42. F.L. Abel and W.H. Newman (eds.): *Functional Aspects of the Normal, Hypertrophied and Failing Heart*. Proceedings of the 5th Annual Meeting of the American Section of the I.S.H.R., held in Hilton Head, S.C., U.S.A. (1983). 1984
ISBN 0-89838-665-9
43. S. Sideman and R. Beyar (eds.): [3-D] *Simulation and Imaging of the Cardiac System*. State of the Heart. Proceedings of the International Henry Goldberg Workshop, held in Haifa, Israel (1984). 1985 ISBN 0-89838-687-X
44. E. van der Wall and K.I. Lie (eds.): *Recent Views on Hypertrophic Cardiomyopathy*. Proceedings of a Symposium, held in Groningen, The Netherlands (1984). 1985
ISBN 0-89838-694-2
45. R.E. Beamish, P.K. Singal and N.S. Dhalla (eds.), *Stress and Heart Disease*. Proceedings of a International Symposium, held in Winnipeg, Canada, 1984 (Vol. 1). 1985 ISBN 0-89838-709-4
46. R.E. Beamish, V. Panagia and N.S. Dhalla (eds.): *Pathogenesis of Stress-induced Heart Disease*. Proceedings of a International Symposium, held in Winnipeg, Canada, 1984 (Vol. 2). 1985 ISBN 0-89838-710-8
47. J. Morganroth and E.N. Moore (eds.): *Cardiac Arrhythmias*. New Therapeutic Drugs and Devices. Proceedings of the 5th Symposium on New Drugs and Devices, held in Philadelphia, Pa., U.S.A. (1984). 1985 ISBN 0-89838-716-7
48. P. Mathes (ed.): *Secondary Prevention in Coronary Artery Disease and Myocardial Infarction*. 1985 ISBN 0-89838-736-1
49. H.L. Stone and W.B. Weglicki (eds.): *Pathobiology of Cardiovascular Injury*. Proceedings of the 6th Annual Meeting of the American Section of the I.S.H.R., held in Oklahoma City, Okla., U.S.A. (1984). 1985 ISBN 0-89838-743-4

50. J. Meyer, R. Erbel and H.J. Rupprecht (eds.): *Improvement of Myocardial Perfusion.* Thrombolysis, Angioplasty, Bypass Surgery. Proceedings of a Symposium, held in Mainz, F.R.G. (1984). 1985   ISBN 0-89838-748-5

51. J.H.C. Reiber, P.W. Serruys and C.J. Slager (eds.): *Quantitative Coronary and Left Ventricular Cineangiography.* Methodology and Clinical Applications. 1986
ISBN 0-89838-760-4

52. R.H. Fagard and I.E. Bekaert (eds.): *Sports Cardiology.* Exercise in Health and Cardiovascular Disease. Proceedings from an International Conference, held in Knokke, Belgium (1985). 1986   ISBN 0-89838-782-5

53. J.H.C. Reiber and P.W. Serruys (eds.): *State of the Art in Quantitative Cornary Arteriography.* 1986   ISBN 0-89838-804-X

54. J. Roelandt (ed.): *Color Doppler Flow Imaging and Other Advances in Doppler Echocardiography.* 1986   ISBN 0-89838-806-6

55. E.E. van der Wall (ed.): *Noninvasive Imaging of Cardiac Metabolism.* Single Photon Scintigraphy, Positron Emission Tomography and Nuclear Magnetic Resonance. 1987
ISBN 0-89838-812-0

56. J. Liebman, R. Plonsey and Y. Rudy (eds.): *Pediatric and Fundamental Electrocardiography.* 1987   ISBN 0-89838-815-5

57. H.H. Hilger, V. Hombach and W.J. Rashkind (eds.), *Invasive Cardiovascular Therapy.* Proceedings of an International Symposium, held in Cologne, F.R.G. (1985). 1987   ISBN 0-89838-818-X

58. P.W. Serruys and G.T. Meester (eds.): *Coronary Angioplasty.* A Controlled Model for Ischemia. 1986   ISBN 0-89838-819-8

59. J.E. Tooke and L.H. Smaje (eds.): *Clinical Investigation of the Microcirculation.* Proceedings of an International Meeting, held in London, U.K. (1985). 1987
ISBN 0-89838-833-3

60. R.Th. van Dam and A. van Oosterom (eds.): *Electrocardiographic Body Surface Mapping.* Proceedings of the 3rd International Symposium on B.S.M., held in Nijmegen, The Netherlands (1985). 1986   ISBN 0-89838-834-1

61. M.P. Spencer (ed.): *Ultrasonic Diagnosis of Cerebrovascular Disease.* Doppler Techniques and Pulse Echo Imaging. 1987   ISBN 0-89838-836-8

62. M.J. Legato (ed.): *The Stressed Heart.* 1987   ISBN 0-89838-849-X

63. M.E. Safar (ed.): *Arterial and Venous Systems in Essential Hypertension.* With Assistance of G.M. London, A.Ch. Simon and Y.A. Weiss. 1987
ISBN 0-89838-857-0

64. J. Roelandt (ed.): *Digital Techniques in Echocardiography.* 1987
ISBN 0-89838-861-9

65. N.S. Dhalla, P.K. Singal and R.E. Beamish (eds.): *Pathology of Heart Disease.* Proceedings of the 8th Annual Meeting of the American Section of the I.S.H.R., held in Winnipeg, Canada, 1986 (Vol. 1). 1987   ISBN 0-89838-864-3

66. N.S. Dhalla, G.N. Pierce and R.E. Beamish (eds.): *Heart Function and Metabolism.* Proceedings of the 8th Annual Meeting of the American Section of the I.S.H.R., held in Winnipeg, Canada, 1986 (Vol. 2). 1987   ISBN 0-89838-865-1

67. N.S. Dhalla, I.R. Innes and R.E. Beamish (eds.): *Myocardial Ischemia.* Proceedings of a Satellite Symposium of the 30th International Physiological Congress, held in Winnipeg, Canada (1986). 1987   ISBN 0-89838-866-X

68. R.E. Beamish, V. Panagia and N.S. Dhalla (eds.): *Pharmacological Aspects of Heart Disease.* Proceedings of an International Symposium, held in Winnipeg, Canada (1986). 1987   ISBN 0-89838-867-8

69. H.E.D.J. ter Keurs and J.V. Tyberg (eds.): *Mechanics of the Circulation.* Proceedings of a Satellite Symposium of the 30th International Physiological Congress, held in Banff, Alberta, Canada (1986). 1987   ISBN 0-89838-870-8

70. S. Sideman and R. Beyar (eds.): *Activation, Metabolism and Perfusion of the Heart.* Simulation and Experimental Models. Proceedings of the 3rd Henry Goldberg Workshop, held in Piscataway, N.J., U.S.A. (1986). 1987   ISBN 0-89838-871-6

71. E. Aliot and R. Lazzara (eds.): *Ventricular Tachycardias. From Mechanism to Therapy.* 1987 ISBN 0-89838-881-3
72. A. Schneeweiss and G. Schettler: *Cardiovascular Drug Therapoy in the Elderly.* 1988 ISBN 0-89838-883-X
73. J.V. Chapman and A. Sgalambro (eds.): *Basic Concepts in Doppler Echocardiography. Methods of Clinical Applications based on a Multi-modality Doppler Approach.* 1987 ISBN 0-89838-888-0
74. S. Chien, J. Dormandy, E. Ernst and A. Matrai (eds.): *Clinical Hemorheology. Applications in Cardiovascular and Hematological Disease, Diabetes, Surgery and Gynecology.* 1987 ISBN 0-89838-807-4
75. J. Morganroth and E.N. Moore (eds.): *Congestive Heart Failure.* Proceedings of the 7th Annual Symposium on New Drugs and Devices, held in Philadelphia, Pa., U.S.A. (1986). 1987 ISBN 0-89838-955-0
76. F.H. Messerli (ed.): *Cardiovascular Disease in the Elderly.* 2nd ed. 1988 ISBN 0-89838-962-3
77. P.H. Heintzen and J.H. Bürsch (eds.): *Progress in Digital Angiocardiography.* 1988 ISBN 0-89838-965-8
78. M.M. Scheinman (ed.): *Catheter Ablation of Cardiac Arrhythmias.* Basic Bioelectrical Effects and Clinical Indications. 1988 ISBN 0-89838-967-4
79. J.A.E. Spaan, A.V.G. Bruschke and A.C. Gittenberger-De Groot (eds.): *Coronary Circulation. From Basic Mechanisms to Clinical Implications.* 1987 ISBN 0-89838-978-X
80. C. Visser, G. Kan and R.S. Meltzer (eds.): *Echocardiography in Coronary Artery Disease.* 1988 ISBN 0-89838-979-8
81. A. Bayés de Luna, A. Betriu and G. Permanyer (eds.): *Therapeutics in Cardiology.* 1988 ISBN 0-89838-981-X
82. D.M. Mirvis (ed.): *Body Surface Electrocardiographic Mapping.* 1988 ISBN 0-89838-983-6
83. M.A. Konstam and J.M. Isner (eds.): *The Right Ventricle.* 1988 ISBN 0-89838-987-9
84. C.T. Kappagoda and P.V. Greenwood (eds.): *Long-term Management of Patients after Myocardial Infarction.* 1988 ISBN 0-89838-352-8
85. W.H. Gaasch and H.J. Levine (eds.): *Chronic Aortic Regurgitation.* 1988 ISBN 0-89838-364-1
86. P.K. Singal (ed.): *Oxygen Radicals in the Pathophysiology of Heart Disease.* 1988 ISBN 0-89838-375-7
87. J.H.C. Reiber and P.W. Serruys (eds.): *New Developments in Quantitative Coronary Arteriography.* 1988 ISBN 0-89838-377-3
88. J. Morganroth and E.N. Moore (eds.): *Silent Myocardial Ischemia.* Proceedings of the 8th Annual Symposium on New Drugs and Devices (1987). 1988 ISBN 0-89838-380-3
89. H.E.D.J. ter Keurs and M.I.M. Noble (eds.): *Starling's Law of the Heart Revisited.* 1988 ISBN 0-89838-382-X
90. N. Sperelakis (ed.): *Physiology and Pathophysiology of the Heart.* Rev. ed. 1988 3rd, revised edition, 1994: see below under Volume 151
91. J.W. de Jong (ed.): *Myocardial Energy Metabolism.* 1988 ISBN 0-89838-394-3
92. V. Hombach, H.H. Hilger and H.L. Kennedy (eds.): *Electrocardiography and Cardiac Drug Therapy.* Proceedings of an International Symposium, held in Cologne, F.R.G. (1987). 1988 ISBN 0-89838-395-1
93. H. Iwata, J.B. Lombardini and T. Segawa (eds.): *Taurine and the Heart.* 1988 ISBN 0-89838-396-X
94. M.R. Rosen and Y. Palti (eds.): *Lethal Arrhythmias Resulting from Myocardial Ischemia and Infarction.* Proceedings of the 2nd Rappaport Symposium, held in Haifa, Israel (1988). 1988 ISBN 0-89838-401-X
95. M. Iwase and I. Sotobata: *Clinical Echocardiography.* With a Foreword by M.P. Spencer. 1989 ISBN 0-7923-0004-1

Developments in Cardiovascular Medicine

96. I. Cikes (ed.): *Echocardiography in Cardiac Interventions.* 1989
ISBN 0-7923-0088-2
97. E. Rapaport (ed.): *Early Interventions in Acute Myocardial Infarction.* 1989
ISBN 0-7923-0175-7
98. M.E. Safar and F. Fouad-Tarazi (eds.): *The Heart in Hypertension.* A Tribute to Robert C. Tarazi (1925-1986). 1989 ISBN 0-7923-0197-8
99. S. Meerbaum and R. Meltzer (eds.): *Myocardial Contrast Two-dimensional Echocardiography.* 1989 ISBN 0-7923-0205-2
100. J. Morganroth and E.N. Moore (eds.): *Risk/Benefit Analysis for the Use and Approval of Thrombolytic, Antiarrhythmic, and Hypolipidemic Agents.* Proceedings of the 9th Annual Symposium on New Drugs and Devices (1988). 1989 ISBN 0-7923-0294-X
101. P.W. Serruys, R. Simon and K.J. Beatt (eds.): *PTCA - An Investigational Tool and a Non-operative Treatment of Acute Ischemia.* 1990 ISBN 0-7923-0346-6
102. I.S. Anand, P.I. Wahi and N.S. Dhalla (eds.): *Pathophysiology and Pharmacology of Heart Disease.* 1989 ISBN 0-7923-0367-9
103. G.S. Abela (ed.): *Lasers in Cardiovascular Medicine and Surgery.* Fundamentals and Technique. 1990 ISBN 0-7923-0440-3
104. H.M. Piper (ed.): *Pathophysiology of Severe Ischemic Myocardial Injury.* 1990
ISBN 0-7923-0459-4
105. S.M. Teague (ed.): *Stress Doppler Echocardiography.* 1990 ISBN 0-7923-0499-3
106. P.R. Saxena, D.I. Wallis, W. Wouters and P. Bevan (eds.): *Cardiovascular Pharmacology of 5-Hydroxytryptamine.* Prospective Therapeutic Applications. 1990
ISBN 0-7923-0502-7
107. A.P. Shepherd and P.A. Öberg (eds.): *Laser-Doppler Blood Flowmetry.* 1990
ISBN 0-7923-0508-6
108. J. Soler-Soler, G. Permanyer-Miralda and J. Sagristà-Sauleda (eds.): *Pericardial Disease.* New Insights and Old Dilemmas. 1990 ISBN 0-7923-0510-8
109. J.P.M. Hamer: *Practical Echocardiography in the Adult.* With Doppler and Color-Doppler Flow Imaging. 1990 ISBN 0-7923-0670-8
110. A. Bayés de Luna, P. Brugada, J. Cosin Aguilar and F. Navarro Lopez (eds.): *Sudden Cardiac Death.* 1991 ISBN 0-7923-0716-X
111. E. Andries and R. Stroobandt (eds.): *Hemodynamics in Daily Practice.* 1991
ISBN 0-7923-0725-9
112. J. Morganroth and E.N. Moore (eds.): *Use and Approval of Antihypertensive Agents and Surrogate Endpoints for the Approval of Drugs affecting Antiarrhythmic Heart Failure and Hypolipidemia.* Proceedings of the 10th Annual Symposium on New Drugs and Devices (1989). 1990 ISBN 0-7923-0756-9
113. S. Iliceto, P. Rizzon and J.R.T.C. Roelandt (eds.): *Ultrasound in Coronary Artery Disease.* Present Role and Future Perspectives. 1990 ISBN 0-7923-0784-4
114. J.V. Chapman and G.R. Sutherland (eds.): *The Noninvasive Evaluation of Hemodynamics in Congenital Heart Disease.* Doppler Ultrasound Applications in the Adult and Pediatric Patient with Congenital Heart Disease. 1990
ISBN 0-7923-0836-0
115. G.T. Meester and F. Pinciroli (eds.): *Databases for Cardiology.* 1991
ISBN 0-7923-0886-7
116. B. Korecky and N.S. Dhalla (eds.): *Subcellular Basis of Contractile Failure.* 1990
ISBN 0-7923-0890-5
117. J.H.C. Reiber and P.W. Serruys (eds.): *Quantitative Coronary Arteriography.* 1991
ISBN 0-7923-0913-8
118. E. van der Wall and A. de Roos (eds.): *Magnetic Resonance Imaging in Coronary Artery Disease.* 1991 ISBN 0-7923-0940-5
119. V. Hombach, M. Kochs and A.J. Camm (eds.): *Interventional Techniques in Cardiovascular Medicine.* 1991 ISBN 0-7923-0956-1
120. R. Vos: *Drugs Looking for Diseases.* Innovative Drug Research and the Development of the Beta Blockers and the Calcium Antagonists. 1991 ISBN 0-7923-0968-5

Developments in Cardiovascular Medicine

121. S. Sideman, R. Beyar and A.G. Kleber (eds.): *Cardiac Electrophysiology, Circulation, and Transport*. Proceedings of the 7th Henry Goldberg Workshop (Berne, Switzerland, 1990). 1991   ISBN 0-7923-1145-0
122. D.M. Bers: *Excitation-Contraction Coupling and Cardiac Contractile Force*. 1991   ISBN 0-7923-1186-8
123. A.-M. Salmasi and A.N. Nicolaides (eds.): *Occult Atherosclerotic Disease*. Diagnosis, Assessment and Management. 1991   ISBN 0-7923-1188-4
124. J.A.E. Spaan: *Coronary Blood Flow*. Mechanics, Distribution, and Control. 1991   ISBN 0-7923-1210-4
125. R.W. Stout (ed.): *Diabetes and Atherosclerosis*. 1991   ISBN 0-7923-1310-0
126. A.G. Herman (ed.): *Antithrombotics*. Pathophysiological Rationale for Pharmacological Interventions. 1991   ISBN 0-7923-1413-1
127. N.H.J. Pijls: *Maximal Myocardial Perfusion as a Measure of the Functional Significance of Coronary Arteriogram*. From a Pathoanatomic to a Pathophysiologic Interpretation of the Coronary Arteriogram. 1991   ISBN 0-7923-1430-1
128. J.H.C. Reiber and E.E. v.d. Wall (eds.): *Cardiovascular Nuclear Medicine and MRI*. Quantitation and Clinical Applications. 1992   ISBN 0-7923-1467-0
129. E. Andries, P. Brugada and R. Stroobrandt (eds.): *How to Face 'the Faces' of Cardiac Pacing*. 1992   ISBN 0-7923-1528-6
130. M. Nagano, S. Mochizuki and N.S. Dhalla (eds.): *Cardiovascular Disease in Diabetes*. 1992   ISBN 0-7923-1554-5
131. P.W. Serruys, B.H. Strauss and S.B. King III (eds.): *Restenosis after Intervention with New Mechanical Devices*. 1992   ISBN 0-7923-1555-3
132. P.J. Walter (ed.): *Quality of Life after Open Heart Surgery*. 1992   ISBN 0-7923-1580-4
133. E.E. van der Wall, H. Sochor, A. Righetti and M.G. Niemeyer (eds.): *What's new in Cardiac Imaging?* SPECT, PET and MRI. 1992   ISBN 0-7923-1615-0
134. P. Hanrath, R. Uebis and W. Krebs (eds.): *Cardiovascular Imaging by Ultrasound*. 1992   ISBN 0-7923-1755-6
135. F.H. Messerli (ed.): *Cardiovascular Disease in the Elderly*. 3rd ed. 1992   ISBN 0-7923-1859-5
136. J. Hess and G.R. Sutherland (eds.): *Congenital Heart Disease in Adolescents and Adults*. 1992   ISBN 0-7923-1862-5
137. J.H.C. Reiber and P.W. Serruys (eds.): *Advances in Quantitative Coronary Arteriography*. 1993   ISBN 0-7923-1863-3
138. A.-M. Salmasi and A.S. Iskandrian (eds.): *Cardiac Output and Regional Flow in Health and Disease*. 1993   ISBN 0-7923-1911-7
139. J.H. Kingma, N.M. van Hemel and K.I. Lie (eds.): *Atrial Fibrillation, a Treatable Disease?* 1992   ISBN 0-7923-2008-5
140. B. Ostadel and N.S. Dhalla (eds.): *Heart Function in Health and Disease*. Proceedings of the Cardiovascular Program (Prague, Czechoslovakia, 1991). 1992   ISBN 0-7923-2052-2
141. D. Noble and Y.E. Earm (eds.): *Ionic Channels and Effect of Taurine on the Heart*. Proceedings of an International Symposium (Seoul, Korea , 1992). 1993   ISBN 0-7923-2199-5
142. H.M. Piper and C.J. Preusse (eds.): *Ischemia-reperfusion in Cardiac Surgery*. 1993   ISBN 0-7923-2241-X
143. J. Roelandt, E.J. Gussenhoven and N. Bom (eds.): *Intravascular Ultrasound*. 1993   ISBN 0-7923-2301-7
144. M.E. Safar and M.F. O'Rourke (eds.): *The Arterial System in Hypertension*. 1993   ISBN 0-7923-2343-2
145. P.W. Serruys, D.P. Foley and P.J. de Feyter (eds.): *Quantitative Coronary Angiography in Clinical Practice*. With a Foreword by Spencer B. King III. 1994   ISBN 0-7923-2368-8

Developments in Cardiovascular Medicine

146. J. Candell-Riera and D. Ortega-Alcalde (eds.): *Nuclear Cardiology in Everyday Practice*. 1994 (in prep.) ISBN 0-7923-2374-2
147. P. Cummins (ed.): *Growth Factors and the Cardiovascular System*. 1993
    ISBN 0-7923-2401-3
148. K. Przyklenk, R.A. Kloner and D.M. Yellon (eds.): *Ischemic Preconditioning: The Concept of Endogenous Cardioprotection*. 1993 ISBN 0-7923-2410-2
149. T.H. Marwick: *Stress Echocardiography*. Its Role in the Diagnosis and Evaluation of Coronary Artery Disease. 1994 ISBN 0-7923-2579-6
150. W.H. van Gilst and K.I. Lie (eds.): *Neurohumoral Regulation of Coronary Flow*. Role of the Endothelium. 1993 ISBN 0-7923-2588-5
151. N. Sperelakis (ed.): *Physiology and Pathophysiology of the Heart*. 3rd rev. ed. 1994
    ISBN 0-7923-2612-1
152. J.C. Kaski (ed.): *Angina Pectoris with Normal Coronary Arteries: Syndrome X*. 1994
    ISBN 0-7923-2651-2
153. D.R. Gross: *Animal Models in Cardiovascular Research*. 2nd rev. ed. 1994
    ISBN 0-7923-2712-8
154. A.S. Iskandrian and E.E. van der Wall (eds.): *Myocardial Viability*. Detection and Clinical Relevance. 1994 ISBN 0-7923-2813-2
155. J.H.C. Reiber and P.W. Serruys (eds.): *Progress in Quantitative Coronary Arteriography*. 1994 . ISBN 0-7923-2814-0
156. U. Goldbourt, U. de Faire and K. Berg (eds.): *Genetic Factors in Coronary Heart Disease*. 1994 ISBN 0-7923-2752-7
157. G. Leonetti and C. Cuspidi (eds.): *Hypertension in the Elderly*. 1994
    ISBN 0-7923-2852-3
158. D. Ardissino, S. Savonitto and L.H. Opie (eds.): *Drug Evaluation in Angina Pectoris*. 1994 ISBN 0-7923-2897-3
159. G. Bkaily (ed.): *Membrane Physiopathology*. 1994 ISBN 0-7923-3062-5
160. R.C. Becker (ed.): *The Modern Era of Coronary Thrombolysis*. 1994
    ISBN 0-7923-3063-3
161. P.J. Walter (ed.), *Coronary Bypass Surgery in the Elderly*. Ethical, Economical and Quality of Life Aspects. 1995 ISBN 0-7923-3188-5
162. J.W. de Jong and R. Ferrari (eds.), *The Carnitine System*. A New Therapeutical Approach to Cardiovascular Diseases. 1995 (forthcoming) ISBN 0-7923-3318-7
163. C.A. Neill and E.B. Clark: *The Developing Heart: A 'History' of Pediatric Cardiology*. 1995 ISBN 0-7923-3375-6

Previous volumes are still available

KLUWER ACADEMIC PUBLISHERS – DORDRECHT / BOSTON / LONDON